Annals of Anthropological Practice

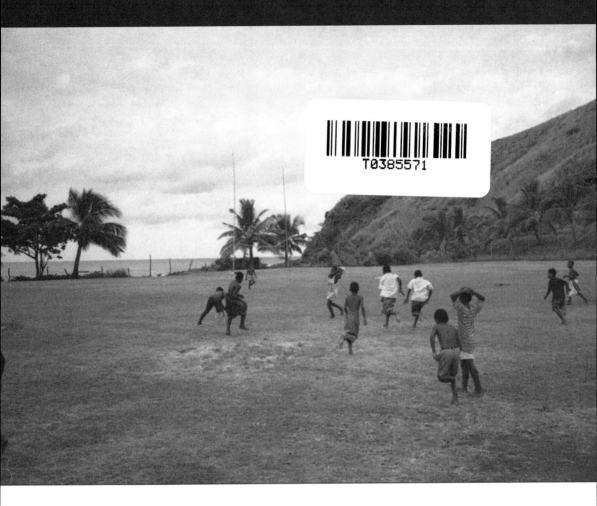

T0385571

Neuroanthropology and Its Applications

Daniel H. Lende and Greg Downey

Volume Coeditors

David Himmelgreen and Satish Kedia

General Editors

NATIONAL ASSOCIATION FOR THE PRACTICE OF ANTHROPOLOGY
A SECTION OF THE AMERICAN ANTHROPOLOGICAL ASSOCIATION

Annals of Anthropological
Practice 36.1

Annals of Anthropological Practice (2153-957X) is published in May and November on behalf of the American Anthropological Association by Wiley Subscription Services, Inc., a Wiley Company, 111 River St., Hoboken, NJ 07030-5774.

Mailing: Journal is mailed Standard Rate. Mailing to rest of world by IMEX (International Mail Express). Canadian mail is sent by Canadian publications mail agreement number 40573520. POSTMASTER: Send all address changes to Annals of Anthropological Practice, Journal Customer Services, John Wiley & Sons Inc., 350 Main St., Malden, MA 02148-5020.

Publisher: Annals of Anthropological Practice is published by Wiley Periodicals, Inc., Commerce Place, 350 Main Street, Malden, MA 02148; Telephone: 781 388 8200; Fax: 781 388 8210. Wiley Periodicals, Inc. is now part of John Wiley & Sons.

Information for Subscribers: Annals of Anthropological Practice is published in two one-issue volumes per year. Institutional subscription prices for 2012 are: Print & Online: US$67 (US), US$65 (Rest of World), €42 (Europe), £34 (UK). Prices are exclusive of tax. Australian GST, Canadian GST and European VAT will be applied at the appropriate rates. For more information on current tax rates, please go to www.wileyonlinelibrary.com/tax-vat. The institutional price includes online access to the current and all online back files to January 1st 2008, where available. For other pricing options, including access information and terms and conditions, please visit www.wileyonlinelibrary.com/access.

Delivery Terms and Legal Title: Where the subscription price includes print issues and delivery is to the recipient's address, delivery terms are Delivered Duty Unpaid (DDU); the recipient is responsible for paying any import duty or taxes. Title to all issues transfers FOB our shipping point, freight prepaid. We will endeavour to fulfil claims for missing or damaged copies within six months of publication, within our reasonable discretion and subject to availability.

Copyright and Photocopying: © 2012 American Anthropological Association. All rights reserved. No part of this publication may be reproduced, stored or transmitted in any form or by any means without the prior permission in writing from the copyright holder. Authorization to photocopy items for internal and personal use is granted by the copyright holder for libraries and other users registered with their local Reproduction Rights Organization (RRO), e.g. Copyright Clearance Center (CCC), 222 Rosewood Drive, Danvers, MA 01923, USA (www.copyright.com), provided the appropriate fee is paid directly to the RRO. This consent does not extend to other kinds of copying such as copying for general distribution, for advertising or promotional purposes, for creating new collective works or for resale. Special requests should be addressed to: permissionsuk@wiley.com

Back Issues: Single issues from current and recent volumes are available at the current single issue price from cs-journals@wiley.com. Earlier issues may be obtained from Periodicals Service Company, 11 Main Street, Germantown, NY 12526, USA. Tel: +1 (518) 537-4700, Fax: +1 (518) 537-5899, Email: psc@periodicals.com.

Journal Customer Services: For ordering information, claims and any inquiry concerning your journal subscription please go to www.wileycustomerhelp.com/ask or contact your nearest office.
Americas: Email: cs-journals@wiley.com; Tel: +1 781 388 8598 or +1 800 835 6770 (toll free in the USA & Canada).
Europe, Middle East and Africa: Email: cs-journals@wiley.com; Tel: +44 (0) 1865 778315.
Asia Pacific: Email: cs-journals@wiley.com; Tel: +65 6511 8000.
Japan: For Japanese speaking support, Email: cs-japan@wiley.com; Tel: +65 6511 8010 or Tel (toll-free): 005 316 50 480.
Visit our Online Customer Get-Help available in 6 languages at www.wileycustomerhelp.com

Associate Editor: Shannon Canney
Production Editor: Sarah J. McKay, Email: napa@wiley.com
Advertising: Kristin McCarthy, Email: kmccarthy@wiley.com

Print Information: Printed in the United States of America by The Sheridan Press.

Online Information: This journal is available online at *Wiley Online Library*. Visit www.wileyonlinelibrary.com to search the articles and register for table of contents e-mail alerts.
Access to this journal is available free online within institutions in the developing world through the AGORA initiative with the FAO, the HINARI initiative with the WHO and the OARE initiative with UNEP. For information, visit www.aginternetwork.org, www.healthinternetwork.org, and www.oarescience.org.

Aims and Scope: The Annals of Anthropological Practice (AAP) is dedicated to the practical problem-solving and policy applications of anthropological knowledge and methods. AAP is peer reviewed and is distributed free of charge as a benefit of NAPA (National Association for the Practice of Anthropology) membership. Through AAP, NAPA seeks to facilitate the sharing of information among practitioners, academics, and students, contribute to the professional development of anthropologists seeking practitioner positions, and support the general interests of practitioners both within and outside the academy. AAP is a publication of NAPA produced by the American Anthropological Association and Wiley-Blackwell. Through the publication of AAP, the AAA and Wiley-Blackwell furthers the professional interests of anthropologists while disseminating anthropological knowledge and its applications in addressing human problems.

Author Guidelines: For submission instructions, subscription and all other information visit: www.wileyonlinelibrary.com

Disclaimer: The Publisher, American Anthropological Association, and Editors cannot be held responsible for errors or any consequences arising from the use of information contained in this journal; the views and opinions expressed do not necessarily reflect those of the Publisher, American Anthropological Association, and Editors, neither does the publication of advertisements constitute any endorsement by the Publisher, American Anthropological Association, and Editors of the products advertised.

ISSN 2153-957X (Print)
ISSN 2153-9588 (Online)

Contents

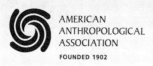
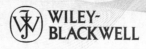

NEUROANTHROPOLOGY AND ITS APPLICATIONS: AN INTRODUCTION

DANIEL H. LENDE
University of South Florida

GREG DOWNEY
Macquarie University

Over the past two decades, the brain sciences have gone through a revolution in theories and methods for understanding neural function and its connections with human cognition, experience, and variation. Today the brain sciences grapple with questions of human development, cross-cultural difference, and neuroplasticity, and scientific thought about the brain plays an increasingly prominent role in public thinking about medical and social problems. In this context, anthropology faces new opportunities for interdisciplinary engagement and cross fertilization. Especially as brain scientists try to move from the lab to positions of advocacy and engagement, anthropological insight should be increasingly valuable to the enterprise, given our field's tradition of cross-cultural research and its ability to analyze how neuroscientific knowledge plays out in society. Anthropologists can also draw on neuroscience to address problems that we face in the field and to develop novel applied approaches, even as we send new questions and important data back to imaging laboratories.

"Neuroanthropology and Its Applications" shows the increasing development of this interdisciplinary field. The articles in this issue demonstrate the combination of theory and application at the core of this emerging area of scholarship, focusing specifically on work in sociocultural arenas, mental and behavioral health, and political-economic influences on human functioning. This special issue together with a new edited volume (Lende and Downey 2012), indicate how rapidly this field is growing (see also Campbell and Garcia 2009; Domínguez et al. 2010; Northoff 2010; Raybeck and Ngo 2011; Reyna 2012a; Roepstorff et al. 2010; Seligman and Brown 2010).[1] We are particularly excited that applied work is playing a formative role in the early stages of neuroanthropological thought. Too often theory and application remain separate in anthropological work, and little crossover occurs between new developments in academia and in nonacademic arenas. This special issue, which includes people actively working in clinical, coaching, and communications settings, demonstrates that a holistic approach to neuroanthropology is possible that includes applied anthropology, critical theory, and interdisciplinary practice. The subfield is being built from the bottom up, from diverse ethnographic and applied problems that have driven researchers across traditional disciplinary boundaries.

ANNALS OF ANTHROPOLOGICAL PRACTICE 36, pp. 1–25. ISSN: 2153-957X. © 2012 by the American Anthropological Association. DOI:10.1111/j.2153-9588.2012.01090.x

In this introduction, we lay out neuroanthropology as a field of anthropology, cover how neuroscience can be drawn into our discipline's distinctive synthetic approach, discuss the increasing influence of brain science, and present a basic framework for applied neuroanthropology. We also review the nine articles in this special issue, organized into three separate clusters: sociocultural issues, mental and behavioral health, and political economy. We finish with a brief account of the roots of neuroanthropology, especially the conversation that arose through collaboration, online discussion, and public engagement, and how this origin helped to make the area applied from its start.

NEUROANTHROPOLOGICAL HOLISM

Neuroanthropology exemplifies the holism that has been a hallmark of anthropology since the work of Franz Boas. The field draws on both biology and culture for data and theory, and embraces both empiricism and critical analysis. Neuroanthropology inherently demands multidisciplinary methods, and—depending on the research problem—can range in approach from one in-depth case study of an idiosyncratic example of human variation to analysis of large data sets. Our emphasis on neurological variation and a comparative approach are foundational for research and application. This breadth of theory and method can challenge any solitary scholar, so neuroanthropology researchers should be open to working on teams or in collaborative efforts to bring the necessary expertise to bear on specific problems and projects.

Neuroanthropology coheres as an area of scholarship in two distinctive ways: first, engagement with neuroscience, especially framed by a "new biology" that emphasizes variation, plasticity, processes, and emerging systems in contrast with older, more mechanistic views of how human biology works (Downey and Lende 2012a; MacKinnon and Fuentes 2012); and second, an insistence that brain function is always embedded in larger, living systems, including the human body, the social field, and the longer-term, larger-scale structures that are the products of human brains yoked into cooperative, cumulative systems. That is, neuroanthropology recognizes that human phenomena are inherently neurological; but at the same time insists that any biological account of the brain that is not sufficiently supple to capture the observable complexity of human life is empirically untenable. To neuroanthropology the brain is inherently plural, both in the sense that there is no single "human brain," and that one of the distinctive traits of the human nervous system is the role of others in shaping it. To bridge brain and culture, neuroanthropology draws on innovations in fields like psychological and medical anthropology that have provided key insights into individual–environment interaction and approaches to addressing problems of human variation. These other subfields have provided examples of ways to study pathology, for example, outside the limits that often come with a western scientific and biomedical view. Without these recent developments, both in neuroscience and in anthropology, neuroanthropology would not be possible.

These specific areas—across neuroscience and biology, and among different strands of anthropology—provide an overall set of ingredients that researchers can develop into different recipes for doing neuroanthropology. No one recipe for doing neuroanthropology will dominate because the human brain itself does not abide by a simple set of rules or consist of only a limited number of processes. Indeed, we believe that neuroanthropology demands an approach that builds theory from research, including applied research, rather than providing a single overarching theoretical narrative in one motion; no one theoretical account can describe the brain because neurological processes vary across different functions, timescales, and contexts. The effort to derive neuroanthropological theory then draws on relevant ideas wherever they might appear, including from both sides of the old opposition between biology and culture or between science and the humanities.

For the practitioners represented in this special edition, neuroanthropology is an analytical response to problems arising from fieldwork. Lende's work on addiction, for example, was inspired by his experiences as a drug counselor. He noticed that what Colombians told him and showed him did not match some of the prevalent biologically based accounts of addiction, especially those that assumed addiction was a behavioral result of a simple brain mechanism (Lende 2005, 2012). Similarly, Downey's work on the perceptual effects of physical training started by taking seriously his expert informants, Afro-Brazilian capoeristas, who told him that training affected how they perceived everyday reality (e.g., Downey 2007). Moving beyond a purely hermeneutical approach to these accounts required asking whether biological evidence supported the potential for physical discipline to alter sensory perception. Neuroanthropologists recognize that our job as researchers is to develop explanations that can match what field research shows us on the ground, and to refine research methods that ferret out the processes that generate human variation.

By responding to problems that arise from fieldwork, and by remaining broadly open to theoretical inspiration from diverse sources, neuroanthropologists appear most likely to contribute to two areas of science and scholarship. First, researchers working within neuroanthropology will contribute to our understanding of how the nervous system works outside of laboratory settings. These contributions to basic brain science can happen through bringing to the study of the brain a greater recognition of human variation, the dynamics of social and environmental interaction, and the profundity of human enculturation, and thus allow the testing of hypotheses in more ecologically valid, natural settings. Second, neuroanthropology can develop sophisticated analyses of human phenomena that are linked with increasing neuroscientific knowledge. Combining critical and cultural theory with a robust understanding of brain function, neuroanthropology will examine the cultural reworkings and social appropriation of knowledge and the political and economic management of neural diversity and difference. Neither approach—basic research or critical analysis—is sufficient on its own for neuroanthropology. Together, they provide the empirical basis to address applied problems as well as the necessary mechanisms for self-correction. This combination of critical and scientific research, augmented by basic lessons learned from applied anthropology, inform the writers collected in this issue, "Neuroanthropology and Its Applications."

Neuroanthropology brings together various strands of anthropology to address complex brain–culture problems in the field and the laboratory. We seek to develop a framework to successfully integrate neuroscience research and methods into our discipline at the same time that we become much better equipped to interrogate and, when necessary, criticize neuroscience from within. Psychological anthropology, biological anthropology, cultural anthropology, and medical anthropology all provide important elements for the research being done by neuroanthropologists.

Psychological Anthropology

Neuroanthropology shares two key themes with psychological anthropology: (1) examining the individual in context and (2) consideration of internal factors. Psychological anthropology has focused on how the individual relates to the environment, in particular sociocultural environments (Levine 2010; Moore and Mathews 2001). A similar framework is crucial for the distinctive contribution of neuroanthropology to our understanding of the brain as so much of neuroscience is oriented to the individual as the operative unit. Neuroscience research often employs methods like neuroimaging that of necessity isolate individuals; from these data, however, neuroscientists often make assertions about social life or cultural patterning without considering the individual–environment interface in the richly informed way of psychological anthropology. For example, studying how individuals inside imaging equipment respond to pictures of members of the opposite sex does not mean that one necessarily understands the much more complex interactive elements of sexuality and attraction. Psychological anthropologists have examined carefully factors internal to the individual, including subjective experience (Willen and Seeman 2012), cognition (Shore 1996; Strauss and Quinn 1998), and emotion (Hinton 1999; Lutz 1988). This foundational work on diverse peoples' meaningful, experiential worlds provides an important background for doing neuroanthropology, from research on phenomenology, embodiment, and the senses to work that has engaged seriously with cognitive science, emotion theory, cognitive linguistics, and metaphor theory. For instance, many current neuropsychological studies of religious sense only explore one facet of the elaborate emotional, perceptual, social, moral and mystical relationships that are routinely described as part of people's varied religious experience (d'Aquili and Newberg 1999; Persinger 1983; Seligman and Kirmayer 2008). As neuroscience increasingly aims to explore human nature, cross-cultural variation, and humans' production of meaning, decades of research by psychological anthropologists provide an important reservoir of rich comparative cases as well as myriad examples of how to successfully draw together quantitative and qualitative data to understand larger questions about human life.

Biological Anthropology

Biological anthropology provides expertise in evolutionary theory, a strong understanding of the mechanisms that underlie behavior and cognition, and an emphasis on comparative analysis and individual variation. Neuroanthropology takes two important lessons from evolutionary theory: first, humans are not infinitely plastic, in spite of some social constructionists' assumptions. Second, our evolutionary history—the phylogeny of our species—is central to understanding patterns of human variation, although by no means does that history alone determine these patterns (Fuentes 2008). Rather, we can better explain phenomena like human sexuality and reproduction (Gettler et al. 2011; Hrdy 2000), vulnerability to addictive drugs (Lende 2007), and our ability to adapt to different environments (Kendal et al. 2011) using the lens of evolutionary adaptation in conjunction with other theoretical approaches, and even identify when a pattern defies what we might expect from evolutionary modeling.

Biological anthropology also provides important comparative data on brain evolution and function from its broad prehistoric and primatological framework (Downey and Lende 2012b; Rilling 2008). By drawing on decades of primate research and paleoanthropology (Hare 2011; MacKinnon and Fuentes 2012; Rilling 2008), neuroanthropologists better position themselves to understand just what the human brain can and cannot do. We know that one persistent problem in both psychology and neuroscience is a widespread sampling bias; making claims about human nature based on the population that winds up in university laboratories can be a precarious exercise (see Henrich et al. 2010). A broad comparative approach—looking among diverse species and into our own evolutionary history—is central to neuroanthropological practice, one of our distinctive contributions to the study of the human brain.

Finally, neuroanthropology borrows from biological anthropology a focus on the mechanisms and processes underlying cognitive functions, virtually all of which are complex assemblages involving parts of the human brain in relations to external elements, such as learned culture, other people, perceptions of the environment, and material culture. Over time, these processes blur the division between internal and external, what is the brain and what is the environment, as experience reshapes the individual's neurological endowment. This focus on the diverse components that shape behavior or that form a functional cognitive system is central to how neuroanthropology analyzes problems and helps us to understand the need for hybrid research expertise, as systems virtually always cross disciplinary territories. Neuroanthropologists recognize that components of "cognitive systems" exist just as well in the environment as in the brain, and processes can function at the organism–environment interface, and not simply internally. This point is crucial because a wide range of disciplines offer insights into dynamic, heterogeneous cognitive systems. For example, because patterns of subjective experience affect brain physiology over time, cognitive "mechanisms" inevitably refuse to obey disciplinary divisions of labor, cutting across science and the humanities, and involve elements on radically different scales, from cellular mechanisms to sociocultural and historical dynamics.

Cultural Anthropology

One formative element of neuroanthropology is ethnography. Ethnographic field work provides evidence of human function and variation that is central to understanding how brains work in the wild, to borrow from Edwin Hutchins (1995). Ethnography can test theories drawn from neuroscience, psychology, or elsewhere against the complexity of the world. Long-term ethnography provides qualitative data that is essential to inform our understanding of human function and enculturation. Moreover, the point of view of our informants can be an important counterbalance to the expertise of lab-based researchers. Although neuroscientists and other researchers possess distinctive and powerful forms of knowledge making without which neuroanthropology would be impossible, their mantle of authority often conceals when their theories have moved beyond the strict purview of the data, smuggling in folk interpretations or culture-based assumptions. For example, the insights that highly skilled practitioners can offer into how they are able to do what they do may provide a level of detail in data that is just not available in university laboratories when college student subjects do not have such highly developed skills. Field research may alert us to specialized neurocultural mechanisms that are not developed by all individuals.

Alongside ethnography, cultural anthropology has developed cross-cultural comparison and relativism, analytical tools ideal to combat consistent problems that crop up when dealing with questions of human nature and variation in the brain sciences (Domínguez 2012; Gelman and Legare 2011; Reyna 2012b; Roepstorff 2011). Psychologists often rely on western undergraduates for their claims about human nature (Henrich et al. 2010); some evolutionary theories view the Pleistocene as formative of a universal human nature (Barkow et al. 1992); extrapolations are made from laboratory results to all times and places that are strikingly inappropriate (Choudhury and Slaby 2012; Turner 2012; Whitehead 2012). Cultural anthropology's emphasis on variation, understanding cultural behavior in context, and using firsthand experience with cultural diversity as leverage to critique one's own cultural and intellectual assumptions, all prove crucial resources in moving neuroscience out of the laboratory and into a much broader consideration of how the human nervous system might function.

Finally, neuroanthropologists pay attention to how processes like enculturation, child rearing, embryonic environment, skill acquisition, socialization, and critical life experiences like ritual shape brain function and development, aligning the field with cultural anthropology's long-standing emphasis on the social and cultural constitution of human beings. We seek to recognize how elements like systems of symbols, systemic inequality, diverse practices, cultural embodiment, ideology, and power can shape the everyday patterning of our nervous systems, and also affect how we conduct neuroscience itself. Political economy and culture are a constitutive part of how brains work, not just an "influence" in the environment. The brain's developmental context does not simply inflect or influence the wiring, firing, and connecting of our brains and bodies; we would not *have* a functioning nervous system without patterned stimulation and behavior, elements that are inherently varied across our species.

Medical Anthropology

Medical anthropology provides important methodological and analytical tools for the project of neuroanthropology. Like neuroscience itself, medical anthropology has consistently investigated determinants of health and well-being, exploring the reality of dysfunction and suffering both as a source of data and as a principle justification for research. Engaging with health problems means that neuroanthropologists can draw on research on the relationship between ability and disability; the cultural construction of illness, normality and deviance; evolutionary biases in health; and other basic anthropological analyses (Antelius 2007; Dumit 2004; Kohrt and Harper 2008; Lende 2007). Moreover, medical anthropology has consistently been critical of biomedicine as an institution, actively questioning how western science constructs the object under study, how politics and economics shape care, and the ways in which medicine acts as a form of power (Lock and Nguyen 2010; Luhrmann 2001). Medical anthropology offers a model for both critical and applied engagement with scientific knowledge, including how technology, institutions, standards of care, and patterns of practice develop in a variety of ways in different societies, even among groups in the same society.

In its critical form, neuroanthropology needs to focus on the laboratories, government institutions, funding bodies, and professional organizations that shape neuroscience knowledge and practice, and then examine how the biomedical industry as well as lay people draw on this knowledge to understand and manage issues related to health and well-being (Choudhury and Slaby 2012; Cohn 2012; Martin 2010; Raikhel 2012; Rees 2010). Neuroanthropology must both collaborate and engage critically with neuroscience, particularly as institutions and our informants increasingly draw on the knowledge offered up by neuroscience in a wide variety of settings.

HOW THE BRAIN REQUIRES NEUROANTHROPOLOGY

The human nervous system is our primary cultural organ. Although our brains are at the center of our nervous system, neuroanthropology embraces a wide view of neural function that includes the system as a whole (Downey and Lende 2012a; Rilling 2008; Worthman 2009). The central nervous system integrates the body and brain and sensory systems and the environment, and mediates our interactions with each other. It guides our reactions to and anticipations of social life (Rilling and Sanfey 2011), underwrites our comprehension of symbolic systems (Deacon 1997), and allows the acquisition of skills and habit formation (Downey 2010; Raybeck and Ngo 2011; Roepstorff et al. 2010). The nervous system brings together consciousness with a host of non- and semiconscious activity that controls the autonomic systems, including cardiovascular functioning, management of hormones, and growth and sexual development, and through development, comes to differently embody social position, gender, race, and other crucial dimensions of experience (Chiao 2010; Gravlee 2009; Hertzman and Boyce 2010; Worthman et al. 2010).

Our understanding of the nervous system has changed radically over the past two decades and will continue to do so over the coming years, which makes us hesitate to propose any grand overarching theories of neuroanthropology. Any theory of brain enculturation that aims to be comprehensive is quite likely to prove either premature or simply impossible at this stage. One of the most dramatic shifts in contemporary neuroscience, however, is the importance of neuroplasticity in our understanding of brain function and structure (Dayan and Cohen 2011; Feldman 2009; Malafouris 2010; Wexler 2011), including in the new field of cultural neuroscience (Ambady and Bharucha 2009; Chiao et al. 2010; Kitayama and Uskul 2011). Many researchers assumed the brain's architecture was fixed by adulthood; we now recognize that it is much more plastic than previously thought, responding to new activities and learning opportunities through functional and structural changes in specific synapses, circuits, and connections.[2]

This recognition has two important implications for cultural theory. First, previous models in cognitive science and evolutionary psychology that relied on metaphors of the brain that failed to recognize this plasticity are now untenable. The view of a hardwired brain structure set down by genetic "blueprint," for example, simply does not match up with the increasingly detailed understanding of gene expression, epigenetics, brain development, skill acquisition, and recovery from brain injury. This research repeatedly highlights that the brain, given the right conditions, is quite plastic (Dayan and Cohen 2011; Wexler 2011), exposing how western cultural and folk assumptions about "innate" cognitive endowments or the irreversibility of brain insult actually became self-fulfilling prognoses, in spite of their dubious empirical basis. Because the mainstream of brain science thought the insult of stroke was irreversible, for example, the forms of therapy that could restore some function were discouraged until both scientific evidence and theory came to recognize that, in some cases, recovery was possible (see Doidge 2007).

Similarly, a view of the mind as a set of encapsulated modules pieced together over our species' evolution—a model used in some strains of evolutionary psychology and cognitive science—increasingly does not match up with data from a wide range of domains, including such diverse research areas as skill acquisition (Downey 2010; Raybeck and Ngo 2011), recovery from brain injury (Doidge 2007), language (Christiansen and Chater 2008; Evans and Levinson 2009), mental calculation (Cantlon and Brannon 2006; Hanakawa et al. 2003; Tang et al. 2006), sensory substitution in the blind and deaf (Downey 2012; Thaler et al. 2011), and even parenting by women and men (Hrdy 2000; Gettler et al. 2011). This research shows that developmental dynamics lead brains to "modularize" as they mature, and may even produce—in most cases—reliable patterns of particular functions localizing in one region of the brain. These patterns, however, are flexible and emergent, rather than innate and preprogrammed. Anthropologists should welcome this new emphasis on brain plasticity and emergent organization because they complement decades of anthropological emphasis on cultural variation and reaffirm the importance of cross-cultural research.

Second, the new "wet-wired" view of brain function, or the idea that structure emerges from organic development, rather than being apportioned into "hard" and "soft" parts, challenges many cultural anthropologists' assumption that they can conveniently set aside biology when studying cognition, perception, or psychology. We now realize that cultural variation and social organization work through biological systems. Culture and social structure literally become anatomy over developmental time. Our anatomical malleability has a role in understanding how variation works (Kanai and Rees 2011), how enculturation happens (Roepstorff et al. 2010), and how political economy creates differential outcomes, such as the effect of poverty and inequality on health and mortality (Worthman et al. 2010). Social and cultural anthropologists cannot hide from biology behind a Cartesian split between the brain and the mind, not because biology determines mind, but because the processes that generate different types of minds also affect brain development.

Research has also challenged any treatment of the brain as isolated from the world, a hardwired computer housed in the skull and filled with cultural software. The body matters in shaping how the brain works. Disease, immune function, nutrition, physical activity, sensory ecologies, and the like have both direct and indirect influence on the nervous system, including the brain. This integrationist view opens up a much wider way to think about how culture shapes the brain, instead of assuming that cultural learning is some type of ideational brain "content" of systems of symbols, ideologies, and class-linked tastes and inclinations. At the same time, research on embodiment has shown how daily experience, body postures, sensory behavior, and other aspects of how we physically interact play a fundamental role in shaping how we perceive the world, think through problems, and react to events. Similarly, work on the "extended mind"—recognizing that not all cognitive function is cleanly encapsulated inside the brain but, rather, engages actively with supports in the environment (Hutchins 1995)— opens up vistas for serious engagement with sociocultural and psychological anthropology (Hutchins 2011). Together, this work challenges neuroanthropology to provide serious accounts of how embodiment, cognition in the wild, ritual, skill acquisition, and sensory learning can shape brain development, structure, and function in different times and places.

Given how the information processing or software metaphor of learning has fallen apart, anthropologists can no longer treat culture merely as software that gets installed on a wholly plastic brain. The brain is plastic, yes, but is still host to a range of specific functions and predilections, often built up over development and sculpted by evolution. Indeed, the brain achieves its plasticity using many innate mechanisms, not in spite of them; recognizing plasticity is not an argument for a "blank slate." For example, the repurposing of neural circuits and the differential activation of particular brain areas both play a role in how the brain can achieve its remarkable flexibility and how much flexibility is possible (Anderson 2010; Westermann et al. 2007). By using a "mix-and-match" approach that draws on different components and processes, some quite evolutionarily old, to meet ongoing demands—some of which are in contrast novel and evolutionarily unprecedented—the brain can repurpose the same resources in diverse ways.[3] This approach is extremely valuable for understanding contextual behavior (such as social roles or vulnerabilities) and also for understanding cultural variation. This model of neural repurposing and marshaling resources into diverse function-based systems represents a fundamentally different way to think about the brain than an older "Swiss army knife" view, where each mental module or region was assumed to have only one function and each function to be reliably locatable to a single brain region.

Taking seriously traits like wet wiring and adaptive repurposing over evolutionary time means that sociality plays a fundamental role in shaping human being, and is not simply a gloss over some basic human nature. Seeking to divide human biological "nature" from variable "culture" at the level of the nervous system is impossible; even the most pervasive brain traits may turn out to be emergent, reconfiguring given the right conditions. Wet wiring means that nurture becomes part of nature, which has important implications for the application of anthropology to the study of childhood, parenting, and development. Through recurring experiences, repeated activities, and daily social interactions, enculturation can create specificity, for example, speaking a specific language. This cultural specificity is not transferable across all situations but, rather, will depend on how specific elements get reactivated in similar and novel situations.

THE APPLICATION OF NEUROSCIENCE

Neuroscience is being pulled into academic fields beyond its traditional domains of laboratory research and clinical application. Economics, politics, philosophy, law, criminology—all are actively drawing on neuroscience, often in ways that may exaggerate the flaws of the basic research and may amount to little more than "neuro-mania" (Legrenzi et al. 2011; Tallis 2011). We must recognize that the limits of science and the problems of laboratory-based research necessarily constrain the claims neuroscientists can make about the brain (Choudhury and Slaby 2012; Downey and Lende 2012a; Whitehead 2012). Outside academia, the use of pharmaceuticals to change and even enhance brain function is a multibillion-dollar industry that at present primarily targets mental and behavioral health problems, although overdiagnosis and patient self-medication has taken neuropharmacology far beyond the strict advice offered on drug packaging (Lakoff 2005; Lock and Nguyen 2010). Questions have arisen about the effectiveness of antidepressants and attention-deficit disorder drugs, at the same time that these pharmaceuticals have become "blockbuster drugs," generating enormous corporate profit and leading to new forms of neurological biopower (Kirsch 2010; Quintero and Nichter 2011). New generations of "cognitive enhancement" drugs raise thorny ethical issues, even as populations like students, soldiers, and others in demanding occupations increasingly use such drugs to enhance their functioning.

Neuroscience is also leading a drive to reshape our understanding of learning, and thus of fields like education, training, and coaching. Educators are reading cognitive neuroscience, and using metaphors about "brain-based training" to enact specific reforms (Sousa 2010), hopes for which sometimes outpace evidence for their effectiveness. Similarly, legal organizations, the military, government, and professional medical societies are influenced by brain research in the work they do and the policies they put into place (Royal Society 2011). Indeed, references to the brain are now a central part of how policy, ideology, and symbolism get debated and justified in modern industrial society (Frazzetto and Anker 2009; Ortega 2009; Rolls 2012). This development necessitates that neuroanthropologists also adopt a critical view of neuroscience (Choudhury and Slaby 2012). Brain-based policy and public debate require us to appreciate that the brain has become the new stand-in for the self, and thus fits into the individualist biases so prevalent in western philosophy (Martin 2010; Ortega 2009).

The quadruple leverage of neuroscience—the authority of science, the power of medical technology, the ability to justify policy, and the rich pool of symbolic meaning—means that its further integration into social institutions around the world is likely to be fast, exceeding the uptake of earlier generations of Western psychological thought. This rapid diffusion will require that neuroanthropologists and allied scholar-practitioners develop equally quickly the research to understand how brains function "in the wild": in other words, do better and more field-based science. The effort should be urgent especially because our informants around the world are more and more likely to adopt "brain-based" languages for understanding themselves. In addition, we want to be positioned to document and interrogate critically how neuroscience increasingly transforms diverse social fields and cultural universes.

Critical approaches to neuroscience already have made a considerable start (Choudhury and Slaby 2012; Dumit 2004). Generally, these scholars examine the political and social uses of neuroscience, and challenge assertions that particular local neurological configurations are timeless, universal, or "natural"; for example, Allan Young (1997) has queried the universality of "post-traumatic stress disorder" (PTSD), documenting the way that traumatic memories and psychiatric practice converged to produce the distinctive profile of PTSD. More recently, critical neuroscientists have argued that greater scrutiny and reflexivity can improve neuroscience research, that the critical approach can feed back to the lab (Choudhury and Slaby 2012). This critical studies approach, buttressed by examinations of biomedicine and technology more broadly (Lock and Nguyen 2010), should be a crucial part of applied neuroanthropology. At the same time, critical approaches have weaknesses, especially for applied neuroanthropology. On the theoretical side, an overly critical stance can limit any contribution to improving brain science, particularly science in field-based settings. Examining the "social, moral, and political implications" of a particular imaging method or theoretical paradigm is not the same as contributing actively to the reform of the basic science or refining neuroscience research techniques. Furthermore, critique is a limited approach to applied anthropology: anthropologists have other ways to make a difference than just critiquing other disciplines, in particular working to develop evidence-based applied programs and advocating for social change.

NEUROANTHROPOLOGICAL INTERVENTION

Applied neuroanthropology builds on general principles of applied anthropology. First, applied neuroanthropology recognizes the importance of human variation in the success (and failure) of projects of all sorts, highlighting that few (if any) universal solutions exist to the problems we face around the globe. Applied neuroanthropology points to patterns of human variation that are often not reducible to either biological or cross-cultural etiology alone; rather, human difference and similarity emerge through interactions across the biology–culture divide. This perspective should clear the ground for more evidence-based approaches to understanding a wide range of problems, like PTSD (Collura and Lende this issue) and stress (Burbank this issue). By undermining the assumption that variation necessarily indicates cultural causes, or that uniformity is evidence of biological innateness, redefining applied issues as explicitly neuroanthropological encourages consideration of diverse causal dynamics. Where brain and culture meet, neuroanthropology-oriented applied approaches are needed either in conjunction with or to replace completely existing biomedical and psychological interventions, and thereby influence political decision making and economic policy.

Like applied anthropology as a whole, applied neuroanthropology advocates a community-based approach to address the problems communities face (Minkler and Wallerstein 2008; Schensul and Trickett 2009). Just as ethnography informs our understanding of the nature of these problems, so community engagement can inform our approach to what we can do. Local expertise will help define the contours of problems beyond what a typical literature review provides. Collaboration can help generate community-based research agendas that engage the research capacities of colleagues in varied disciplines. Community feedback, as well as practical knowledge about what has and hasn't worked previously, will buttress critiques of existing efforts and foster an evidence-based approach to making recommendations. Neuroanthropology, in conjunction with the communities in which we work, can set novel research questions, apply basic neuroscience and anthropology to practical problem solving, and advocate for change and solutions to local problems.

Finally, neuroanthropology recognizes that applied research is different from traditional scholarly endeavors (Low and Merry 2010; Rylko-Bauer et al. 2006; Sabloff 2011). Too often researchers unfamiliar with the challenges of applied research assume that theory leads directly to application in an unproblematic fashion. Neuroanthropologists will need to advocate developing knowledge about a problem *and* knowledge about how to make a difference. That how-to knowledge can include applied theory, familiarity with local resources for change, and an awareness not just of a community's needs but also what social structures might limit or appropriate any plans for a program or policy change. Application of knowledge—brain science research, for instance—often requires its own separate theoretical bases; to help transform scientific findings into effective programs requires practical knowledge of what works in the target setting, and feedback on the strengths and limits of a variety of approaches. Ongoing innovation and testing ideally involves the following: (1) a concern with application from the outset of the project so that application is not an afterthought, a consideration added on only after research is completed; (2) ongoing testing both in terms of the theory we apply and our modes to intervene to generate change in dynamic systems, because engagement will require a broader empirical basis for understanding how systems and communities function; (3) recognition that, as with all dynamic systems, an intervention that works at one point in time may not have the same effect as the systems reconfigure and change; and (4) the social, political, and cultural savvy to get initial results so that a community's resources, including its trust, can be invested in later stages of applied research. Although fully applied research will embrace all these stages, we recognize that much basic research and theory development remains to be done in neuroanthropology. Most applied work will fall on a continuum from normal academic research to complete engagement in the

TABLE 1. Neuroanthropology and Its Applications: Finding and Filling the Gaps

"Aiming at the Gaps"	Neuroanthropology	Societal Dynamics	Example	Approach
Vulnerabilities	Vulnerable individuals and groups	Social dynamics that worsen outcomes	Addiction and availability of treatment	Address vulnerabilities and negative social dynamics
Communications	Complex science	Public misunderstanding	Brain development and learning	Translational communications
Policies	Advancing knowledge	Mistaken expert thinking	Coaching and skill acquisition	Evidence-based policy development
Programs	Individual/environment interactions	Unidimensional programs	Immigrant mental health	Program change and development

development of new applications, which can range from advocacy and public communication to the piloting of novel programs.

The more researchers recognize that their work can have an applied dimension, especially from its earliest stages, and that we can propose novel social interventions or projects that might make a difference as part of an overall scholarly trajectory inside or outside the academy, the more applied work will simply become part of what it means to do neuroanthropology. Getting data and ideas relevant to applied outcomes as part of an overall research process is particularly important, given how much field research anthropologists do and the inherent difficulties we often have in going back to our research sites. Neuroanthropology from the beginning should gather useful, applicable data and develop the sorts of novel insights that can lead to policy innovation, based on field observation, community engagement, and our own practical experience.

Identifying Gaps

One key approach for doing applied neuroanthropology is to identify gaps between the local dynamics revealed by ethnographic or community-based research and existing superlocal programs, policies, and public understandings about a particular domain or arena (see Table 1). For example, addictive behavior emerges at the intersection of neurobiological and sociocultural processes (Lende 2005, 2007, 2012). Government policies and biomedical treatment approaches can exist at odds with the neuroanthropological dynamics of addiction, and may even worsen problems for those most vulnerable in some contexts (Hansen and Skinner this issue). Thus, neuroanthropology, by synthesizing neuroscience and anthropology, provides an evidence-based approach that can generate innovative, finely tailored approaches to local variants of larger social problems. At the same time, using more critical and sociocultural analyses, neuroanthropologists can examine how large-scale dynamics in society might interact with the formative processes at the level of the individual's nervous system, and look for pernicious interactions between these levels—from the way inequality can exacerbate educational or health problems to the role of public misunderstandings of research findings in blocking good policy. These gaps between phenomena at different levels of analysis can affect the ongoing development of the individual, resulting in poor outcomes, increased vulnerability in particular groups, and ineffective policy.

We perceive four general points where neuroanthropologists might address the causal structures underlying specific problems in health, development, psychological well-being, education, or other areas.

One: Vulnerabilities

As our understanding of neurocultural dynamics advances, we will perceive more accurately how people might be vulnerable to particular pathologies, problems, and negative social interactions. In ways similar to evolutionary medicine's recognition of mismatches—that evolved predispositions can be at odds with rapid social and technological change in our modern world—neuroanthropology can identify particular vulnerabilities in the mismatch between neurological resources and environmental demands. For example, toxic stress during childhood can deflect or impede childhood brain development. Neuroanthropology can inform our approach to redressing the social forces that generate stress and how we train children to cope with stress (Lende this issue). Similarly, the processes that promote addiction to synthetic drugs as well as the institutions that manage treatment (incl. pharmaceuticals) intersect to produce differential vulnerability for the urban poor and more affluent city dwellers (Hansen and Skinner this issue). Diverging outcomes—such as disproportionate morbidity, higher rates of psychological problems, and lower average achievements in schools—can alert us to the intersection of underlying neurological diversity and sociocultural institutions that translate diversity into disparity.

Two: Communications

Neuroanthropology, as a science that bridges the biology–culture gap, is complicated. The field draws on research in neuroscience, human development, psychology, and sociology. The wider public often has views at odds with the latest scientific findings, and these mistaken understandings can undermine individual decision making and institutional policy. Finding effective ways to communicate complex ideas to a wider public is one important way neuroanthropology can have an applied impact (Lindland and Kendall-Taylor this issue). By drawing on ideas about learning, cultural models, metaphors, and framing, neuroanthropologists can better strategize about how to communicate to a broad audience, and then refine these communication strategies as necessary. We can highlight problems with existing metaphors, such as the double-edged implications of the "poverty poisons the brain" approach that is increasingly prominent in science journalism and policy development (Lende this issue). Finally, our emerging specialty can also draw on the popularity of brain-based understandings to persuade the public that social and cultural dynamics matter because of the ways that they influence brain development. For example, Sarah Mahler's (2012) *Culture as Comfort: The Many Things You Already Know About Culture (But Might Not Realize)* uses neuroanthropology to present one of the most basic ideas of anthropology, ethnocentrism, to a broad audience: why does the familiar come to seem natural and "comfortable" while other ways of life make us uncomfortable?

Three: Policies

One arena where neuroanthropologists can contribute substantially is to the basic knowledge that informs policy improvements. This approach takes doing "basic research" one step further by explicitly considering the applied dimensions while designing projects, including working with experts, getting data relevant to applied outcomes, and testing policy-oriented ideas where possible. For example, as outlined by Downey (this issue), high-level coaches in sport often carry erroneous assumptions about skill acquisition, player variation, and training modalities. Neuroanthropology research can provide evidence-based recommendations for improving what athletes and coaches do. Neuroanthropological knowledge provides a cultural and social corrective to more narrow research in a language that other experts and policy makers understand.

Four: Programs

Neuroanthropologists can help to transform existing programs and develop novel proposals to address pressing social, behavioral, and mental health problems. These initiatives will often focus more on a micro- or individual level than most centrally initiated, large-scale policy efforts, because neuroanthropology places an emphasis on the practices and experiences that lie between embodied biology and social dynamics. For example, Kohrt and colleagues (this issue) describe how they use neuroanthropology, ethnographic research, and clinical expertise to adapt treatment approaches for dealing with immigrant mental health. Similarly, Myers (this issue) calls for an approach to schizophrenia that addresses the daily practices and rituals that shape healing and well-being, rather than resorting to existing options like incarceration or powerful medications. Existing programs often assume a "one size fits all" approach that does not address the inherent variation at multiple levels that shapes health as well as social problems like binge drinking, high risk behavior, and violence. Neuroanthropologists should assertively move to test their own best ideas for positively affecting community health and, at the same time, capture crucial feedback about what works and what does not, as they attempt to design novel applied programs.

At the heart of the "identifying gaps" approach is a commitment to examine both the neuroanthropology of phenomena and what we can do to address problems. At present, our field can sometimes divide these two, employing an integrated biocultural perspective when seeking to understand problems and deploying a critical and sociocultural approach to examine policy, intervention, and program development. However, as neuroanthropology continues to develop, and the evidence base of neuroanthropology at the brain, individual, and social levels grows, the overall integration of analysis and application should become a more seamless whole.

ORGANIZATION OF THE ISSUE

This issue of *Annals of Anthropological Practice* consists of three sets of three articles each. The first group of articles uses neuroanthropology and psychological anthropology to engage in basic research, critical analysis, and applied work on the sociocultural realm. The second cluster of articles examines mental and behavioral health problems, from immigrant mental health to schizophrenia and PTSD. In the final section, the authors use neuroanthropology to examine political economy and social inequality.

SOCIOCULTURAL ANALYSES AND ENGAGEMENT

In the opening section, the three articles examine how analyses of culture, meaning, and practice can inform applied approaches within anthropology. By focusing on variation, the gaps between research and public beliefs, and the importance of taking into account cultural theory and ethnographic research, these articles show that critical engagement with neuroscience and cognitive science can yield innovative analyses, plans for applied research, and theoretically driven and empirically tested communication strategies.

Greg Downey in "Cultural Variation in Rugby Skills: A Preliminary Neuroanthropological Report" shows how important understanding variation is to providing evidence-based recommendations for athlete development programs. Highly skilled individuals, specifically different national playing styles in rugby, provide evidence for the existence of diverse ways to be expert. To understand this variation, Downey explores a synthesis of enskilment as a model for enculturation and the potential role of "degenerate" brain structures—multiple structures that can serve the same function—in underwriting diverse skill in athletes at individual and group levels. Using the "natural laboratory" of the Pacific nations for his research, Downey suggests how a mixed-method approach with neuroanthropology at its core can use consultation with experts, participant-observation, interview, and quantitative methods to produce empirical evidence on variation in cognitive playing styles. Two key applied dimensions stand out from this work: anthropologists can (1) point to mismatches between training and the actual game, and then provide a more accurate inventory of the cognitive demands and skills needed to match the exigencies of play; and (2) directly confront obsolete, even contradictory assumptions of uniformity among players and a conviction that a preordained form of "talent" exists that prevails among coaches, scouts and commentators on sports, as seen in discussions about race, innate talent, and "talent identification" as a form of expertise.

Eric Lindland and Nathaniel Kendall-Taylor in "Sensical Translations: Three Case Studies in Applied Cognitive Communications" address the work of the FrameWorks Institute, especially how researchers apply psychological anthropology to problems in communications. Lindland and Kendall-Taylor draw on cultural models research as well as metaphor and framing theory as part of an overall communication analysis strategy. This article shows how decades of research in psychological anthropology can successfully make the transition to an applied setting, and provides an important example for how neuroanthropology can successfully develop, not just in applied settings, but in consultancy and advocacy. Their article stands out for its empirical approach to developing a communications strategy, as well as to testing the strategy to make sure that it works. Moreover, Lindland and Kendall-Taylor clearly outline a theoretical rationale for the project's impact, in contrast to much of social science theory (which focuses on explaining "why," rather than "how"). Their emphasis on bringing latent cognitive models to the foreground, filling in gaps of understanding through extending expert models, and providing common sense models that better match expert knowledge through accurate simplification and targeted improvement provides a set of common elements—a theory—that applied approaches in other domains should aim to emulate. Finally, as this introduction also argues, Lindland and Kendall-Taylor's case study of education shows how much brain-based discourse is already part of how experts and parents think about children's mental health, and represents an important area where neuroanthropological research could clarify the issues at stake and suggest viable ways to address public deficits of understanding and thinking about the brain.

Katie Glaskin in "Empathy and the Robot: A Neuroanthropological Analysis" examines how robotics engineers are designing for empathy, trying to take into account the neural and interactive components of humans' relationship with robotic technology. Glaskin argues that their design approach, largely focused on neuroscience, leaves to one side the cultural dimensions of interaction, emotion, and empathy. In addressing the work of roboticists, Glaskin presents a broader argument about how we are increasingly anthropomorphizing technology. She takes roboticists to task for failing to recognize how their own approach to design, utilizing a reductionist and largely noncultural view of emotion, is in itself culture producing. Her work thus presents a twofold dynamic, critiquing directly the scientific basis of emotion research that roboticists use as inaccurate, and raising central, underaddressed questions about how design and technology produce both practices and objects that define what counts as human or not.

MENTAL AND BEHAVIORAL HEALTH

The three articles in the second section show how neuroanthropologists approach mental health and well-being in diverse contexts, and point to new, more integrated approaches to address these problems on the ground. Strikingly, all the articles share parallel approaches, focusing on the techniques, relationships, objects, and practices that lie between embodied biology, cultural meaning, and social inequality as key to applying neuroanthropology in the field of mental and behavioral health. Rather than simply drawing on techniques from outside anthropology, each article focuses on how neuroanthropologists can adapt, develop, and invent new approaches to address mental and behavioral health jointly through individual interactions, social interventions, and institutional change.

Brandon Kohrt, Sujen Maharjan, Damber Timsina, and James Griffith, in "Applying Nepali Ethnopsychology to Psychotherapy for the Treatment of Mental Illness and Prevention of Suicide among Bhutanese Refugees," use ethnography, therapeutic work, and applied neuroanthropology to address mental health issues among Nepali refugees from Bhutan. Ethnographic work with Nepali Bhutanese living in camps in southeastern Nepal provided an account of how these people interpret mental health and illness; this knowledge, in turn, informed work with refugees in the United States. Kohrt and colleagues review step-by-step how cognitive behavioral, interpersonal, and dialectal behavior forms of therapy can be applied to the Bhutanese once the therapist recognizes how both local ethnopsychologies and therapeutic effects match up with neuroanthropological dynamics.

Neely Myers, in "Toward an Applied Neuroanthropology of Psychosis: The Interplay of Culture, Brains and Experience," argues that psychosis and schizophrenia are best understood by examining the interplay of culture, brains, and experience. Myers presents experience as a crucial mediating factor between the neuropsychological foundations underlying psychosis and the cultural contexts that promote or inhibit vulnerability to psychosis. Using the case study of "Leroy," a 32-year-old African American man living in New York City, Myers sketches how institutional forces, local social relations, and embodied vulnerability powerfully shape Leroy's entry into psychosis and then undermine his ability to manage and recover from schizophrenia. Myers finishes by examining the structural forces in Leroy's life that arrayed themselves in opposition to what we know of healing, and how social factors could have helped him better negotiate his lived experience of psychosis. She appeals for an applied neuroanthropology that directly examines those practices and rituals that can help people dealing with psychosis and other mental health maladies.

Gino Collura and Daniel Lende, in "Post-Traumatic Stress Disorder and Neuroanthropology: Stopping PTSD before It Begins," discuss the neuroanthropology of stress, trauma, and PTSD among U.S. soldiers serving in combat zones. They critique the biomedical approach to PTSD, arguing that it disregards the formative effects that institutional and social contexts have on trauma, adaptation, and recovery. Collura and Lende focus on how concepts of resilience and trauma can be better understood by including the meaningful dimensions of people's lives, recognizing the diversity of individuals who enter into military service, and the dislocations in identity that can occur while deployed, which can also increase vulnerability to trauma. On the applied side, they address the ethics of work with the military, describing how they strive to be on the side of soldiers and to address the inevitable trauma that comes from deployment and combat. They propose specific approaches to enhancing resilience among soldiers, while also calling for more research to better outline the neuroanthropology of trauma and recovery.

POLITICAL ECONOMY AND CRITICAL ANALYSES

Most neuroanthropology research to present has focused on the intersection of neuroscience and culture, and less on how neuroscience intersects with political economy, inequality, and social structure, all of which shape human development, neural enculturation, and human variation. The authors of the articles in the final section highlight how neuroanthropology is equally amenable to the sort of work in biocultural anthropology that has focused on human biology, adaptation, political economy, and structural inequality (Goodman and Leatherman 1998). The authors also seek to position neuroanthropology to advance specific critical insights, pragmatic recommendations, and potential interventions to deal with today's pressing social problems.

Victoria Burbank, in "Life History and Real Life: An Example of Neuroanthropology in Aboriginal Australia," examines how history, ethnography, and the neurobiology of stress and pregnancy help us understand the tremendous differences in mortality between Indigenous and non-Indigenous Australians. Using the case study of the remote Arnhem Land community of Numbulwar, Burbank looks at how environmental stressors, particularly coming from the social dynamics of inequality and discrimination, can have intergenerational effects. We increasingly realize how life history theory, developmental origins research, and the neuroanthropology of stress allow us to better explain entrenched health disparities in marginalized communities. Burbank argues that this type of "considered etiology" can correct and even contradict policy and public discourse, working against media stereotypes and political decisions often justified by erroneous accounts of history, biology, and difference. In particular, Burbank's approach encourages neuroanthropologists to consider the long-term consequences of past history, including how that history biases current policy decisions.

Helena Hansen and Mary E. Skinner in "From White Bullets to Black Markets and Greened Medicine: The Neuroeconomics and Neuroracial Politics of Opioid Pharmaceuticals" describe how synthetic opiates, and the treatment of the health problems that result from these powerful pharmaceuticals, have created new economies and politics for many individuals in the addiction treatment industry. Contrasting the differing histories of methadone clinics and physician-prescribed buprenorphine (a new maintenance opioid), Hansen and Skinner demonstrate the existence of a two-tiered approach to addiction treatment that follows existing social, gender, and racial discrepancies. Using the lens of neuroanthropology, they argue that these enduring social inequalities, coupled with the powerful neurological impact of the pharmaceuticals, actually exaggerates the biological, political and economic dependence of the urban poor on synthetic opioids, both illegal and legal. Hansen and Skinner highlight the importance of addressing the structural differences that in both cases (but particularly for the poor) drive people's addicted involvement in markets of access to drugs and treatment.

Daniel Lende in "Poverty Poisons the Brain" examines emerging research that links poverty and social inequality, with a focus on toxic stress during childhood and subsequent negative health, educational, and behavioral outcomes. This model of "poverty poisons the brain" is increasingly popular in both the media and in policy-making institutions like the American Academy of Pediatrics, and has important lessons for neuroanthropology about how social experience gets under the skin. However, the same model works to hide the social conflicts that drive the overall system by narrowly focusing questions about poverty on proximate factors and individual neurobiology, effacing the larger-scale social forces from sustained consideration. Lende examines how the concepts of social embodiment, the dynamics of stress, and the production of inequality can transform "poverty poisons the brain" research and lead to more robust policy recommendations in the future.

CONCLUSION

For the editors, this issue, as well as neuroanthropology more generally, had its origins in a weblog. We founded Neuroanthropology.net in December 2007; this online forum then became one of the primary means to develop the ideas and professional connections that fed the growth of this new area of research. Alongside traditional means, such as departmental interactions, panels at professional meetings, a specialized conference, and our 2012 edited volume, neuroanthropology has emerged into a field through its electronic presence.

From early on, we used the weblog to address public controversies, discuss applied work, reflect on teaching, and document what we were doing in more closed settings like conferences or scholarly articles in ways that a much broader public could access. The platform provided by the blog, and the transparency and engagement it facilitated, helped make neuroanthropology explicitly applied and public from the beginning. We could take risks on the blog that might not fly in a 15-minute conference paper at a once-a-year gathering; we could challenge existing research, critique prominent public figures, and hold accountable science journalists with a much larger audience and faster reaction cycle. These efforts taught us much about how to apply neuroanthropology in ways that made sense to a broader public and to competing expert opinions. Although online writing is not recognized by many measures of academic achievement, for us, working in a fast-changing, emerging research area, this genre was essential to nurture a new area of expertise. We did not know who, or what, was beyond our disciplinary field as we ventured into uncharted areas. By writing about these issues online, we learned more quickly, bumping up against a range of researchers and issues in the dark as we sought to apply neuroanthropological thinking to a range of questions.

We believe that this same sort of engagement can happen in multiple ways as the neuroanthropology community grows in breadth and size. Applied engagement will happen in the field, in the classroom, out in the community, in reported research, and online. We found that being online facilitated engagement for us in particular, but we want to emphasize that there are numerous ways to be applied and that we should aim for a diversity of approaches that matches the diversity of the world. The articles presented here deliver on that simple point—let's get started on neuroanthropology and its applications because the engagement itself is such a productive generator of new ideas, refined research methods, and the anthropological imagination.

NOTES

1. The volume, *The Encultured Brain: An Introduction to Neuroanthropology* (Lende and Downey 2012), lays out the scholarly bases of neuroanthropology, including theoretical foundations, methodological considerations, biological background, and ten case studies of neuroanthropological research. The editors and other collaborators have especially sought to encourage wide-ranging collaboration and interdisciplinary inspiration through new electronic media on the Neuroanthropology weblog (http://blogs.plos.org/neuroanthropology/).

2. For an excellent account of how applied work can be influenced by theoretical work on the brain and, at the same time, influence neuroscientific theory, see Schwartz and Begley (2002). Schwartz's insights from using "guided neuroplasticity" in working with obsessive compulsive disorder are remarkable, even if his use of "quantum theory" is highly idiosyncratic.

3. Alongside "mix and match," another metaphor to understand how neural plasticity and enculturation come together is "plug and play": where the brain plugs in the needed processes to be able to play with ongoing demands.

REFERENCES CITED

Ambady, Nalini, and Jamshed Bharucha
    2009 Culture and the Brain. Current Directions in Psychological Science 18(6):342–345.

Anderson, Michael L.
    2010 Neural Reuse: A Fundamental Organizational Principle of the Brain. Behavioral and Brain Sciences 33:245–266.

Antelius, Eleonor
    2007 The Meaning of the Present: Hope and Foreclosure in Narrations about People with Severe Brain Damage. Medical Anthropology Quarterly 21(3):324–342.

Barkow, Jerome H., Leda Cosmides, and John Tooby, eds.
    1992 The Adapted Mind: Evolutionary Psychology and the Generation of Culture. New York: Oxford University Press.

Campbell, Benjamin C., and Justin R. Garcia
    2009 Neuroanthropology: Evolution and Emotional Embodiment. Frontiers in Evolutionary Neuroscience 1(4). http://www.ncbi.nlm.nih.gov/pmc/articles/PMC2841818, accessed 14 December 14, 2009.

Cantlon, Jessica F., and Elizabeth M. Brannon
    2006 Adding Up the Effects of Cultural Experience on the Brain. Trends in Cognitive Sciences 11(1):1–4.

Chiao, Joan Y.
    2010 Neural Basis of Social Status Hierarchy across Species. Current Opinion in Neurobiology 20(6):803–809.

Chiao, Joan Y., Ahmad R. Hariri, Tokiko Harada, Yoko Mano, Norihiro Sadato, Todd B. Parrish, and Tetsuya Iidaka
    2010 Theory and Methods in Cultural Neuroscience. Social, Cognitive and Affective Neuroscience 5(2–3):356 361.

Choudhury, Suparna, and Jan Slaby, eds.
    2012 Critical Neuroscience: A Handbook of the Social and Cultural Contexts of Neuroscience. Madden, MA: Wiley Blackwell.

Christiansen, Morten H., and Nick Chater
    2008 Language as Shaped by the Brain. Behavioral and Brain Sciences 31(5):489–509.

Cohn, Simon
    2012 Disrupting Images: Neuroscientific Representations in the Lives of Psychiatric Patients. *In* Critical Neuroscience: A Handbook of the Social and Cultural Contexts of Neuroscience. S. Choudhury and J. Slaby, eds. Pp. 179–194. Malden, MA: Wiley Blackwell.

d'Aquili, Eugene G., and Andrew B. Newberg
    1999 The Mystical Mind. Minneapolis: Fortress.

Dayan, Eran, and Leonardo G. Cohen
    2011 Neuroplasticity Subserving Motor Skill Learning. Neuron 72(3):443–454.

Deacon, Terrence
    1997 The Symbolic Species: The Co-Evolution of Language and the Brain. New York: W. W. Norton.

Doidge, Norman
    2007 The Brain That Changes Itself; Stories of Personal Triumph from the Frontiers of Brain Science. New York: Penguin.

Domínguez Duque, Juan F.
    2012 Neuroanthropology and the Dialectical Imperative. Anthropological Theory 12(1):5–27.

Domínguez Duque, Juan F., Robert Turner, E. Douglas Lewis, and Gary Egan
    2010 Neuroanthropology: A Humanistic Science for the Study of the Culture–Brain Nexus. Social, Cognitive and Affective Neuroscience 5(2–3):138–147.

Downey, Greg
    2007 Seeing without a "Sideways Glance": Visuomotor "Knowing" and the Plasticity of Perception. *In* Ways of Knowing: New Approaches in the Anthropology of Knowledge and Learning. Mark Harris, ed. Pp. 222–241. New York: Berghahn.

2010 "Practice without Theory": A Neuroanthropological Perspective on Embodied Learning. Journal of the Royal Anthropological Institute 16(supp. 1):22–40.

2012 Balancing across Cultures: Sensory Plasticity. *In* The Encultured Brain: An Introduction to Neuroanthropology. Daniel H. Lende and Greg Downey, eds. Pp. 169–194. Cambridge, MA: MIT Press.

Downey, Greg, and Daniel H. Lende

2012a Neuroanthropology and the Encultured Brain. *In* The Encultured Brain: An Introduction to Neuroanthropology. Daniel H. Lende and Greg Downey, eds. Pp. 23–65. Cambridge, MA: MIT Press.

2012b Evolution and the Brain. *In* The Encultured Brain: An Introduction to Neuroanthropology. Daniel H. Lende and Greg Downey, eds. Pp. 103–137. Cambridge, MA: MIT Press.

Dumit, Joseph

2004 Picturing Personhood: Brain Scans and Biomedical Identity. Princeton: Princeton University Press.

Evans, Nicholas, and Stephen C. Levinson

2009 The Myth of Language Universals: Language Diversity and its Importance for Cognitive Science. Behavioral and Brain Sciences 32(5):429–492.

Feldman, Daniel E.

2009 Synaptic Mechanisms for Plasticity in Neocortex. Annual Review of Neuroscience 32:33–55.

Fuentes, Agustín

2008 Evolution of Human Behavior. New York: Oxford University Press.

Frazzetto, Giovanni, and Suzanne Anker

2009 Neuroculture. Nature Reviews Neuroscience 10:815–821.

Gelman, Susan A., and Christine H. Legare

2011 Concepts and Folk Theories. Annual Review of Anthropology 40:379–398.

Gettler, Lee T., Thom W. McDade, Alan B. Feranil, and Christopher W. Kuzawa

2011 Longitudinal Evidence that Fatherhood Decreases Testosterone in Human Males. Proceedings of the National Academy of Sciences 108(39):16194–16199.

Goodman, Alan H., and Thomas Leatherman

1998 Building a New Biocultural Synthesis: Political-Economic Perspectives on Human Biology. Ann Arbor: University of Michigan Press.

Gravlee, Clarence C.

2009 How Race Becomes Biology: Embodiment of Social Inequality. American Journal of Physical Anthropology 139(1):47–57.

Hanakawa, Takashi, Manabu Honda, Tomohis Okada, Hidenao Fukuyama, and Hiroshi Shibasaki

2003 Neural Correlates Underlying Mental Calculation in Abacus Experts: Functional Magnetic Resonance Imaging Study. Neuroimage 19(2):296–307.

Hare, Brian

2011 From Hominoid to Hominid Mind: What Changed and Why? Annual Review of Anthropology 40:293–309.

Henrich, Joseph, Steven J. Heine, and Ara Norenzayan

2010 The Weirdest People in the World? Behavioral and Brain Sciences 33(2–3):61–83.

Hertzman, Clyde, and Tom Boyce

2010 How Experience Gets under the Skin to Create Gradients in Developmental Health. Annual Review of Public Health 31(1):329–347.

Hinton, Alexander L., ed.

1999 Biocultural Approaches to the Emotions. New York: Cambridge University Press.

Hrdy, Sarah

2000 Mother Nature: Maternal Instincts and How They Shape the Human Species. New York: Ballantine Books.

Hutchins, Edwin

1995 Cognition in the Wild. Cambridge, MA: MIT Press.

2011 Enculturating the Supersized Mind. Philosophical Studies 152(3):437–446.

Kanai, Ryota, and Geraint Rees
  2011 The Structural Basis of Inter-Individual Differences in Human Behaviour and Cognition. Nature Reviews Neuroscience 12(4):231–242.
Kendal, Jeremy, Jamshid J. Tehrani, and John Odling-Smee
  2011 Human Niche Construction in Interdisciplinary Focus. Philosophical Transactions of the Royal Society B: Biological Sciences 366(1566):785–792.
Kirsch, Irving
  2010 The Emperor's New Drugs: Exploding the Antidepressant Myth. New York: Basic Books.
Kitayama, Shinobu, and Ayse K. Uskul
  2011 Culture, Mind, and the Brain: Current Evidence and Future Directions. Annual Review of Psychology 62:419–449.
Kohrt, Brandon A., and Ian Harper
  2008 Navigating Diagnoses: Understanding Mind-Body Relations, Mental Health, and Stigma in Nepal. Culture, Medicine and Psychiatry 32(4):462–491.
Lakoff, Andrew
  2005 Pharmaceutical Reason: Knowledge and Value in Global Psychiatry. New York: Cambridge University Press.
Legrenzi, Paolo, Carlo Umilta, and Frances Anderson
  2011 Neuromania: On the Limits of Brain Science. New York: Oxford University Press.
Lende, Daniel H.
  2005 Wanting and Drug Use: A Biocultural Approach to the Analysis of Addiction. Ethos 33(1):100–124.
  2007 Evolution and Modern Behavioral Problems. In Evolutionary Medicine and Health: New Perspectives. Wenda Trevathan, E. O. Smith, and James J. McKenna, eds. Pp. 277–291. New York: Oxford University Press.
  2012 Addiction and Neuroanthropology. In The Encultured Brain: An Introduction to Neuroanthropology. Daniel H. Lende and Greg Downey, eds. Pp. 339–362. Cambridge, MA: MIT Press.
Lende, Daniel H., and Greg Downey, eds.
  2012 The Encultured Brain: An Introduction to Neuroanthropology. Cambridge, MA: MIT Press.
Levine, Robert A., ed.
  2010 A Reader in Psychological Anthropology. Malden, MA: Wiley Blackwell.
Lock, Margaret, and Vinh-Kim Nguyen
  2010 An Anthropology of Biomedicine. Malden, MA: Wiley Blackwell.
Low, Setha, and Sally E. Merry
  2010 Engaged Anthropology: Diversity and Dilemmas. Current Anthropology 51(supp. 2):203–226.
Luhrmann, Tanya M.
  2001 Of Two Minds: An Anthropologist Looks at American Psychiatry. New York: Vintage.
Lutz, Catherine A.
  1988 Unnatural Emotions: Everyday Sentiments on a Micronesian Atoll and Their Challenge to Western Theory. Chicago: University of Chicago Press.
MacKinnon, Katherine, and Agustín Fuentes
  2012 Primate Social Cognition, Human Evolution, and Niche Construction: A Core Context for Neuroanthropology. In The Encultured Brain: An Introduction to Neuroanthropology. Daniel H. Lende and Greg Downey, eds. Pp. 67–102. Cambridge, MA: MIT Press.
Mahler, Sarah J.
  2012 Culture As Comfort: The Many Things You Already Know about Culture (But May Not Realize). New York: Pearson Education.
Malafouris, Lambros
  2010 Metaplasticity and the Principles of Neuroarchaeology. Journal of Anthropological Sciences 88:49–72.
Martin, Emily
  2010 Self-Making and the Brain. Subjectivity 3(4):366–381.
Minkler, Meredith, and Nina Wallerstein, eds.
  2008 Community-Based Participatory Research for Health: From Process to Outcomes. San Francisco: Jossey Bass.

Moore, Carmella C., and Holly F. Mathews, eds.

  2001 The Psychology of Cultural Experience. Cambridge: Cambridge University Press.

Northoff, Georg

  2010 Humans, Brains and Their Environments: Marriage between Neuroscience and Anthropology? Neuron 65(6):748–751.

Ortega, Francisco

  2009 The Cerebral Subject and the Challenge of Neurodiversity. BioSocieties 4(4):425–445.

Persinger, Michael A.

  1983 Religious and Mystical Experiences as Artifacts of Temporal Lobe Function: A General Hypothesis. Perceptual and Motor Skills 57(3f):1255–1262

Quintero, Gilbert, and Mark Nichter

  2011 Generation RX: Anthropological Research on Pharmaceutical Enhancement, Lifestyle Regulation, Self-Medication and Recreational Drug Use. In A Companion to Medical Anthropology. Merrill Singer and Pamela Erickson, eds. Pp. 339–355. New York: John Wiley and Sons.

Raikhel, Eugene

  2012 Radical Reductions: Neurophysiology, Politics and Personhood in Russian Addiction Medicine. In Critical Neuroscience: A Handbook of the Social and Cultural Contexts of Neuroscience. Suparna Choudhury and Jan Slaby, eds. Pp. 227–252. Malden, MA: Wiley Blackwell.

Raybeck, Douglas, and Paul Y. L. Ngo

  2011 Behavior and the Brain: Mediation of Acquired Skills. Cross-Cultural Research 45(2):178–207.

Rees, Tobias

  2010 Being Neurologically Human Today: Life and Science and Adult Cerebral Plasticity (An Ethical Analysis). American Ethnologist 37(1):150–166.

Reyna, Stephen P.

  2012a Introduction: Special Issue—Neuroanthropology. Anthropological Theory 12(1):3–4.

  2012b Neo-Boasianism, A Form of Critical Structural Realism: It's Better than the Alternative. Anthropological Theory 12(1):73–99.

Rilling, James K.

  2008 Neuroscientific Approaches and Applications within Anthropology. Yearbook of Physical Anthropology 51:2–32.

Rilling, James K., and Alan G. Sanfey

  2011 The Neuroscience of Social Decision-Making. Annual Review of Psychology 62:23–48.

Roepstorff, Andeas

  2011 Culture: A Site of Relativist Energy in the Cognitive Sciences. Common Knowledge 17(1):37–41.

Roepstorff, Andreas, Jörg Niewöhnerc, and Stefan Beck

  2010 Enculturing Brains through Patterned Practices. Neural Networks 23(8–9):1051–1059.

Rolls, Edmund T.

  2012 Neuroculture: On the Implications of Brain Science. New York: Oxford University Press.

Royal Society

  2011 Neuroscience and the Law. London: The Royal Society.

Rylko-Bauer, Barbara, Merrill Singer, and John van Willigen

  2006 Reclaiming Applied Anthropology: Its Past, Present, and Future. American Anthropologist 108(1):178–190.

Sabloff, Jeremy A.

  2011 Where Have You Gone, Margaret Mead? Anthropology and Public Intellectuals. American Anthropologist 113(3):408–416.

Schensul, Jean J., and Edison Trickett

  2009 Introduction to Multi-Level Community Based Culturally Situated Interventions. American Journal of Community Psychology 43(3–4):232–240.

Schwartz, Jeffrey M., and Sharon Begley

  2002 The Mind and the Brain: Neuroplasticity and the Power of Mental Force. New York: Regan Books.

Seligman, Rebecca, and Ryan A. Brown

2010 Theory and Method at the Intersection of Anthropology and Cultural Neuroscience. Social, Cognitive and Affective Neuroscience 5 (2–3):130–137.

Seligman, Rebecca, and Laurence Kirmayer

2008 Dissociative Experience and Cultural Neuroscience: Narrative, Metaphor and Mechanism. Culture, Medicine and Psychiatry 32(1):31–64.

Shore, Bradd

1996 Culture in Mind: Cognition, Culture, and the Problem of Meaning. New York: Oxford University Press.

Sousa, David A.

2010 Mind, Brain, and Education: Neuroscience Implications for the Classroom. Bloomington, IN: Solution Tree Press.

Strauss, Claudia, and Naomi Quinn

1998 A Cognitive Theory of Culture. New York: Cambridge University Press.

Tallis, Raymond

2011 Aping Mankind: Neuromania, Darwinitis, and the Misrepresentation of Humanity. Durham: Acumen.

Tang, Yiyuan, Wutian Zhang, Kewei Chen, Shigang Feng, Ye Ji, Junxian Shen, Eric M. Reiman, and Yijun Liu

2006 Arithmetic Processing in the Brain Shaped by Cultures. Proceedings of the National Academy of Science 103(28):10775–10780.

Thaler, Lore, Stephen Arnott, and Melvyn Goodale

2011 Neural Correlates of Natural Human Echolocation in Early and Late Blind Echolocation Experts. PLoS ONE 6(5):e20162. doi: 10.1371/journal.pone.0020162, accessed March 20, 2012.

Turner, Robert

2012 The Need for Systematic Ethnopsychology: The Ontological Status of Mentalistic Terminology. Anthropological Theory 12(1):29–42.

Westermann, G., Denis Mareschal, Mark H. Johnson, Sylvain Sirois, Michael W. Spratling, and Michael S. C. Thomas

2007 Neuroconstructivism. *Developmental Science* 10(1):75–83.

Wexler, Bruce E.

2011 Neuroplasticity: Biological Evolution's Contribution to Cultural Evolution. *In* Culture and Neural Frames of Cognition and Communication. Shihui Han and Ernst Pöppel, eds. Pp. 1–17. Heidelberg: Springer Berlin Heidelberg.

Whitehead, Charles

2012 Why the Behavioural Sciences Need the Concept of the Culture-Ready Brain. Anthropological Sciences 12(1):43–71.

Willen, Sarah, and Donald Seeman

2012 Introduction: Experience and Inquietude. Ethos 40(1):1–23.

Worthman, Carol M.

2009 Habits of the Heart: Life History and the Developmental Neuroendocrinology of Emotion. American Journal of Human Biology 21(6):772–781.

Worthman, Carol M., Paul M. Plotsky, Daniel S. Schechter, and Constance A. Cummings

2010 Formative Experiences: The Interaction of Caregiving, Culture, and Developmental Psychobiology. New York: Cambridge University Press.

Young, Allan

1997 The Harmony of Illusions: Inventing Post-Traumatic Stress Disorder. Princeton: Princeton University Press.

CULTURAL VARIATION IN RUGBY SKILLS:
A PRELIMINARY NEUROANTHROPOLOGICAL REPORT

GREG DOWNEY
Macquarie University

Cultural differences in sports playing styles may be the result of players possessing diverging cognitive–perceptual strategies, with resulting differences in the underlying neurological correlates of skilled behavior. The chapter describes the preliminary stages of an applied project with national rugby unions to understand how different developmental environments for skill acquisition may effect cognitive variation by making use of "degenerate" neurological structures, or the ability of multiple neurological structures to produce similar outcomes. Neurocognitive differences in skill have implications for talent identification, appropriate training, and the difficulty of capturing skilled action in laboratory settings, which artificially narrow players' potential to use diverse problem solving strategies. [skill acquisition, neuroanthropology, sports, rugby, cognitive variation, neural degeneracy]

Just south of downtown Sydney, across the street from the Football Stadium and historic Cricket Ground, fit young men (and an occasional young woman) come together three times weekly to train under the watchful eye of some of Australia's most highly respected developmental coaches. Singled out for their athletic prowess, the "high performance" group of the Australian Rugby Union meets for an hour, working through a range of drills, simulations, and training exercises. Outside of these sessions, the players practice with their local rugby clubs and school teams, in some cases playing for the elite private colleges of Sydney that are the breeding ground of most of the Wallabies, the members of the Australian national rugby team.

The session often begins with warm-up exercises: players stand in groups of three or four and pass the ball to each other, practicing the sport's distinctive underarm, two-handed technique, or they do some light stretching and running. As training begins in earnest, exercises become more complex and demanding. Players face each other in small groups—two-on-two or four-on-three or some other configuration—learning to work together, run the best "lines" to draw defenders out of position, and contain an offense. They drill basic skills like passing, tackling, and contesting the ball in the "ruck," when players from both sides struggle for possession of the ball on the ground following a tackle. Drills are punctuated with instruction. Coaches intervene to point out problems or suggest changes in technique.

Moments of the fluctuating action of a rugby match are generally abstracted and drilled out of context. The "forwards," for example, may be pulled out to rehearse repeatedly the "set pieces" that define their positions: the "scrum," when eight players

ANNALS OF ANTHROPOLOGICAL PRACTICE 36, pp. 26–44. ISSN: 2153-957X. © 2012 by the American Anthropological Association. DOI:10.1111/j.2153-9588.2012.01091.x

bind together to try to push the opposing forwards off the ball as it is returned to play, and the "lineout," when the ball is restarted by a throw from the sideline, and teams vie for the ball in the air by lifting a teammate. Other specialists may be called aside to refine their kicking technique or their defense against kicks, or practice attacking swiftly by sweeping and passing laterally across field.

Rarely, players scrimmage in larger numbers, seldom approaching the massed 15-against-15 of the full rugby side, and never with all of the hallmarks of a formal game. Training is invariably fragmented, punctuated with frequent intervals of rest, instruction, and sips from water bottles. The contest seldom approaches the intensity of a real game.

In Tonga and Fiji, the young men who will someday face the Wallabies are engaged in quite different forms of "training." These athletes mostly play informal games, some virtually every afternoon with their brothers, cousins, and neighbors in villages on local fields. In these informal settings, without the structured training that Sydney's elite young athletes have come to expect, boys participate regardless of age or expertise, and they play without the intervention of a coach, trainer, or referee. Australian players who have toured in the Pacific Islands speak with grudging respect of local pick-up games played on fields of cut cane and mud, at times without shoes, even when the sweltering air dripped with humidity. Some shake their heads as they recall trips, marveling when they talked about the intimidating, brutal tackling and shoulder charging endured by the Tongan and Fijian youth, in contrast to the constrained contact during training at Sydney; a player injured in Sydney training might not be able to recover in time for a valuable club game. Rugby aficionados often argue that village rugby creates a distinctive style of play among Islander teams: aggressive, creative, but with a tendency to get caught out in defense or commit ill-timed forward passes for penalties at inopportune moments. Coaches have suggested that, if Fiji or Tonga could develop more disciplined play and pick representative teams purely on merit without regard to group loyalties, they would perform even better on the international stage.

This article reports preliminary field observations, as well as both theoretical and practical issues that have arisen at the start of an applied neuroanthropology project currently under way by the author and Dr. John Evans of the University of Sydney. Working in partnership with a number of rugby organizations, especially the Australian Rugby Union during the preliminary phase, we are seeking to better understand diversity among highly skilled individuals. That is, using a mixed method approach, we examine the developmental influences on players identified as "talented" or high performing, including specialized coaching, informal practice, and linked nonrugby activities, such as participation in other sports. Our goal is to document and analyze distinctive playing styles because we believe that they may be underwritten by diverse cognitive and perceptual strategies leading to distinctive patterns of decision making, group coordination, and strategic maneuvering.

Using a mixture of ethnographic, videographic, and quantitative methods, we are analyzing variation in play. The project seeks to advise coaches and scouts how to apply neuroanthropological insights to their practice, especially tailoring training to diverse forms of expertise, recognizing promising players from unfamiliar cultural backgrounds, and better matching training environments to the demands of training (see also Evans in press). Although focused specifically on sport, the project has implications for how training programs, in complex or high-pressure decision making take account of cognitive diversity.

THE RESEARCH PROBLEM: CULTURAL VARIATION IN SKILL

The Pacific provides an ideal "natural laboratory" for studying cultural differences in rugby skills because the region is a stronghold for elite expertise in the sport; New Zealand is the current Rugby World Cup holder, and Australia and various Pacific nations all compete well in international competition in spite of lower populations than rival countries like France and England. Highly skilled players flow out of this region for lucrative contracts with better financed European and Asian clubs; some fans of the sport argue that even Samoa, a tiny island nation of less than 200,000 people, could contend for world champion if so many of the country's best players were not on contract in the European professional leagues or playing for New Zealand.

Although the level of achievement is high across the region, the training contexts in these countries vary significantly. For example, rugby union in Australia was the last football code to become professional in the 1990s, and the sport is still associated with elite secondary schools and high social status. The competing rugby league code (referred to in Australia as "league" or "rugby league," whereas rugby union is called "union" or "rugby"), with significant differences in rules and playing dynamics, by contrast, is considered a more "working-class" sport, having been professional for most of the 20th century. In contrast, rugby union is the popular sport of choice broadly in New Zealand and among indigenous peoples of Pacific Island communities (except Papua New Guinea, where rugby league is dominant). All of these settings, including social dynamics, stylistic preferences, and local ethnic associations in the sport, shape distinctive approaches to training and talent identification.

Commentators, coaches, athletes, and sports fans alike all recognize that the "same" sports can be played in quite distinct fashions; in fact, one of the great attractions of international events like the Rugby World Cup is the confrontation among national styles, a resource that the International Rugby Board (IRB) recognizes (see IRB 2004). Much like the Maōri *haka*, performed by New Zealand's All-Blacks prior to rugby matches, the confrontation of cultures, not just national teams, helps to make each competition distinctive. The IRB has included increasing the international competitiveness of the Pacific Island rugby teams—especially Fiji, Tonga, and Samoa—among its strategic goals for the coming decade in part because of their charismatic playing style (IRB 2010).

The internationalization of the sport, however, has created challenges for maintaining national distinctiveness and managing players of diverse backgrounds, as coaches and even high-level players change countries for professional reasons. The appointment of New Zealander Robbie Deans to the head coaching position of the Australian national team, the Wallabies, was welcomed by most fans of the sport although many call for a return to an Australian coach when Deans's contract expires. The concern is not simply nationalism but a worry that foreign-born coaches may not be able to work well with local athletic talent and tactics.

Anthropologists and other cultural researchers have highlighted how important the stylistic distinctiveness of athletes can be for the nationalist imagination, in association football (soccer), boxing, and a range of other sports, including rugby (e.g., Black and Nauright 1998; Chandler and Nauright 1999; Diné 2001; Maguire and Tuck 1998; Tuck 2003). The national pride invested in playing style, and the sheer volume and occasional elegance of sports commentary, has allowed cultural historians to document how the nation is "imagined" in soccer, cricket, and boxing (e.g., Appadurai 1997; Archetti 1999; Bairner 2001; Lever 1983; Sugden 1996). The late sociologist, Pierre Bourdieu (1990) identified subnational differences in "styles" of playing the same sport as crucial for understanding class-based relations of individuals to their own bodies.

But the clash of playing styles at events like the World Cup is also an opportunity to study the cultural configuration of skill from a neuroanthropological perspective, especially the way that different developmental environments might produce diversity in skilled performance. A cultural constructivist study of athletic style can remain agnostic about whether stylistic differences actually exist; most cultural and anthropological research focuses on public discourse *about* differences in playing style or native theories about how a people's distinctive way of playing arises, but does not explore the potential biocultural reality of differing techniques. If stylistic differences really do exist, and if they are the result of distinctive neurological strategies in skill, then various coaching and training techniques may not work equally well with all players.

CULTURE AS SKILL–ENSKILMENT AND NEUROPLASTICITY

Anthropologist Tim Ingold (2000) advocates treating enculturation in general as "enskilment" to overcome conceptual problems produced by a model of culture as shared internalized knowledge or group belonging (see also Marchand 2010). Learning culture, according to Ingold (2000:416), as anthropologists typically understand it, "entails an internalisation of collective representations or, in a word, *enculturation*. 'Understanding in practice,' by contrast, is a process of *enskilment*, in which learning is inseparable from doing, and in which both are embedded in the context of a practical engagement in the world—that is, in dwelling." The conceptual move to reframe enculturation as enskilment privileges practice over abstract understanding, situated and perceptual ability over meaning or interpretation, as the central accounts of how people live through diverse cultures.

The shift to a model of enskilment also benefits neuroanthropology because the model highlights the combined biocultural processes that make up enculturation; in contrast, treating "culture" as shared information can reinscribe a pernicious opposition between culture and biology by conceptually separating mental content from the brain. The "shared information" definition can suggest that culture is ideational content, rather than (simultaneously) cognitive and physiological change. Elsewhere (Downey 2010b:318), I have argued that we find "the boundary between culture and biology erased in the developmental emergence of skill," that the "biocultural consequences of skill acquisition collapses clear distinctions between 'learning,' 'development,' and 'phenotypic adaptation.'" Ingold (1998:26) likewise points out "that throughout life, the body undergoes processes of growth and decay, and that as it does so, particular skills, habits, capacities and strengths, as well as debilities and weaknesses, are enfolded into its very constitution—in its neurology, musculature, even its anatomy." Through comparison with skills, we can better understand how culture takes hold of the body and nervous system, remodeling and allocating physiological resources, deeply enculturing the human organism (see Ericsson and Lehmann 1996; Sands 1999).

Ideology and explicit discourse are still part of culture, of course, even at this biocultural level, such as the way theories about motor learning, images of idealized bodies, or ideals for good coaching shape the drills in which young athletes must engage at rugby training three nights a week in my Sydney field site. But what psychologists Zajonc and Markus (1984) call the "hard" interface between culture and the nervous system in the enskilment model is mundane bodily techniques, practices, and habits. Physical training makes it clear that cultural "embodiment" is not a theoretical metaphor or purely phenomenological fact. Especially for a study of sport, in which explicit and semiotic elements may be impoverished relative to extraordinary practical proficiency and physiological adaptation, this model of culture as enskilment is particularly attractive (see also Ingold 2001).

Modeling enculturation as enskilment also allows neuroanthropologists to draw on empirical evidence for physiological adaptation during skill acquisition to better understand how cultural regimes of training might involve changes in neural architecture (see Downey 2012). Highly skilled populations like musicians (Bengtsson et al. 2005; Gaser and Schlaug 2003; Münte et al. 2002), typists (Cannonieri et al. 2007), taxicab drivers (Maguire et al. 2000), and jugglers (Draganski et al. 2004; Draganski and May 2008) all evidence distinctive patterns of practice-dependent neurological development (for review, see May 2011). From sports in particular, a range of neuropsychology experiments demonstrate that high proficiency individuals have distinctive neuroanatomical features, such as increased cortical thickness or gray matter density in functionally relevant regions. Support has come from studies of a range of athletes, including divers (Wei et al. 2011), basketball players (Park et al. 2011), recreational golfers (Bezzola et al. 2011), and judo and tai chi practitioners (Jacini et al. 2009; Kerr et al. 2008).

As exciting as these results are, however, they also demonstrate that an account of neural enculturation cannot be assembled solely from imaging data, nor can skill be predicted on the basis of cortical specialization alone. Jäncke and colleagues (2009), for example, found that golfers' handicaps, a measure of their proficiency, correlated with a quantitative shift in neuroanatomy. However, the transformation was not incremental: golfers achieving handicaps around 15 strokes demonstrated a marked reorganization and increased gray matter volume in cortical areas associated with sensorimotor control and planning processes. Further practice and greater expertise, in contrast, did not result in additional reorganization. Jäncke's team suggests that the cortical reorganization occurred relatively early in training, between approximately 800 and 3,000 practice hours, and that further proficiency may arise from greater functional efficiency, not increased cortical density (Jäncke et al. 2009:4–5).

In research by the same team based on ballet dancers, Hänggi and colleagues (2010) found that some specialized white and gray matter volume *decreased* in expert dancers compared to control subjects. As Hänggi and colleagues discuss (2010:1202), in some case studies, expertise appears to result in *lower* levels of neural activity in areas associated with control (see also Del Percio et al. 2008; Draganski et al. 2006; Maguire et al. 2000; Meister et al. 2005). Although the results were unexpected to the team, the pattern of evidence suggests that our understanding of how skills sculpt neuroplasticity needs to appreciate the complexity of developmental processes (for reviews, see Dayan and Cohen 2011; Kelly and Garavan 2005). Not all increases in skill necessarily correlate to increased cortical recruitment or neuroanatomical expansion; some stages of expertise might have their own patterns, such as a streamlining of control functions, a paring down of extraneous neural activity, or a shift of the cognitive "load" of a task from one brain region to another.

For example, anthropologists and psychologists recognize that visual behavior—the pattern of where a person looks—changes as he or she becomes more proficient at visual tasks (see Duffy et al. 2009). Tim Ingold (2000) argues that a crucial dimension of enculturation is what ecological psychologist James Gibson called an "education of attention" (Gibson 1979:254). To gain proficiency is not merely to learn a semiotic code or develop movement capacities, but also to move from being a naive observer to a proficient agent, one who recognizes what parts of the environment yield up crucial information (see also Downey 2007; Grasseni 2004, 2009).

Certainly, empirical studies of athletes have found that highly skilled individuals adopt efficient visual search patterns, concentrating on key features of a scene. For example, eye-tracking studies of tennis players, cricket batsmen, and soccer goalkeepers demonstrate that, as players' expertise grow, they reliably focus on particular parts of an opponent's wind-up to anticipate where a serve, a pitch, or penalty kick will go (see Land and MacLeod 2000; Savelsbergh et al. 2002; Singer et al. 1996; Williams et al. 2002). As Williams (2000:745) writes in a review of the research on soccer: "Skilled and less-skilled performers can be differentiated on the basis of their visual search behaviours, their ability to distinguish evolving patterns of play and to discern key postural cues signifying opponents' future actions" (for review, see Vickers 2007). Behavior and habits, like a refined visual scanning pattern, may allow expert practitioners to more effectively extract necessary information or reduce non-task-related neural activity, so the expert brain may actually be less metabolically active given the same perceptual–cognitive challenge (e.g., Gobel et al. 2011).

ENCULTURED SKILLS AND NEUROCOGNITIVE DIVERSITY

The psychological research on elite skills, however, often does not consider the possibility that variation in styles of play or cognitive–perceptual strategies may exist at the highest levels of achievement. That is, the research on "elite performance" often presumes that expertise is marked by convergence; although novices may be inept in a variety of ways, experts are assumed to share a single optimal solution strategy (Downey 2010a). For example, psychological exploration of highly skilled chess players' performance by de Groot (1965) and Simon and Chase (1973) argued that their superior performance was based on recall strategies for chess-specific patterns, which allowed them to perceive larger meaningful patterns in the placement of pieces. All chess masters were assumed to be refining the same or quite similar cognitive mechanisms. The presumption of uniformity—what Lonner (1993) calls an implicit "absolutism"—is a hallmark of cognitive neuroscience (see also Henrich et al. 2010). Vogel and Awh (2008:171) explain: "variability across individuals is typically treated as a nuisance or as error variance" (see also Kanai and Rees 2011).

Landmark theoretical and empirical work by Anders Ericsson and diverse colleagues, for example, take for granted that expertise is "maximal adaptation" to "task constraints," implying that the structure of the task determines the ideal configuration for neurological resources and practical strategies (see, e.g., Ericsson and Lehmann 1996). In fact, Ericsson's work on "deliberate practice" does not require that expertise be uniform, I would argue. Many of the tasks chosen to study, however, are tightly constrained and may allow only one neurological solution. For highly canalized tasks, increasing expertise likely produces convergence, if human neurological potential affords only one possible solution. But for a variety of tasks, multiple ways may exist to be an expert. The question of expert variation is an empirical one and, in the case of rugby, prima facie evidence supports the hypothesis that experts at the same positions may accomplish what they do in diverse ways (see Downey 2010a).

Suggestively, recent research in cross-cultural psychology and cultural neuroscience both demonstrate that different groups have diverging strategies for achieving similar functions, even quite basic skills, in areas such as reading (Siok et al. 2004), empathy (Cheon et al. 2011), object processing (Goh and Park 2009), self-perception (Zhu et al. 2007), and attentional control (Duffy et al. 2009). For example, research with diverse national groups finds that they employ different strategies in computer-based problems, and that these strategies make use of dissimilar cognitive resources (see Güss et al. 2009; Strohschneider and Güss 1998, 1999). Neuroimaging research often corroborates behavioral and psychological evidence for cultural diversity.

One of the clearest examples of cultural influence on skill is in the area of mental arithmetic, where psychological researchers have long recognized that training can lead to substantially different ways of realizing mental calculations (e.g., Stigler 1984). Tang and colleagues (2006) discuss how children from China and the United States, faced with the same math problem—such as, "3 + 4 = ?"—activate different brain areas. The research team suggests a number of different developmental factors that may influence how numbers are handled neurologically, such as elementary school pedagogy and writing systems (although both use Arabic numbers; see Tang et al. 2006:10778). But one clear candidate for causing divergent forms of neural enculturation is the use of the abacus in calculation. Neural imaging has found that "abacus-based mental calculation" enlists visuospatial imagery-related areas of the brain not involved in verbal-based calculation, and that persistent finger-based abacus training increases fractional anisotropy, a measure of brain connectivity, between the areas being used, possibly explaining these subjects' higher working memory capacity for digits and letters (Hanakawa et al. 2003; Hu et al. 2011; Tang et al. 2006).

These studies of cultural differences in the cognitive and neurological resources underlying the same or similar functions suggests that neurological enculturation may not simply involve differential development of specialized brain areas; because of the brain's structure, the same or similar functions may be accomplished using diverse mechanisms or underlying structures. This potential form of "similar-in-appearance-but-different-in underlying-function" neural enculturation can arise because of the brain's *degeneracy*, a term used in biological theory to describe a system that can obtain the same outcome using various means.[1]

NEURAL DEGENERACY AS FOUNDATION FOR BRAIN ENCULTURABILITY

Complex neurological systems tend to be extraordinarily "degenerate" in the biological sense, demonstrating a wide variety of ways to produce similar functions: "structurally different circuits within the degenerate repertoires are each able to produce a particular output leading to repetition or variation of a given mental or physical act" (Edelman 1998:54; see also Edelman 2006:57; Edelman and Gally 2001; Mason 2010; Price and Friston 2002). Gerald Edelman describes how degeneracy in neuroanatomy serves a crucial role: assuring stability of performance in a complex organic system:

> Besides guaranteeing association, the property of degeneracy also gives rise to the robustness or stability of memorial performance. There are large numbers of ways of assuring a given output. As long as a sufficient population of subsets remains to give an output, neither cell death, nor intervening variables competitively removing a particular circuit or two, nor switches in contextual aspects of input signals will, in general, be sufficient to extirpate a memory. [1998:54]

Degeneracy in the brain means that a given output cannot be definitively linked to a single neural circuit or pattern of activity; a "consistent" memory, for example, may be summoned by a shifting network of neurological activity because the brain itself is constantly changing (Edelman 1998:53). Nor can similar function be taken to prove that different individuals' brains are similar. Edelman and Gally (2001:13765) cite the example of individuals who lack the corpus callosum, the major fiber tract connecting the brain hemispheres. This significant abnormality cannot be detected at times without subtle testing because these individuals compensate with other neurological structures. Degeneracy is not the same as redundancy, as Friston and Price (2003) explain; degenerate structures are not exact duplicates, but can substitute and perform the same function, accomplishing the same or quite similar outcome.

Particularly important for anthropologists, degenerate neural structures may underlie even widespread "universals" of human behavior, perception, or psychology (e.g., Brown 1991), not just across different cultures, but even within a single cultural group. Growing appreciation of neural malleability and degeneracy, and subtle research techniques are even revealing cultural differences in brain functioning not visible in psychological studies, so often based on explicit self-report (see Fiske 2002:81–82). Ironically, even though cultural anthropologists criticize psychologists for assuming homogeneity, any approach to cognition based on explicit discussion or social discourse might commit similar errors if we do not recognize that shared symbolic or semiotic behavior might mask underlying intragroup neural diversity.

Of course, not all cognitive functions will be subserved by equally degenerate structures; some skills may be highly canalized, their achievement only possible using specific or rare neural resources (see Price and Friston 2002). Neural plasticity is not evenly distributed in the brain, and some types of plasticity can only be achieved in specific circumstances, such as the sensory or stimulus deprivation brought about by disability or profound neurological insult.[2] In some cases, however, we might be able to observe the hallmarks of degeneracy in the behaviors themselves, when function—although shared—is not identical under all conditions.

The example of abacus-based mental calculation and the presence of high levels of structural degeneracy in the brain should encourage neuroanthropologists to search specifically for candidate cultural variations in neural dynamics underlying shared function. Degeneracy may be a hallmark of especially "enculturable" brain systems: those parts of human neural architecture or types of cognitive function with the greatest degeneracy would be especially prone to diverse configurations, both between and within cultures. For example, studies of attentional control across cultures show that, although groups may possess similar, multiple systems for control, groups vary in the ease with which they can employ them. Culturally "non-preferred" tasks take more effort than those behaviors that are culturally encouraged (see Hedden et al. 2008). Because of the complexity and late developmental emergence of elite athletic skills, I suspect that these skills may be an excellent candidate site to search for culturally inflected degeneracy.

But degeneracy should also caution us to be wary of dismissing or obstructing methodologically the possibility of substantial interindividual variation, even within a group. Kanai and Rees (2011) encourage neuroscientists to make use of variation, rather than treat it as annoyance, to better understand the links between brain anatomy and variation in cognition and behavior; anthropologists should do the same when we study culture. For example, our research team believes that we can make use of exceptional individuals and interindividual variation to better understand the forces of enculturation in part because our subjects are such behavioral outliers.

ATHLETES AS TARGETS OF ENCULTURATION

At first blush, sport and coaching may appear odd subjects for the application of neuroanthropology, and not just because sport is more generally neglected in anthropology (see Sands 1999). Participants in our research frequently joke that studying cognition in rugby is itself an oxymoron given the brute nature of the sport.[3] In fact, sport, especially esoteric skills like handling an oblong ball, juggling with one's feet, or hitting a near-imperceptible fastball with a narrow piece of wood, are an ideal forum to study the enculturation of the nervous system because the activities are simultaneously so evolutionarily unprecedented and yet pursued with such extraordinary discipline. On the one hand, utterly pointless and without pragmatic value, and, on the other hand, supremely demanding and culturally valorized, especially when played at the level we are discussing, sports demonstrate in dramatic terms how cultural values can shape individual development, including physiology.

Elite athletes, by definition, are statistical outliers. They are selected for their unusual ability, subjected to extreme training regimens, supported by a powerful sporting bureaucracy and industry, feted for their achievements, and encouraged on by the promise of fame, professional sporting contracts, and even a kind of secular glory. The "high performance" squad of the Australian Rugby Union may seem to be a rarefied community in which to study enculturation. But, as Daniel Ansari (2012:93) points out, animal models and laboratory studies of neuroplasticity likely underrepresent the magnitude of the brain's enculturability: "Although these studies have enhanced our understanding of the 'changeable brain,' neither animal models nor studies of basic sensorimotor plasticity in the human brain can provide insights into the plasticity associated with uniquely human learning and experiences." If a short regimen of juggling instruction can produce observable neurological change (Draganski et al. 2004), how much more so will years of arduous training. Athletes, like professional musicians, meditators, and London cab drivers, engage in profound, long-term projects of neural and physical self-manipulation, demonstrating the potential of human self-fashioning (see Downey 2010b; Ericsson and Lehmann 1996). Moreover, athletes stand against a trend among what Henrich and colleagues (2010) remind us are quite "weird" subjects in psychological research: the contemporary Western trend toward more sedentary lives, and an accompanying constellation of sensory and physiological traits, such as quietism, disproportionately elaborate language skills, perceptual biases, obesity, and relative muscular and skeletal frailty.

A skills-based, processual model of enculturation in neuroanthropology allows us to see elite athletes' nervous systems, not just as statistical outliers, but as extremely refined products of widespread training mechanisms within a culture. Culturally diverse elite athletes can serve as the test case for the neuroanthropological study of enculturation because experts may make evident in exaggerated form divergent cultural developmental trajectories (see Rogoff 2003). If elite athletes or other highly skilled individuals from a range of backgrounds and training regimens closely resemble each other, we can conclude that a skill is highly canalized or has uniform impact on practitioners. But if different training regimens produce diverse cognitive strategies, or make use of degenerate neural structures, we have concrete examples of cultural variation across the "same" activity.

COGNITION "ON THE PITCH": MAKING DECISIONS WHILE PLAYING

Preliminary discussions and ethnographic observation with local experts—commentators, coaches and former players—are our starting point to generate hypotheses about cognitive and perceptual diversity among rugby athletes (Downey 2008). The research team is focusing especially on Rugby Sevens, the IRB sanctioned seven-a-side form of the sport, for a number of practical and methodological reasons. First, because "Sevens" is less thoroughly professionalized and high profile than the 15-player form of rugby union, barriers to accessing players and coaches are lower. Second, as Sevens is played on a full-sized field, much more of the game is spent in running, passing, and kicking; virtually all players have to make decisions constantly and must perceive the shifting configuration of the defense and their own teammates. Specialized roles and elaborate set pieces, like the scrum and lineout, are much less pronounced in the faster-flowing Sevens competition. Third, IRB-sanctioned Sevens events bring together national teams at tournaments several times a year, where short-format games are played in rapid succession, resolving the entire tournament (with more than 40 matches typically) among multiple countries in several days. In contrast, a Rugby World Cup is played only every four years and takes months to progress from the pool through the elimination stages of the tournament to the final. The data generated at a single tournament is enormous and, in the current series, offers samples of athletes from 16 countries. From an applied perspective, the complex perceptual-strategic skills—sometimes referred to almost mystically as a player's "vision" or "sense of the game"—are considered among the most difficult to coach.

Based on initial conversations with coaches and experts, we are focusing on two key situations for studying cultural differences in skill: decisions to pass or kick while running in open field and positioning while in the fullback position, the last line of defense. We suspect that the defensive skill may be a highly canalized one, affording little possible variation in cognitive strategy, whereas the open-field attacking role may be liable to at least four types of strategies (one of which is also potentially quite variable). From preliminary consultation, we are hypothesizing that players in open-field decision making may rely on the following strategies:[4]

1 pattern recollection and execution of rehearsed sequences arising from high-coached familiarity with predesignated plays;
2 perceptual-responsive tactics that depended heavily on perceiving idiosyncratic opportunities and using broad motor-perceptual skills with much less need to recall preordained patterns of attack;
3 concentration on a small repertoire of highly perfected pivot sequences that are idiosyncratic to the individual player (and thus narrow the defense's possible responses); and
4 socially dispersed expertise depending on long-term familiarity with one's teammates and shared anticipation of collective action.

We hope that, at a future stage of the research, we will be able to employ mobile forms of brain imaging to directly trace brain metabolic processes during practice; at this stage, the technology is not yet available (but see Leff et al. 2011).

Because skills like the complex decision-making processes involved in rugby are so context dependent, attempting to remove them to the laboratory would likely undermine completely the ecological validity of normal skilled behavior (Dicks et al. 2010). For instance, the third and fourth hypothetical strategies—a player actively provoking a set of defense responses or working with familiar teammates—would both be impossible to simulate in a laboratory setting with virtual reality, rendering these forms of expertise invisible to examination outside the context of play. That is, because a rugby player is active and moving in a decision-making situation, able to shift his or her actions to narrow an adversary's response, and because skill may depend heavily on ability to collaborate and combine with teammates, experimental protocols may make it impossible for some players to act skillfully. The laboratory setting itself may force some players to resort to less preferred cognitive strategies, essentially becoming "less skilled" because of the experimental environment. Moreover, differences in expertise become most obvious only in the most complex decision-making settings, not in artificially simplified situations (see Ripoll et al. 1995).

For this reason, our project design follows the model provided by Edwin Hutchins (1995) for close anthropological study of cognition through mixed methods, including participant-observation, quantitative observation through video, and consultation with local experts. Although our interest in cognitive diversity is grounded especially in a neuroanthropological recognition of degeneracy in brain structures and the consequences of developmental dynamics for neuroplasticity, Hutchins's model demonstrates why the study of the brain must move to embrace ethnographic methods as well as laboratory-based research. In his studies of navigation, Hutchins showed compellingly that problem solving made use of elements of the environment, including other individuals, so that cognition needed to be caught "in the wild" to be understood.

We also seek to use eye-tracking technology in an open, exploratory fashion. As Henderson discusses, "because attention plays a central role in visual and cognitive processing, and because eye movements are an overt behavioral manifestation of the allocation of attention in a scene, eye movements serve as a window into the operation of the attentional system" (2003:498; see also Liversedge and Findlay 2000). Research on expert practitioners has revealed that increasing skill correlates with changes in visual search patterns to more effective strategies and fixations on key perceptual landmarks, even when athletes are not conscious of what they are doing (Land and Tatler 2009).

To gain greater cross-cultural purchase, through close analysis of game tapes from international tournaments, we are seeking to find whether certain players or national teams demonstrate distinctive patterns of decision making. We will be drawing on "native" informants as well, including testing to see if specific patterns are more likely to be treated as promising or "talented" by scouts and those responsible for choosing which athletes get access to specialized coaching. That is, as neuroanthropologists, we take seriously both quantitative data on playing patterns as well as the qualitative differences in playing styles perceived by local experts, commentators, and coaches. If, in fact, expert observations turn out to be empirically well founded, as we believe some are, we will be able to shorten the distance from hypothesis to testing by consulting with "indigenous" experts.

But sport needs neuroanthropology, I would argue, as much as anthropologists need elite skills as an object of study. Ironically, sports commentary and coaching are strongholds of obsolete and essentialist thinking—racism and faith in "talent" which borders on genetic predestinationism. Essentialism reigns precisely because the processes through which human experience, social interaction, and behavior patterns become our physiological and neurological condition are so opaque and, frankly, incredible to most observers (see also Williams and Ericsson 2005). The gap between the ability of the Australian Wallabies and that of the average young athlete yawns so wide that we often cannot imagine how that divide could be closed; surely such profound difference must already be present, in some inchoate form, at the onset of a person's life. We foresee that our research will have concrete applications in coaching practice, talent identification, and quantifying cultural differences.

First, as our research team has begun an activity survey of training techniques and a video-based analysis of international Sevens competition, especially examining the perceptual and cognitive demands placed on players, we have almost immediately observed a number of marked discrepancies: the demands of training do not appear to coincide well with the exigencies of the game. Players are being asked to confront challenges in games with virtually no training in comparable situations. Ironically, the behavioral–cognitive mechanisms that might make a player excel at the routinized forms of training—diligence, predictability, docility, tolerance for boredom, and the ability to follow instructions— may militate against expert performance at the highest level. Coaches, however, can be suspicious of researchers, resistant to change, and averse to risk, as Richard Light (2001) found in an ethnographic study of an attempt to change a school's rugby style in Australia. To fail while doing what is expected is potentially less dangerous for a coach than to attempt change. Neuroanthropological analysis can help to clarify how the brain and nervous system as a whole can be better trained for the demands of high pressure decision making and skill execution.

Second, the effort to analyze the relationship among players' emerging skills, cultural variation in cognition, and coaching methods is especially imperative, because rugby union is growing more socially and ethnically diverse in Australia and striving to be inclusive. At the same time, the field of "talent identification" is undergoing its own change and professionalization, hardening prematurely, in our opinion, an overly simple and uniform understanding of what expertise looks like early in its development (see Phillips et al. 2010 for a critique). Aboriginal Australians, for example, are underrepresented in rugby union, especially compared to their extraordinarily disproportionate levels of participation in the professional Australian Football League and the National Rugby League, the two competing codes. An appreciation of cultural variation is a latecomer to sports psychology (e.g., Schinke and Hanrahan 2009), but interest has recently begun to grow, especially as coaches in the United States are forced to contend with greater diversity among their players. A similar recognition of how culture affects the development of skill needs to be introduced to the field of "talent identification."

In fact, we believe that one of the most important applied outcomes of this research may be an evidence-based argument that uniform coaching and training methods may not provide all variations of expertise with equal developmental opportunity. Local understandings of "talent" may be biased to recognize and nurture some variants of elite skill, and training techniques may seek to impose problem-solving or performance strategies on players regardless of their own capacities.

Developmental coaches share with anthropologists an interest in diversity. For talent scouts, understanding what makes individuals perform differently is crucial to assessing a player's potential and appropriate training. In contrast, Vogel and Awh (2008:171) suggest, "Most cognitive neuroscientists are interested in understanding how everyone thinks, not trying to catalog and characterize the entire range of abilities across the population or understand how and why a given individual thinks differently from another." The sorts of outlying individuals who might be scrubbed from a pool of psychological subjects for being so unusual are precisely the people that might be of special interest to both neuroanthropologists and scouts for elite athletics program, although for quite different reasons. Developing the research tools to be able to identify and quantify in some meaningful way the differences among cultures in cognitive approach to a shared activity, like a sport, may help us to translate our cultural research into improved, more inclusive, training and recruiting. In the extraordinary skills of the highly trained athlete, we see both a frontier for research on human variation and a horizon for human achievement.

NOTES

1. Paul Mason introduced me to the biological concept of "degeneracy" and Gerald Edelman's work on the subject. In spite of my resistance to the term, I am grateful for Paul's persistence, although he cannot be blamed for any error in interpretation of the theoretical material in this work.

2. See also Luria (1966) for a classic study of the effects of neurological lesions.

3. I typically respond that I am not studying first- or second-rowers, the burly players responsible for the notoriously physical "scrum" to decide possession of the ball. In fact, ethnographic observation as well as my own research on the skills involved in fight sports leads to the conclusion that physical exertion itself is enormously difficult, and the body must be fine-tuned to accomplish virtually any athletic task. Proprioception, tactile sensation, and pain perception can undergo sophisticated and subtle forms of cultural fine-tuning, leading to profoundly encultured sensory systems (see Downey 2007, 2012).

4. For a more extensive discussion of these strategies, including paradigmatic athletes said to represent these styles, see Downey 2010a.

REFERENCES CITED

Ansari, Daniel
    2012 Culture and Education: New Frontiers in Brain Plasticity. Trends in Cognitive Sciences 16(2):93–95.
Appadurai, Arjun
    1997 Playing With Modernity: The Decolonization of Indian Cricket. In Modernity at Large. Pp. 89–113.
        New York: Oxford University Press.
Archetti, Eduardo P.
    1999 Masculinities: Football, Polo and the Tango in Argentina. Oxford: Berg.

Bairner, Alan

2001 Sport, Nationalism, and Globalization: European and North American Perspectives. Albany: State University of New York Press.

Bengtsson, Sara L., Zoltán Nagy, Stefan Skare, Lea Forsman, Hans Forssberg, and Fredrik Ullén

2005 Extensive Piano Practicing Has Regionally Specific Effects on White Matter Development. Nature Neuroscience 8(9):1148–1150.

Bezzola, Ladina, Susan Mérillat, Christian Gaser, and Lutz Jäncke

2011 Training-Induced Neural Plasticity in Golf Novices. Journal of Neuroscience 31(35):12444–12448.

Black, David R., and John Nauright

1998 Rugby and the South African Nation: Sport, Culture, Politics and Power in the Old and New South Africa. Manchester: Manchester University Press.

Bourdieu, Pierre

1990 In Other Words: Essays Towards a Reflexive Sociology. Translated by Matthew Adamson. Stanford, CA: Stanford University Press.

Brown, Donald E.

1991 Human Universals. New York: McGraw-Hill.

Cannonieri, Gianna C., Leonardo Bonilha, Paula T. Fernandes, Fernando Cendes, and Li M. Li

2007 Practice and Perfect: Length of Training and Structural Brain Changes in Experienced Typists. Neuroreport 18(10):1063–1066.

Chandler, Timothy J. L., and John Nauright

1999 Making the Rugby World: Race, Gender, Commerce. New York: Frank Cass.

Cheon, Bobby K., Dong-mi Im, Tokiko Harada, Ji-Sook Kim, Vani A. Mathur, Jason M. Scimeca, Todd B. Parrish, Hyun Wook Park, and Joan Y. Chiao

2011 Cultural Influences on Neural Basis of Intergroup Empathy. Neuroimage 57(2):642–650.

Dayan, Eran, and Leonardo G. Cohen

2011 Neuroplasticity Subserving Motor Skill Learning. Neuron 72(3):443–454.

de Groot, Adriaan D.

1965 Thought and Choice in Chess. The Hague, Netherlands: Mouton.

Del Percio, Claudio, Paolo M. Rossini, Nicola Marzano, Marco Iacoboni, Francesco Infarinato, Pierluigi Aschieri, Andrea Lino, Antonio Fiore, Giancarlo Toran, Claudio Babiloni, and Fabrizio Eusebi

2008 Is There a "Neural Efficiency" in Athletes? A High-Resolution EEG Study. Neuroimage 42(4):1544–1553.

Dicks, Matt, Chris Button, and Keith Davids

2010 Examination of Gaze Behaviors under in situ and Video Simulation Task Constraints Reveals Differences in Information Pickup for Perception and Action. Attention, Perception, and Psychophysics 72(3):706–720.

Diné, Philip

2001 French Rugby Football: A Cultural History. New York: Berg.

Downey, Greg

2007 Seeing with a "Sideways Glance": Visuomotor "Knowing" and the Plasticity of Perception. *In* Ways of Knowing: New Approaches in the Anthropology of Knowledge and Learning. Mark Harris, ed. Pp. 222–241. New York: Berghahn.

2008 Coaches as Phenomenologists: Para-Ethnographic Work in Sports. Proceedings of the 2006 Annual Conference for the Australasian Association for Theatre, Drama and Performance Studies (ADSA), Being There: Before, During and After. Sydney: ADSA.

2010a Cultural Variation in Elite Athletes: Does Elite Cognitive-Perceptual Skill Always Converge? *In* ASCS09: Proceedings of the 9th Conference of the Australasian Society for Cognitive Science. W. Christensen, E. Schier, and J. Sutton, eds. Pp. 72–80. Sydney, Australia: Macquarie Centre for Cognitive Studies. doi: 10.5096/ASCS200912, accessed November 17, 2010.

2010b Throwing Like a Brazilian: On Ineptness and a Skill-Shaped Body. *In* Anthropology of Sport and Human Movement. Robert R. Sands and Linda R. Sands, eds. Pp. 297–326. Lanham, MD: Lexington.

2012 Balancing across Cultures: Sensory Plasticity. *In* The Encultured Brain: An Introduction to Neuroanthropology. Daniel H. Lende and Greg Downey, eds. Pp. 169–194. Cambridge, MA: MIT Press.

Draganski, Bogdan, Christian Gaser, Volker Busch, Gerhard Schuierer, Ulrich Bogdahn, and Arne May
2004 Neuroplasticity: Changes in Grey Matter Induced by Training. Nature 427(6972):311–312.

Draganski, Bogdan, Christian Gaser, Gerd Kempermann, H. Georg Kuhn, Jürgen Winkler, Christian Büchel, and Arne May
2006 Temporal and Spatial Dynamics of Brain Structure Changes during Extensive Learning. Journal of Neuroscience 26(23):6314–6317.

Draganski, Bogdam, and Arne May
2008 Training-Induced Structural Changes in the Adult Human Brain. Behavioural Brain Research 192:137–142.

Duffy, Sean, Rie Toriyama, Shoji Itakura, and Shinobu Kitayama
2009 Development of Cultural Strategies of Attention in North American and Japanese Children. Journal of Experimental Child Psychology 102(3):351–359.

Edelman, Gerald M.
1998 Building a Picture of the Brain. Daedalus 127(2):37–69.
2006 Second Nature: Brain Science and Human Knowledge. New Haven: Yale University Press.

Edelman, Gerald M., and Joseph A. Gally
2001 Degeneracy and Complexity in Biological Systems. Proceedings of the National Academy of Sciences (USA) 98(24):13763–13768.

Ericsson, K. A., and Andreas C. Lehmann
1996 Expert and Exceptional Performance: Evidence of Maximal Adaptation to Task Constraints. Annual Review of Psychology 47(1):273–305.

Evans, John
In press Specificity and Cognitive Demand: Beating a Path to Game Centred Coaching in Rugby. *In* University of Sydney Papers in HMHCE, vol. 1. Wayne Cotton and Donna O'Connor, eds. Sydney: University of Sydney.

Fiske, Alan P.
2002 Using Individualism and Collectivism to Compare Cultures—A Critique of the Validity and Measurement of the Constructs: Comment on Oyserman et al. (2002). Psychological Bulletin 128(1):78–88.

Friston, Karl J., and Cathy J. Price
2003 Degeneracy and Redundancy in Cognitive Anatomy. Trends in Cognitive Science 7(4):151–152.

Gaser, Christian, and Gottfried Schlaug
2003 Brain Structures Differ between Musicians and Non-Musicians. Journal of Neuroscience 23(27):9240–9245.

Gibson, James J.
1979 The Ecological Approach to Visual Perception. Boston: Houghton Mifflin Harcourt.

Gobel, Eric W., Todd B. Parrish, and Paul J. Reber
2011 Neural Correlates of Skill Acquisition: Decreased Cortical Activity during a Serial Interception Sequence Learning Task. NeuroImage 58(4):1150–1157.

Goh, Joshua O., and Denise C. Park
2009 Culture Sculpts the Perceptual Brain. Progress in Brain Research 178:95–111.

Grasseni, Cristina
2004 Skilled Vision: An Apprenticeship in Breeding Aesthetics. Social Anthropology 12(1):41–55.

Grasseni, Cristina, ed.
2009 Skilled Visions: Between Apprenticeship and Standards. New York: Berghahn.

Güss, C. Dominik, Ma. Teresa Tuason, and Christiane Gerhard
2009 Cross-National Comparisons of Complex Problem-Solving Strategies in Two Microworlds. Cognitive Science 34(3):489–520.

Hanakawa, Takashi, Honda, Manabu, Okada, Tomohis, Fukuyama, Hidenao, and Shibasaki, Hiroshi
2003 Neural Correlates Underlying Mental Calculation in Abacus Experts: Functional Magnetic Resonance Imaging Study. Neuroimage 19(2):296–307.

Hänggi, Jürgen, Susan Koeneke, Ladina Bezzola, and Lutz Jäncke

  2010 Structural Neuroplasticity in the Sensorimotor Network of Professional Female Ballet Dancers. Human Brain Mapping 31(8):1196–1206.

Hedden, Trey, Sarah Ketay, Arthur Aron, Hazel Rose Markus, and John D. E. Gabrieli

  2008 Cultural Influences on Neural Substrates of Attentional Control. Psychological Science 19(1):12–17.

Henderson, John M.

  2003 Human Gaze Control during Real-World Scene Perception. Trends in Cognitive Science 7(11):498–504.

Henrich, Joseph, Steven J. Heine, and Ara Norenzayan

  2010 The Weirdest People in the World? Behavioral and Brain Sciences 33(2–3):61–135.

Hu, Yuzheng, Fengji Geng, Lixia Tao, Nantu Hu, Fenglei Du, Kuang Fu, and Feiyan Chen

  2011 Enhanced White Matter Tracts Integrity in Children With Abacus Training. Human Brain Mapping 32(1):10–21.

Hutchins, Edwin

  1995 Cognition in the Wild. Cambridge, MA: MIT Press.

Ingold, Tim

  1998 From Complementarity to Obviation: On Dissolving the Boundaries between Social and Biological Anthropology, Archaeology and Psychology. Zeitschrift für Ethnologie 123(1):21–52.

  2000 The Perception of the Environment: Essays on Livelihood, Dwelling and Skill. New York: Routledge.

  2001 From the Transmission of Representations to the Education of Attention. In The Debated Mind: Evolutionary Psychology versus Ethnography. Harvey Whitehouse, ed. Pp. 113–153. New York: Berg.

International Rugby Board (IRB)

  2004 Strategic Plan. http://www.irb.com/mm/document/aboutirb/0/041207irbstrategicplan_772.pdf, accessed January 6, 2012.

  2010 Strategic Plan 2010–2020. Dublin: International Rugby Board.

Jacini, Wantuir F. S., Gianna C. Cannonieri, Paula T. Fernandes, Leonardo Bonilha, Fernando Cendes, and Li M. Li

  2009 Can Exercise Shape Your Brain? Cortical Differences Associated with Judo Practice. Journal of Science and Medicine in Sport 12(6):688–690.

Jäncke, Lutz, Susan Koeneke, Ariana Hoppe, Christina Rominger, and Jürgen Hänggi

  2009 The Architecture of the Golfer's Brain. PLoS ONE 4(3):e4785.

Kanai, Ryota, and Geraint Rees

  2011 The Structural Basis of Inter-Individual Differences in Human Behaviour and Cognition. Nature Reviews Neuroscience 12(4):231–242.

Kelly, A. M. Clare, and Hugh Garavan

  2005 Human Functional Neuroimaging of Brain Changes Associated with Practice. Cerebral Cortex 15(8):1089–1102.

Kerr, Catherine E., Jessica R. Shaw, Rachel H. Wasserman, Vanessa W. Chen, Alok Kanojia, Thomas Bayer, and John M. Kelley

  2008 Tactile Acuity in Experienced Tai Chi Practitioners: Evidence for Use Dependent Plasticity as an Effect of Sensory-Attentional Training. Experimental Brain Research 188:317–322.

Land, Michael F., and Peter McLeod

  2000 From Eye Movements to Actions: How Batsmen Hit the Ball. Nature Neuroscience 3(12):1340–1345.

Land, Michael F., and Benjamin W. Tatler

  2009 Looking and Acting: Vision and Eye Movements in Natural Behaviour. Oxford: Oxford University Press.

Leff, Daniel Richard, Felipe Orihuela-Espina, Clare E. Elwell, Thanos Athanasiou, David T. Delpy, Ara W. Darzi, and Guang-Zhong Yang

  2011 Assessment of the Cerebral Cortex during Motor Task Behaviours in Adults: A Systematic Review of Functional Near Infrared Spectroscopy (fNIRS) Studies. NeuroImage 54(4):2922–2936.

Lever, Janet

    1983 Soccer Madness. Chicago: University of Chicago Press.

Light, Richard

    2001 "Open It up a Bit": Competing Discourses, Physical Practice, and the Struggle over Rugby Game Style in an Australian High School. Journal of Sport and Social Issues 25(3):266–282.

Liversedge, Simon P., and John M. Findlay

    2000 Saccadic Eye Movements and Cognition. Trends in Cognitive Sciences 4(1):6–14.

Lonner, Walter J.

    1993 Foreward. In Cognition and Culture: A Cross-Cultural Approach to Cognitive Psychology. Jeanette Altarriba, ed. Pp. v–viii. Amsterdam: North-Holland.

Luria, A. R.

    1966 Human Brain and Psychological Processes. Translated by Basil Haigh. New York: Harper and Row.

Maguire, Eleanor A., David G. Gadian, Ingrid S. Johnsrude, Catriona D. Good, John Ashburner, Richard S. J. Frackowiak, and Christopher D. Frith

    2000 Navigation-Related Structural Change in the Hippocampi of Cab Drivers. Proceedings of the National Academy of Science (USA) 97(8):4398–4403.

Maguire, Joseph, and Jason Tuck

    1998 Global Sports and Patriot Games: Rugby Union and National Identity in a United Sporting Kingdom since 1945. Immigrants and Minorities 17(1):103–126.

Marchand, Trevor H. J.

    2010 Making Knowledge: Explorations of the Indissoluble Relation between Minds, Bodies, and Environment. Journal of the Royal Anthropological Institute 16:S1–S21.

Mason, Paul H.

    2010 Degeneracy at Multiple Levels of Complexity. Biological Theory 5(3):277–288.

May, Arne

    2011 Experience-Dependent Structural Plasticity in the Adult Human Brain. Trends in Cognitive Science 15(10):475–482.

Meister, Ingo, Timo Krings, Henrik Foltys, Babak Boroojerdi, Mareike Müller, Rudolf Töpper, and Armin Thron

    2005 Effects of Long-Term Practice and Task Complexity in Musicians and Nonmusicians Performing Simple and Complex Motor Tasks: Implications for Cortical Motor Organization. Human Brain Mapping 25:345–352.

Münte, Thomas F., Eckhart Altenmüller, and Lutz Jäncke

    2002 The Musician's Brain as a Model of Neuroplasticity. Nature Reviews Neuroscience 3(6):473–478.

Park, In Sung, Kea Joo Lee, Jong Woo Han, Nam Joon Lee, Won Teak Lee, Kyung Ah Park, and Im Joo Rhyu

    2011 Basketball Training Increases Striatum Volume. Human Movement Science 30(1):56–62.

Phillips, Elissa, David Keith, Ian Renshaw, and Marc Portus

    2010 Expert Performance in Sport and the Dynamics of Talent Development. Sports Medicine 40(4):271–283.

Price, Cathy J., and Karl J. Friston

    2002 Degeneracy and Cognitive Anatomy. Trends in Cognitive Sciences 6(10):416–421.

Ripoll, Hubert, Yves Kerlirzin, Jean-Fraçois Stein, and Bruno Reine

    1995 Analysis of Information Processing, Decision Making, and Visual Strategies in Complex Problem Solving Sport Situations. Human Movement Science 14(3):325–349.

Rogoff, Barbara

    2003 The Cultural Nature of Human Development. Oxford: Oxford University Press.

Sands, Robert R., ed.

    1999 Anthropology, Sport and Culture. Westport, CT: Bergin and Garvey.

Savelsbergh, Geert J. P., A. Mark Williams, John van der Kamp, and Paul Ward

    2002 Visual Search, Anticipation, and Expertise in Soccer Goalkeepers. Journal of Sports Sciences 20(3):279–287.

Schinke, Robert J., and Stephanie J. Hanrahan
  2009 Cultural Sport Psychology. Champaign, IL: Human Kinetics.
Simon, Herbert A., and William G. Chase
  1973 Skill in Chess. American Scientist 61(4):393–403.
Singer, Robert N., James H. Cauraughab, Dapeng Chenab, Gregg M. Steinbergab, and Shane G. Frehlich
  1996 Visual Search, Anticipation, and Reactive Comparisons between Highly-Skilled and Beginning Tennis Players. Journal of Applied Sport Psychology 8(1):9–26.
Siok, Wai Ting, Charles A. Perfetti, Zhen Jin, and Li Hai Tan
  2004 Biological Abnormality of Impaired Reading Is Constrained by Culture. Nature 431:71–76.
Stigler, James W.
  1984 "Mental Abacus": The Effects of Abacus Training on Chinese Children's Mental Calculation. Cognitive Psychology 16(2):145–176.
Strohschneider, Stefan, and Dominik Güss
  1998 Planning and Problem Solving: Differences between Brazilian and German Students. Journal of Cross-Cultural Psychology 29(6):695–716.
  1999 The Fate of the Moros: A Cross-Cultural Exploration of Strategies in Complex and Dynamic Decision Making. International Journal of Psychology 34(4):235–252.
Sugden, John
  1996 Boxing and Society: An International Analysis. New York: Manchester University Press.
Tang, Yiyuan, Wutian Zhang, Kewei Chen, Shigang Feng, Ye Ji, Junxian Shen, Eric M. Reiman, and Yijun Liu
  2006 Arithmetic Processing in the Brain Shaped by Cultures. Proceedings of the National Academy of Science USA 103(28):10775–10780.
Tuck, Jason
  2003 Making Sense of Emerald Commotion: Rugby Union, National Identity and Ireland. Identities: Global Studies in Culture and Power 10(4):495–515.
Vickers, Joan N.
  2007 Perception, Cognition, and Decision Training: The Quiet Eye in Action. Champaign, IL: Human Kinetics.
Vogel, Edward K., and Edward Awh
  2008 How to Exploit Diversity for Scientific Gain: Using Individual Differences to Constrain Cognitive Theory. Current Directions in Psychological Science 17(2):171–176.
Wei, Gaoxia, Yuanchao Zhang, Tianzi Jiang, and Jing Luo
  2011 Increased Cortical Thickness in Sports Experts: A Comparison of Diving Players with the Controls. PLoS ONE 6(2):e17112.
Williams, A. Mark
  2000 Perceptual Skill in Soccer: Implications for Talent Identification and Development. Journal of Sports Sciences 18(9):737–750.
Williams, A. Mark, and K. Anders Ericsson
  2005 Perceptual-Cognitive Expertise in Sport: Some Considerations When Applying the Expert Performance Approach. Human Movement Science 24(3):283–307.
Williams, A. Mark, Paul Ward, John M. Knowles, and Nicholas J. Smeeton
  2002 Anticipation Skill in a Real-World Task: Measurement, Training, and Transfer in Tennis. Journal of Experimental Psychology: Applied 8(4):259–270.
Zajonc Robert B., and Hazel Markus
  1984 Affect and Cognition: The Hard Interface. In Emotion, Cognition, and Behavior. Carroll E. Izard, Jerome Kagan, and Robert B. Zajonc, eds. Pp. 73–102. London: Cambridge University Press.
Zhu, Ying, Li Zhang, Jin Fan, and Shihui Han
  2007 Neural Basis of Cultural Influence on Self-Representation. NeuroImage 34(3):1310–1316.

SENSICAL TRANSLATIONS: THREE CASE STUDIES IN APPLIED COGNITIVE COMMUNICATIONS

ERIC H. LINDLAND
FrameWorks Institute

NATHANIEL KENDALL-TAYLOR
FrameWorks Institute

The FrameWorks Institute applies cultural models and metaphor theory from cognitive anthropology to develop communications devices that reframe public understandings and discourses on social problems. This article traces three case studies, in the areas of child mental health, budgets and taxes, and environmental health, where substantial gaps between scientific and public knowledge were identified, and describes the research process to develop "explanatory metaphors" to close those gaps and cultivate more accurate and expansive patterns of public thinking. Three distinct cognitively attuned communications tasks are described: (1) foregrounding an extant but recessive cognitive model prominent among the public; (2) filling a domain-specific "cognitive lacuna" in public thinking by introducing a modified version of an existing model from a kindred cognitive domain; and (3) building off or working around an existing dominant cognitive model that is consistent with expert knowledge but incomplete. The article concludes with observations on how the practice of applied communications has challenged and strengthened our theory of culture and cognition. [cultural models, communications research, applied research, metaphor, science translation]

Western anthropologists have long been keen to explore the boundaries between everyday and specialized knowledge: between cultural knowledge that is broadly distributed among members of a population, and that knowledge that is more exclusively the domain of specialists who, by whatever means, have come to see and think differently about some aspect of the world. When anthropology's focus was more squarely trained on non-Western cultures, this line of exploration often delved into the study of shamans and diviners, and on the means, purposes, and functions of esoteric knowledge and ritual practice in socioreligious contexts (Benedict 1922; Boas 1902; Lévi-Strauss 1963). As the discipline's lens has turned increasingly on Western society and knowledge, the same impulse has led to explorations on the margins between everyday "common sense" notions of the world and those derived from the specialized pursuit of scientific knowledge (Kempton 1987; McCloskey 1983).

ANNALS OF ANTHROPOLOGICAL PRACTICE 36, pp. 45–67. ISSN: 2153-957X. © 2012 by the American Anthropological Association. DOI:10.1111/j.2153-9588.2012.01092.x

At the FrameWorks Institute—a nonprofit, interdisciplinary, social science research group—we work in this zone between common sense and scientific knowledge. Since 1999, the FrameWorks Institute has been investigating how Americans think about social issues—from early child development to climate change to criminal justice reform—to help scientists, policy experts, and advocates more effectively engage the public in thinking about public policy solutions to these issues. FrameWorks has developed an approach to communications research and practice called Strategic Frame Analysis™, which integrates theory and methods from the cognitive and social sciences to describe and explain how communications in general, and media in particular, influence public support for social policies. FrameWorks defines framing as "the way a story is told—its selective use of particular symbols, metaphors, and messengers, for example—and to the way these cues, in turn, trigger the shared and durable cultural models that people use to make sense of their world" (Bales and Gilliam 2004:15).

FrameWorks undertakes this work with support from foundations, groups of scientists and policy experts, and a range of other nonprofit organizations. Our goal is to deliver a communications strategy that is grounded in research and has the potential to broaden the public debate. On any given issue, our work is twofold: descriptive in characterizing both commonsense and scientific understandings of an issue, and prescriptive in developing communications devices that translate expert perspectives to the public in ways that are accessible and can effect shifts in thinking.

In both our descriptive and prescriptive work, we employ the theory and language of "models." Grounded in psychological anthropology, we describe the public's commonsense patterns of thinking as cultural models, those "presupposed, taken-for-granted models of the world that are widely shared . . . by the members of a society and that play an enormous role in their understanding of the world and their behavior in it." (Quinn and Holland 1987:4). In this view, cultural models are constituent features of both culture and cognition, realized both in the world and in the mind via what Bradd Shore (1991:22) calls "two moments of birth." As features of cognition, cultural models are "a community's conventional resources for meaning making" (Shore 1996:47) and organize perspectives, interpretations, and understandings of what is both real and ideal in the world. As Keesing (1987:374) writes: "Such models comprise the realms of (culturally constructed) common sense. They serve pragmatic purposes; they explain the tangible, the experiential (hence perspectivally egocentric), the probable; they assume a superficial geology of causation; they hold sway in a realm in which exceptions prove rules and contradictions live happily together." This approach builds off attention to the well-recognized limitations of cognitive capacity and our need as humans to create mental shortcuts to function amid a tremendous volume and complexity of environmental and sensory inputs (Bruner 1990; Hastie and Park 1986; Schank 1995; Sherman et al. 1989).

Two further assumptions guide our work. The first is that people operate with multiple models in mind, often about the same domains of experience, and that the operational salience of any given model varies and alternates according to context (Shore 1996). For example, a person who on a Tuesday marches to "get government off our backs" might, following a tornado on Wednesday, seek aid from that same government. The model of government as oppressor that informed Tuesday's march is different from the model of government as assister invoked in Wednesday's appeal. This is not to say that alternate cognitive models always contrast in such strong terms, but only that they can.

The second assumption is that people construct and employ models at varying degrees of specificity and generality in making meaning—that cognition is layered. Following Shore (1996), we find it useful to distinguish between models that are more concrete, focused, and linked to specific domains of human experience, and more abstract and comprehensive models, called "foundational schemas," that structure cognition across a range of domains (see also Bennardo 2011). Often, specific models will be "nested" in more generalized models, which can in turn be nested in even more comprehensive and foundational ones. In our research across issue domains we have identified a set of foundational schemas that underlie and organize cognition on social issues in U.S. society, a topic we will return to in our conclusion.

We also use the language of "models" to characterize scientists' and experts' conventionalized understandings of a given issue, describing these as expert models that constitute a scientific sense that typically differs from those commonsense understandings in broader circulation (Kempton 1987; Linde 1987). That is not to say that scientists and experts do not themselves participate in "common sense," for they most assuredly do (D'Andrade 1995; Keesing 1987). What it does suggest is that the body of knowledge that emerges from a scientific perspective is typically differentiated in key ways from knowledge derived from everyday processes of meaning-making. As such, it comes as no surprise that, alongside areas of more shared understandings, our work has identified substantial differences between public and expert models.

Accurately identifying these differences represents the first task around which our work revolves. It requires describing the predominant patterns of shared thinking that characterize both the U.S. public's common sense and experts' scientific sense of a given social issue, and then analytically "mapping the gaps" to characterize how they overlap and diverge. Once this landscape has been mapped, our second task emerges—developing communications devices that translate some targeted body of expert knowledge in ways that are "easy to think" and can be fluidly integrated into public discourse and thinking, bringing both into greater alignment with scientific and expert perspectives. As our case studies will show, this second task is anything but straightforward.

Over the course of many research projects, this second task has pushed FrameWorks researchers to characterize with increasing specificity our own theory of mind in response to several key questions: How do we characterize the cognitive landscape in which cultural models are held and organized? What is the relationship among models in mind? How do communications, especially linguistic ones, enter into this interplay of models and to what effect? What kinds of shifts in cognitive modeling can be predicted, targeted, and instigated in communications? Although our efforts to address these questions have been grounded in psychological anthropology and communications theory, we believe there are larger lessons in our research for applied efforts across the cognitive sciences, including emergent research fields like neuroanthropology. In this way, we hope our work can serve as one model for how to harness cognitive theory to address applied problems.

To help establish this theory-to-practice model, we present three case studies below from our applied communications research, each of which demonstrates a unique cognitively attuned communications challenge. But first, a brief description of our methods and theory.

RESEARCH METHODS

Recognizing that cognitive models come in many forms—spatial, temporal, visual, auditory, and otherwise—our research methods, collectively called Strategic Frame Analysis[TM], have consistently focused on linguistic modeling. This reflects the importance of language as a central communications device across the spectrum of modern media and the strength and facility of using interviews, focus groups, and other forms of talk research as a way to access people's patterns of thinking (Quinn 2005).

Descriptive

Early on in the research process, FrameWorks conducts semistructured, one-on-one, two-hour cultural models interviews with members of the public to elicit "chunks" of talk (Quinn 2005) that allow for identification and analysis of the deep and implicit patterns of understanding that inform how members of a culture approach and understand a specific issue. As a set of 20 to 30 interviews, typically distributed across three or four geographic locations in the country, they are conducted by a team of anthropologists trained in cognitive theory and cultural models interviewing and analysis. Analysis seeks to identify and characterize those models that are most broadly shared across the sample, and deemphasizes those variations, complexities, and idiosyncrasies that are observed.

We then select a sample of thought leaders in the specific area of expertise targeted for translation. We use a mixed-methods approach to ascertain how these experts understand and define the target issue, including one or more of the following methods: (1) one-on-one phone interviews with a range of experts, typically drawn from academia, advocacy, and public service; (2) materials reviews of organizational literature, websites, pamphlets, white papers, etc. to ascertain content and messaging strategies; (3) literature reviews; and (4) professional conference attendance by one or more ethnographers. Using data from these sources, we conduct a thematic analysis using grounded theory (Strauss and Corbin 1990) to identify how experts define and understand the issue area and its challenges, and the policy and program solutions they point to as ways forward.

We then compare these two bodies of data to identify both congruities and incongruities between expert and public conceptualizations and models. The incongruities, or "gaps in understanding" as we call them, represent areas where understandings are likely to break down as members of the public interpret and make sense of expert and scientific messaging. These gaps, therefore, become the primary targets to address in prescriptive reframing research. As described in the case studies below, these gaps can take many forms, with models diverging simply by level of detail or degree of elaboration, or because they are based on entirely different underlying premises and assumptions.

To appreciate the way that public discourse is patterned and disseminated (Gamson and Modigliani 1989), FrameWorks often conducts media content analyses to review and analyze the framing of an issue across a variety of news media, including network and cable television channels, national and regional newspapers, news radio programs, and online news and blog sites. We code these materials to identify and quantify the frames and models used within that coverage (Iyengar 1991), as well as important thematic patterns like reporting style, content, and allocation of news time. By comparing patterns in news coverage with those from cultural models interviews, we begin to see whether and how cultural models are propagated and reinforced in news (Goffman 1974).

To round out the descriptive research, we conduct six to eight peer discourse sessions, similar to focus groups, in two or three geographic locations to explore intragroup negotiations around an issue. Typically consisting of nine people, sessions are designed to open a space for discussion and debate to see the discursive life of models and frames as they are articulated in and shaped by peer-to-peer social interactions and expectations. Demographic criteria vary by issue, but are often differentiated across sessions by education, race, age, or political affiliation. The sessions also serve as an opportunity to experiment with early versions of prescriptive strategies as potential reframing devices are inserted into conversations and subsequently analyzed to determine their effects.

Prescriptive

FrameWorks develops and tests a range of tools and strategies that communicators can use to reframe public understandings of an issue. Among them, two stand out as the most consistent and foundational to our work: values and explanatory metaphors. We understand values to be an important subset of cultural models that are imbued with heightened degrees of salience and sentiment and constitute an important feature of cognition They often act to mediate cognition in important ways by preferencing, filtering, grouping, or otherwise organizing relations among models in mind (Jennings 1991; Rokeach 1973; Schwartz 1994). In the social and public policy areas where we do research, we develop and test values to assess whether and how they provide answers to questions such as, "Why does this matter?" or "What is at stake?" and in so doing shift people's orientation to the issue domain.

Explanatory metaphors are created to concretize and clarify technical concepts and processes in terms that are easily understood and highly communicable.[1] Numerous studies in the cognitive sciences, as well as a growing body of FrameWorks research, have established that people's ability to reason about complex, abstract, or technical concepts relies heavily on metaphor and analogy (Collins and Gentner 1987; Lakoff and Johnson 1980; Ortony 1993; Shore 1996). We develop, test, and refine simple and concrete metaphorical devices to help people organize information in new ways, fill in missing understandings, and shift attention away from problematic defaults. We pay close attention to the entailments that accompany specific metaphors and whether and how they direct peoples' thinking and talk. We recognize that some can be effective in achieving instrumental translation goals, but that others may reinforce default models or direct thinking in novel but counterproductive directions. By the end of the research process on any given project, most of the candidate, most of the candidate metaphors will have been put aside as either problematic or insufficiently effective, and only the one or two that have been validated as effective will be recommended as reframing devices. The three case studies that follow focus specifically on the research process and criteria through which explanatory metaphors are developed and tested.

National Experimental Surveys are used to quantitatively test the relative efficacy of reframing elements (Iyengar 1991; Iyengar and Kinder 1987). These are large-N (2,000–7,000), web-based, random assignment experiments in which respondents are exposed to either a control or one of a set of framed messages built around values, metaphors, or other frame elements. Each respondent is then asked a series of questions to assess their attitudes and support for a variety of related policies and programs. Using this method, we demonstrate the effects of exposure to particular frames on policy preferences. For candidate explanatory metaphors, experimental surveys are adapted to test the effects of each metaphor on issue understanding, application, and metaphor-to-concept fit.

To test the utility and user-friendliness of an explanatory metaphor, FrameWorks conducts short, 10–15 minute on-the-street interviews. Recruited in public places, informants are asked to reason about an issue unaided by a metaphor, are then introduced orally to a single explanatory metaphor, and are then asked to talk further about the target issue. Those metaphors that emerge as potentially effective undergo a second round of qualitative testing in Persistence Trials, a research version of the game of telephone. In sequence, pairs of research participants take turns learning a metaphor as a way to talk about an issue area and then teaching the metaphor to subsequent pairs of participants, allowing researchers to evaluate how well a given metaphor holds up in social interaction as it is used and shared across generations of paired users.

CASE STUDIES

The three case studies presented below demonstrate the complexity of reframing, and the utility of a cognitive and cultural models perspective in creating communications strategies. Each case study identifies a different cognitive task toward which our prescriptive communications research has been or is being applied. Although the summary of each case study provided here is necessarily abridged, PDF copies of all research reports for each case study can be accessed at the FrameWorks Institute website.[2]

Study One: Foregrounding Recessive Cognitive Models to Translate the Science of Child Mental Health

Between 2008 and 2010, with funding from the Center on the Developing Child at Harvard University and the Endowment for Health (NH), FrameWorks conducted research to explore and broaden the U.S. public's understanding of child mental health (CMH). The project aimed to make messaging about the science of CMH more accessible to the public and in so doing increase support for policies and programs this research suggests are effective in improving child outcomes.[3]

FrameWorks's research on CMH illustrates both a communications challenge we commonly encounter and a cognitively attuned strategy for addressing this challenge. The challenge comes when a set of dominant cultural models is persistently applied in ways that occlude more science-based or comprehensive understandings of the issue. The strategy emerges when we are able to identify, as we often are, a set of more backgrounded or "recessive" cultural models that is available for thinking about the target issue, models that are in greater consonance with expert models. In these cases, as described below, we focus on developing strategies that pull these backgrounded models to the forefront of cognition in a way that can upstage those dominant models that block engagement with the target content. This is essentially a model-shifting strategy.

Descriptive research

FrameWorks began the project by reviewing various academic literatures on CMH, paying careful attention to the multidisciplinary nature of this work (Kendall-Taylor and Mikulak 2009). This review was supplemented with a set of eight one-on-one phone interviews conducted with what the literature review suggested were leading experts in the field. These two streams of data were synthesized to produce a set of key expert messages about CMH. These were further winnowed, built out, and refined as FrameWorks researchers attended, as participant-observers, several key multidisciplinary meetings of CMH experts. FrameWorks subsequently participated in the design and facilitation of a two-day summit, Healthy Development: A Summit on Young Children's Mental Health, designed specifically to arrive at a final set of messages that would serve as the content to be communicated in reframing efforts (see Society for Research on Child Development 2009).

Research continued with 20 cultural models interviews conducted in Dallas and Cleveland and eight peer discourse sessions in Boston, Phoenix, and Chicago. Across both research methods, participants were asked a cascading series of open-ended questions about CMH, analysis of which demonstrated key contours of a broadly distributed and generalized public understanding:

> In general, Americans rely on different sets of assumptions to think about mental health than they do to think about mental illness. The former is largely defined in terms of "feelings" over which an individual is responsible for exerting control, while the latter is characterized in terms of chemical imbalances in the brain resulting from faulty but immutable genetic factors. This bifurcated modeling applies to both children and adults.
>
> Public thinking about mental health in children is strongly mediated by two generalized models of "children." In one, children lack basic emotional capacities like memory and "strong" emotions, leading informants to doubt whether young children can even have mental health. In the second, contradictory, model, children are "really just little adults," as one informant put it, and therefore, "of course" experience emotional states just as do adults. In this case, comparable diagnostic criteria and treatments should apply.
>
> Across these various ways of thinking about child mental health or illness, a developmental perspective was weak or lacking altogether. The genetic model of

chemical imbalances was highly deterministic and largely lacking developmental process, while the "feelings" model of mental health was largely framed in terms of personal control and responsibility. Sensitivity to environmental and developmental factors, if extant, was subsumed in talk about the parental role and the importance of upbringing.

These patterns are dramatically different from the explanations experts wish to advance, which emphasize (1) the reality of mental health in even very young children; (2) the importance of understanding the developing brain as the location for mental health; (3) the importance of environmental factors both in and out of the home; and (4) the deleterious effects of chronic and severe stressors on brain development. These contrasts lay open key features of the communications challenge, as the public's most readily accessible and practiced ways of modeling mental states in children run counter to the messages that experts believe are essential for the public to understand if they are to support a new set of public policies. In short, thinking the science through the public's dominant, or foregrounded, cultural models renders key parts of the science of CMH hard to think.

At the same time, however, lay interviews also evidenced a set of less top-of-mind, more backgrounded assumptions and understandings about CMH that are more consonant with expert thinking: (1) that the community that surrounds a child is an important determinant in their mental state; (2) that prolonged and severe stress can negatively affect mental health; (3) that poor foundations of health and development cause poor mental health; and (4) that CMH is about a child's ability to function. In terms of translating the science to the public, these backgrounded models represent promising targets for communication efforts.

By this point in the research process, the communications task was becoming clear: to develop messaging strategies that could foreground these more promising recessive models, and background the less productive dominant ones, and in so doing help make the science easier to think. More specifically, the work of the reframing strategy was to (1) foreground an ecological perspective regarding the factors that shape and remediate mental health while backgrounding more individualistic assumptions of responsibility over mental states; (2) foreground a model of CMH as linked to the brain and development, while backgrounding assumptions that mental health "is just about feelings"; (3) pull a sense of pragmatism and solvability to the foreground, while backgrounding deterministic orientations; (4) activate and preference the linkage model between a child's mental health and notions of functioning; and (5) foreground the recessive understanding that ongoing and severe stress threatens a child's development and mental health, and supplant notions that stress is a necessary and useful feature of those processes.

With clarity on these specific goals, we began to design and test communications tools that could be deployed to accomplish these background-to-foreground cognitive shifts.

Prescriptive research

As described in our methods section, values and explanatory metaphors are two key reframing tools employed by FrameWorks. In this article, we focus our attention on the development and testing of explanatory metaphors and their cognitive effects. That said, coming out of the descriptive research, FrameWorks researchers hypothesized that values could be effective in doing some of the cognitive shifting work just identified, as they have in previous research areas (Gilliam 2007; Simon and Davey 2010). More specifically, we hypothesized that values could background individualist orientations to causation and remediation, while foregrounding more latent ecological systems and collective conceptions. We also thought that values might be effective in pushing senses of fatalism and determinism into the background by pulling forward a sense that CMH issues could, in fact, be addressed and improved. We return briefly at the end of this case study to describe our values results, but now focus on the development and testing of explanatory metaphors.

Drawing on over a decade of framing research on early childhood development, FrameWorks first looked to two metaphors that have proven effective in helping Americans think about child development more generally (see Erard et al. 2009) as potentially useful tools in communicating about CMH. The first is *brain architecture,* or the notion that brain development can be compared to building a house from the ground up. The second is *toxic stress,* or the notion that some types of stress (severe and ongoing) can disrupt developmental processes and damage stress-response and connected systems. Results of qualitative research confirmed the utility of brain architecture in pushing dominant models of mental health as "just feelings" into the background and foregrounding latent connections between mental health and developmental processes. Research also confirmed that toxic stress, when employed in conversations about CMH, backgrounded the ideas that genes are the only concrete determinant of mental states and that stress is beneficial to development, and instead foregrounded the recessive cultural model that stress can have negative impacts on health and development (Simon 2010a).

Recruiting these two metaphors from earlier research left two key reframing tasks unaddressed: (1) to shift people off the models that children do not have mental health or that it is primarily about controllable feeling-states, and instead foreground models of its reality and functional importance; and (2) to promote a sense of preventative and remedial agency. Ideally, we would also identify a metaphor that reinforced and worked in concert with the values in accomplishing the individualist-to-collective and determinist-to-solvability shifts. With these tasks in mind, FrameWorks designed and tested a new set of 12 potential metaphors, with titles like engine, electricity, roadway, game plan, roots, cornerstone, brain health, exposure, signature, and levelness. Over the course of more than a year, candidate metaphors were tested, culled, and refined through on-the-street interviews ($\times$49), Quantitative Testing ($N = 2,000$), and Persistence Trials ($\times$6), from which one metaphor, the comparison of CMH to the levelness of a table or piece of furniture, emerged as most successful (Erard et al. 2010b). This was a surprising result for FrameWorks researchers, as early on in the design process levelness was considered one of the weaker candidate metaphors. Its success across the research methods highlights the importance of rigorous empiricism in this form of applied work and shows that the only way to know what a metaphor will actually do and how it will "behave" is to empirically test its effect.

One way to think about child mental health is that it is like the levelness of a piece of furniture, say, a table. The levelness of a table is what makes it usable and able to function, just like the mental health of a child is what enables him or her to function and do many things. [See Erard et al. 2010b for full version.]

The levelness metaphor, which proved both readily understandable and communicable, was powerful in foregrounding two of the extant but recessive models—that environments are important determinants of CMH, and that CMH is connected to a child's functioning more generally. The metaphor also helped people to locate mental health in the brain, rather than in vague feeling states, and to think about degrees of mental health, rather than use a bifurcated model of health or illness. In getting people to think about the relationship between a table and the ground it rests on, and about the multiple ways one can address an unlevel table, the levelness metaphor also helped people consider the range of factors that can influence CMH, and opened up thinking about multiple intervention strategies. In the process, the metaphor also effectively pushed more problematic cultural models into the background—including models of mental health as the exclusive product of emotional states, of individuals as responsible for controlling their emotions, and of senses of genetic determinism.

The final suite of reframing recommendations included a set of tools that could be deployed to push dominant but unproductive cultural models about the mental states of children into the background of cognition while pulling extant but more latent models to the forefront. This suite included two values that emerged as useful from Quantitative Testing. The first was a call to national prosperity, which backgrounded individualist orientations about CMH and foregrounded a more ecological, systemic, and collective perspective. The second was the value of ingenuity, which backgrounded notions of futility associated with CMH and foregrounded pragmatic, innovative ways of thinking about the issue. These values were recommended for use in concert with three metaphors: brain architecture, to bring connections between CMH and development to the forefront; toxic stress, to recruit the recessive model of stress as having negative impacts on mental health; and levelness, to push a host of unproductive dominant definitional models of children's mental states into the background and pull forward latent understandings of functioning, of connections between development and mental health, and of the importance of ecologies, resources, and populations. These reframing tools were combined in a messaging toolkit, as well as in a multimedia presentation that includes examples of effective applications of the communications strategies.

Study Two: Filling in a Cognitive Lacuna on Budgets and Taxes by Recruiting Models from Kindred Domains

Starting in 2008, with funding from the DEMOS Center for the Public Sector, Kansas Action for Children, and the John D. and Catherine T. MacArthur Foundation, FrameWorks has examined ways that Americans think and talk about budgets and taxes. The research was designed to ascertain whether and how Americans understand the relationship between taxes and the public goods and services they make possible, as well as the process by which priorities are set for the allocation of public resources. The research sought to identify evidence-based framing strategies that could be used to communicate to Americans a more deliberate, realistic, and informed view of the relationship between budgets and taxation and their role in achieving collective services and goals for the country (Davey and Bales 2010).

In this project, FrameWorks identified and addressed a second kind of cognitively attuned communications challenge. This involved developing an explanatory metaphor that could fill a domain-specific cognitive lacuna by recruiting an existing model (or models) from a kindred domain. By "cognitive lacuna," we mean a domain of cognition where the public has very weak or nonexistent models for thinking about some process, relationship, role, or other feature that is defined by experts as necessary to understanding the reality of that domain (see also Levy 1984). In short, cognitive lacunae exist when a key feature in the expert model is conspicuously absent or "un-modeled" for members of the public. In translating scientific and expert knowledge, such absences represent a core challenge.

In the CMH research just described, the communications challenge was to develop a metaphoric device that could foreground recessive models and enhance their cognitive salience in and connection to the target issue domain. In our work on budgets and taxes, the task was to recruit a dominant model from another, more familiar, domain and use a metaphoric device to fill the existing conceptual void.

To begin this research, FrameWorks conducted 25 cultural models interviews in Baltimore, Philadelphia, and Cleveland and six peer discourse sessions in Phoenix, Charlotte, and Kansas City. In both interviews and peer sessions, participants were asked to engage general questions and topics about budgets, taxes, and the relationship between the two. Unlike most of our research projects, we did not conduct interviews with experts on this topic, but instead relied on a comprehensive report written by the National Research Council and the National Academy of Public Administration, entitled "Choosing the Nation's Fiscal Future" (www.ourfiscalfuture.org). This document was analyzed to distill the set of messages toward which our communications research was directed and to which our strategies and tools were held accountable.

Descriptive research

FrameWorks used both the cultural models interviews and peer discourse sessions to draw conclusions about the cultural models used by Americans to think about budgets and taxes, and whether and how they are related to the larger work of government. Four findings stand out:

> An ill-defined and monolithic model of "government" as a large, bureaucratic, and often corrupt "other" whose functions are too vast, complex, and mysterious to comprehend was dominant among the public. Faced with questions about public functions, this model provides a ready-made cognitive "shortcut" that mutes attention to specific government functions, processes, or services (see also Aubrun and Grady 2004).

The public largely uses a consumer, rather than a civic model to define taxes and their purpose. Informed by this model, individuals who pay taxes should "get their money's worth" in identifiable and measurable services within a short-term timeframe.

Most members of the public appear to lack a well-articulated model of large-scale public budgets. Given this domain-specific absence, or "cognitive lacuna," when asked to speak to public budgets, our informants recruited a model from another familiar domain—that of the monthly personal or household budget, a small-scale model where planning is relatively short term and success is defined by outputs never exceeding inputs.

Budgets and taxes are largely unconnected concepts for most members of the public. Initially this was a surprising finding for us, but with time the reasons for this disconnect became increasingly apparent. Lacking a clear model of public budgets, and using a consumer rather than a civic model to think about taxation, informants struggled to cognize a relationship between budgets and taxes, the processes that relate the two, or their combined relationship to public services and structures. Without such an integrative model, the implications of both budgets and taxes and the public's role in either were poorly conceptualized, and public services were largely taken for granted.

By the end of this descriptive research we had a good understanding of the problem, and were positioned to define the key cognitive work for an explanatory metaphor to accomplish: to fill the cognitive lacuna about public budgets—what they are, how they function in time, and the collective purposes toward which they are directed—and in so doing, model a structural and temporal relationship between taxes, budgets, and resultant public services. Ideally, the metaphor would also facilitate a collective rather than individualist framing of these relationships.

We hypothesized that values could be effective in cultivating civic rather than consumer orientations and help shift people's thinking toward more collectivist notions of budgets and taxes. Ideally, one or more values could be identified to work in parallel with an explanatory metaphor to help people see themselves as citizens in the give-and-take of a larger social contract (see Kendall-Taylor and Bales 2009).

Prescriptive research

We used the last question in the cultural models interviews to begin experimenting with potential reframing strategies. Each informant was presented with two possible ways to think about "taxes"—"taxes as investments," which represents an argument frequently made in advocacy materials, and "taxes as exchanges," an idea derived in part from Marcel Mauss's seminal work *The Gift* (1990). Informants were then guided through a discussion to explore whether and how each idea might open up new ways of thinking about the relationship between budgets and taxes. As will be discussed below, the "taxes as exchanges" idea generated several productive directions, while the idea of "taxes as investments" was largely unproductive. Informants' dominant model of investments, as long-term processes that carry risk, conflicted with a model of taxation as payments that should result in quick and predictable benefits in which taxpayers get their "money's worth." These conflicting base models quickly suggested an unproductive reframing analogue.

Based on these results, and drawing from previous FrameWorks research on government, peer discourse sessions were designed to explore the effectiveness of several prospective reframing devices (see Kendall-Taylor and O'Neil 2009). Of the ideas explored, three were metaphors—"household budgets," "prosperity grid," and "exchanges"—and one was a concept entitled "pay now or pay later," which focused on the savings incurred by taking a preventative, rather than a remedial approach to intervention.

The "household budgets" and "prosperity grid" metaphors were generally unsuccessful in structuring thinking and talking in the desired directions. Discussions of the former were undermined by talk about how public budgets are not like household budgets because of their scale, while "prosperity grid" frequently led to critiques of unfair efforts to "spread the wealth." The "exchanges" metaphor demonstrated more promising, if still mixed, results. It helped participants talk about the otherwise taken-for-granted services that government budgets provide, through an assumed reciprocal process and obligation of "give and take." It also led, however, to problematic discussions of "unfairness" and the idea that some pay more or less than their "fair" share. This moved talk away from public purposes and social responsibility and toward ideas of taxes as unfair involuntary exchanges with distorted cost–benefit ratios.

Productively, the "pay now or pay later" concept shifted talk away from a short-term consumer model of "getting one's money's worth" and toward discussions of long-term goals and purposes. Conversation shifted from "what I need to get from my taxes," or "what budgets do for me" toward the need for taxes to support "our country" or "our society." The concept also connected budgets with taxes, helping participants explicitly recognize that the services and infrastructure that budgets provide and on which citizens rely have to be funded, and that this funding typically comes from public taxes. This more explicit talk about the goal of taxes led to more pragmatic discussions about the need to fund public services and infrastructure for the long term.

In the months that followed, FrameWorks developed and tested a total of nine candidate metaphors to evaluate their capacity to fill in people's understanding about the relationship between budgets, taxes, and public structures, and to cultivate more supportive ways of thinking and talking about those relationships (see Erard et al. 2010a). These metaphors were run through our standard sequence of evaluative and experimental methods, with each method serving both a winnowing function—as some metaphors performed well while others did not—and a refining function—as each iterative source of data was used to change the execution of the metaphors to address specific conceptual problems. The methods also allowed for evaluation of each metaphor's functionality with an eye toward eventual deployment in concert with values and other framing recommendations. Space does not permit a discussion of the findings from each of those methods and subsequent analyses, although reports from each method are available at the FrameWorks Institute (n.d.a).

The result of this research trajectory was development and refinement of an explanatory metaphor that built off two strong cultural models that were already part of public thinking, but that were not typically applied to thinking about budgets and taxes.

Future Planning: The idea that it is a good idea to plan ahead and to put aside the funds necessary to realize plans and visions

Exchange: The idea that much of human social and economic life is structured by relationships of giving and receiving where bonds of expectation and obligation are created and sustained

On its own, neither model succeeded in filling the public's cognitive lacuna on public budgets, nor helped structure an improved understanding of the relationship between budgets, taxes, and services, and the collective benefits of that relationship. The exchange model lacked sufficient temporal perspective, while the planning model failed to structure the relationship between taxes and services. Combining the two models, however, produced a powerful effect, borne out in subsequent quantitative testing (Erard et al. 2010a). The result was an explanatory metaphor entitled "forward exchange," which read as follows:

> Public budgets and taxes make up a system of forward exchange. Budgets give us a schedule for paying taxes forward in time for public goods whose importance we all agree on. The public goods we have today weren't paid for by taxes we just paid or are about to pay. They were paid for in the past, by taxes that were budgeted then to meet our needs now. So, a good public budget is one that plans for the future and for the unexpected. And good taxes are those that allow us to pay for public goods and services that we've planned for.

Combined with the value of prevention, which also tested well (Simon 2010b), forward exchange helped people think about the common goals to which budgets and taxes are the central means. Together, these tools helped shift people away from short-term, consumerist thinking and toward a notion of shared priorities for a common future. Thought of in terms of a forward exchange, budgets and taxes became means to a now visible end, not ends in themselves.

Study Three: Addressing a Productive but Narrow Dominant Model of Environmental Health

A project on environmental health provides insight into a third kind of cognitively attuned communications challenge. This involves the effort to develop an explanatory metaphor that builds off or works effectively around a dominant cultural model that is aligned with the science and is productive, but remains too narrow in scope.

Starting in 2010, FrameWorks began research on environmental health (EH) on behalf of the American Public Health Association, the Association of Public Health Laboratories, and the Association of State and Territorial Health Officials with funding from the CDC's National Center for Environmental Health. The goal of the research was to develop communications strategies to help those working in EH policy, practice, research, and advocacy speak with a more consistent and strategic voice to both public and policy audiences about their field and its work. The larger goal is to build the social and political will required to support efforts to reduce harm associated with environmental hazards, and to help build a strong and enduring infrastructure for EH communication.

Four research methods were employed to generate a summary of the expert view of environmental health: (1) ten one-on-one phone interviews with expert practitioners and academics; (2) a literature review; (3) participant-observation at an EH professional meeting; and (4) a FrameWorks-hosted online webinar with 14 experts from the field, consisting of a structured Q-and-A session and solicited response to and critique of an initial summary of "the expert view" derived from the first three methods.

To map public understandings of the issue, FrameWorks conducted 21 cultural models interviews with members of the public in Dallas; Cleveland; South Bend, Indiana; and Boulder, Colorado. Informants were asked a series of open-ended questions designed to elicit implicit understandings associated with the terms and work of EH (Lindland and Kendall-Taylor 2011).

Descriptive research

The phrase "environmental health" was unfamiliar to most of our informants, even as a majority were able to correctly guess that it referred to some form of environmental impact on human health. A minority understood it to refer instead to the health of the environment. That said, once a correct definition of the topic was established, broader patterns of public modeling emerged, concerned largely with EH threats and structured by a dominant model of what constitutes such threats—contaminants, especially those that threaten the safety of food, water, air, and household environments. The strength and broad distribution of this contaminant model was evidenced in consistent talk about fears of exposure to chemicals, particulates, artificial hormones and steroids, heavy metals, pollen, plastics, and the like.

Although informants' talk revealed a robust model of contaminant threats, it showed a very weak and fragmented model for thinking about EH work. When primed, informants were able to articulate basic knowledge about prevention efforts in sanitation ("garbage men" and dumps) and food safety (hairnets and inspectors), but were unfamiliar with the broader scope of work in these areas, and unable to discuss EH work in other arenas, like chemical and radiation exposure. Unpracticed in thinking about the contours and scope of EH work overall, members of the public struggled to identify the key agencies, institutions, hierarchies, professions, and skill sets of the field, and consistently defaulted to the more familiar arenas of environmentalism and health care.

Notably however, over the course of interviews, as informants engaged in discussions of EH threats and what can be done about them, they quickly and consistently changed their tune and began speaking to the criticalness of basic EH functions like sanitation, air and water quality, and food safety work. In other words, once pulled into active thinking, these functions shifted from absent and taken for granted to present and very important. From a cognitive perspective, it seemed that actively talking about contaminant threats served to foreground and bring onstage a model of salience that otherwise lived mostly in the cognitive background—offstage, if you will—where it failed to structure people's thinking about and understanding of the domain.

In addition to the dominant contaminant model, informants employed a series of more recessive or "backgrounded" models about EH impacts, including understandings that social relationships, economic conditions, and the organization of built environments can have profound health effects. These models represented promising targets for communications development and testing.

Although we do not attempt a full summary of expert perspectives of EH here, there are key features that stand out relative to the patterns in public thinking. Experts agree that EH's work is to assure the conditions of human health and provide healthy environments for people to live, work, and play. This work is accomplished through two parallel emphases: (1) risk assessment, prevention, and intervention efforts aimed at reducing or eliminating contaminant and contagion threats to human health via air, water, food, soil, vector, and animal exposures; and (2) health promotion efforts that address large-scale systemic factors and construct wellness-friendly environments at the population level. This two-pronged mission depends on publicly funded research, communications, surveillance, epidemiology, subject matter expertise, and policy efforts that address the full scope of environmental impacts on health from the local to global scales.

In comparing the expert and public views, two areas stand out, regarding (1) the relationship between threats and work, and (2) the factors recognized as having EH impacts. In both areas, a significant gap and overlap between expert and public thinking can be identified. In the first, while experts demonstrated a consistent awareness of, and commitment to, the importance of EH work, the public often took this work for granted and failed to consider its ongoing nature and critical importance. This represents a key gap for communications to address. Yet, once the public's thinking was activated through questioning from the interviewer, talk about EH work was generally consistent with expert positions, asserting that preventative, proactive approaches to EH threats are ideal. This represents an important overlap. The second notable area concerns EH factors. Both experts and the public agree that contaminants and contagions represent a real and pervasive threat to human health. This also represents an important overlap. Yet, experts emphasized a broader set of interconnected factors that affect human health at the population level, including social, economic, infrastructural, and climatic factors. Although several of these factors were evident as backgrounded or recessive cultural models among members of the general public, they were minor themes in a larger story focused overwhelmingly on toxic exposures at the individual and household level. This represents a key gap.

COGNITIVE COMMUNICATIONS IMPLICATIONS

As of the writing of this article, FrameWorks has yet to begin the next phases of prescriptive research to develop and test metaphors, values, and other framing devices to evaluate their potential to align public thinking with expert opinion and build public support for EH efforts. The overlaps identified suggest an avenue for moving forward by deliberately engaging those patterns in public thinking that are consistent with the expert story, including attention to social, economic, and infrastructural factors.

The challenge is what to do about the contaminant model. It is clear that the public has a robust model of contaminant threats to human health, one that is consistent with expert thinking. It is also clear that many people have a well-developed pattern of avoiding engagement with the broader scope of those threats, thereby keeping thoughts about the work required to address them offstage. Finally, it is clear that the strength of the contaminant model as a source of threat provides a cognitive pathway for an offstage model of EH work to quickly emerge onstage as salient, even critical. In this respect, the contaminant model serves an important function.

With all of this said, the communications strategy for the EH field might seem clear: construct messaging that triggers the contaminant model, and in so doing raise the public profile for EH work. If raising issue salience was the only goal for our partners in the field, that would likely be an effective strategy. However, there is another key goal held by many in the EH field, including our partners in this research: to help the public think more broadly about EH impacts, to move their thinking "upstream" to consider the broader, macrolevel factors that result in downstream contaminant and contagion threats to human health—factors like urban and infrastructure planning, built environments, patterns of transportation and energy use, and social and economic factors, like poverty, that create differential susceptibility to negative EH impacts. For EH experts and advocates, making the public smarter about this broader set of factors is a major goal—one that many feel will translate into building support for the kind of policy initiatives that can have the greatest impact.

In light of this larger communications agenda, the advantages of triggering the "contaminant model" become less clear. Does the activation of this highly available way of thinking constitute a building block for constructing a more elaborated and expansive vision of EH, including increased attention to social, economic, cultural, infrastructural, and climactic factors? We have seen that some of these factors exist as recessive public models, so perhaps the strength of the contaminant model can be harnessed to bolster them. Or, is the contaminant model so dominant that its invocation will crowd out other ways of thinking about EH as it takes people to a satisfying, ready-made cognitive moment that says "I know what this is about—contaminants"? Or, worse yet, will triggering the contaminant model invoke the avoidance pattern that has already been evidenced, thereby reinforcing the default pattern of not thinking about EH work, efforts, and solutions in the first place?

Future research will work to develop and test one or more explanatory metaphors that can address these questions while accomplishing two critical tasks: (1) heightening awareness of the importance of publicly funded EH work, and (2) moving people's thinking "upstream" toward more macro- and population-level EH causal factors. Considering how the contaminant model both dominates and constrains people's thinking, even as it serves to bring EH work "on-stage" in thinking, it remains for future prescriptive communications research to ascertain the model's utility or liability as a referent in a broader communications strategy.

CONCLUSION: THEORY TO PRACTICE AND BACK AGAIN

Our experience in doing applied cognitive research has compelled us to engage theory with increasing specificity even as we find our applied work pushing that theory in new directions. Our work has both been informed by and confirmed many core features of cognitive theory more generally, and cultural models theory more specifically. These include the hierarchical nature of modeling (D'Andrade 1984; Kronenfield et al. 2011; Shore 1996); the contextual nature of cognition generally and modeling more specifically (Ewing 1990; LeVine 1984; Kempton 1987); and the extent to which people typically hold multiple, sometimes conflicting, models in reasoning about complex issues (Ewing 1990; Quinn and Holland 1987; Shore 1996; Strauss and Quinn 1997). At the most basic level, our work affirms that many of the cognitive constructs brought to bear in making meaning operate largely at the implicit level, even as there are also more explicit cultural constructs or "cultural theories" (D'Andrade 1984, 1995; Quinn and Holland 1987; Shore 1996). Our research also affirms the integral relationship between metaphoric reasoning, cultural models, and meaning making (Collins and Gentner 1987; Lakoff and Johnson 1980; Shore 1996), as we have found repeatedly that metaphors are powerful tools in communicating ideas, in large part because of their ability to tap into and orchestrate movements among cultural models in mind.

Two key assertions likewise inform and are confirmed by our applied work. The first is the general assertion, which has been more fully developed by others (Bales and Gilliam 2004; Carey 1988), that culture matters in communication. The second, more specific, assertion is that communications practice benefits from a concrete and workable theory of culture that provides a unit of analysis that can be operationalized both analytically and in subsequent messaging efforts. We have attempted to show that cultural models theory is an effective theoretical and methodological framework through which to conceptualize and articulate the mediating role of culture, allowing researchers to describe and map the assumptions, representations, and propositions that shape the way people understand issues and information and, in turn, to create more effective means of communicating. Like any model of reality, the linguistic representations of the cultural models that we identify are by necessity simplifications of reality (Shore 1996), but we are convinced that they serve as viable representations of the key features and contours of that underlying cognitive and conceptual reality we seek to describe.

So, too, are the spatial metaphors we employ to account for both cognitive processing and the potential effects of communications on that processing. As have others, we find it useful to think of cognition as a landscape (Sayre 1997), with features of cognition (models) that are more or less foregrounded or backgrounded, or as a theater stage, with models that are coming and going on-stage and off-stage based on contextual cues. In many respects, these metaphors mirror notions of explicit and implicit, and of conscious and unconscious, yet in our view carry less binary and more gradated and processual associations. In fact, what we have seen in our work is that the right metaphor can serve to bring off-stage models on-stage, and even upstage otherwise dominant models. We have seen how typically backgrounded models can become increasingly foregrounded, especially when a value or metaphor carries entailments that facilitate that shift. This language of spatiality suggests a dynamic perspective on models—in terms of their relative positioning in mind and the extent to which communications or other factors can serve to mediate their repositioning. It also raises key questions—about the relationship among models and their relative effects on reasoning, and about the relationship between any given model's position and the reasoning process. Our hope is that some of these questions will prove provocative for others working at the intersections of the behavioral and brain sciences.

To conclude, we point to a central challenge in our work, one that emerges at the intersections of our research findings, our organizational goals, cognitive theory, and the confluence of neuroanthropology and applied work that characterizes this volume. Across the scope of our research, we have repeatedly identified a strong and pervasive pattern in public thinking that attributes primary, if not exclusive, responsibility for social problems to individuals. Whether the topic is levels of crime, educational disparities, health and fitness, sexual violence, or immigration, the model of the individual as the self-determining, responsible agent emerges over and over again as the dominant perceptual lens through which Americans define, diagnose, and think about solutions to social problems. In our CMH research, this was manifest in people's talk about helping children gain control over their emotions as the most effective intervention. In our budgets and taxes research, it was evident in talk about individual consumers getting their money's worth for their tax dollars paid. Finally, in our EH research, it could be seen in talk about individuals taking responsibility at the household level, as the first and most important line of defense, to protect themselves and their families from contaminant threats.

In our view, this pervasive pattern is rooted in what can be best described as an underlying foundational schema of individualism in U.S. culture. This foundational schema underlies and informs a series of more domain-specific, person-centered models that are dominant, foregrounded, and easy to think, and that run directly counter to efforts to help people think about policy interventions at the social and population levels. As such, one of FrameWorks's central tasks is figuring out ways to help people widen the scope of their thinking, to see a bigger picture defined not by the actions of individual agents, but by systems that both shape and are shaped by their actions—social, economic, political, and otherwise—and that can be addressed through public policy. On any given research issue, we seek to widen the lens on that issue, even as we recognize that our work across all issues confronts a larger challenge in shifting the foundations of how we as Americans understand and think about improving our collective life and future together. We feel that attention to this widening task is central not only for communications with the general public but also for scientists doing similar applied work, especially for neuroanthropologists seeking to widen perspectives about the complex intersections between human nervous systems and the social and cultural systems that people inhabit.

We hope that this article has made the case for the relevance of cognitive theory for communications practice, and of that practice for cognitive theory. We hope, too, that this discussion can contribute to a larger theoretical effort to address the relative strength and dynamic interplay of mental models and their role in cognition and reasoning, as well as the effects of media and communications on that interplay. Finally, we hope that it might contribute to the work of others seeking to integrate theory and practice within the larger emerging field of neuroanthropology. Our experience in conducting applied cultural research has strengthened in us the conviction that theory-driven applied research is a critical tool in creating effective communications about social and scientific issues in the service of improved public policy. It has also strengthened our belief that creating effective communications is an empirical endeavor that turns on a set of propositions and questions about which social scientists know a great deal. Above all else, we hope that this piece has made it clear that effective public policy communication is anything but simple "common sense."

NOTES

Acknowledgments. Thanks to Susan Nall Bales and Bradd Shore for their insights and contributions to earlier drafts of this article. This piece reflects many years of mentorship and intellectual guidance from each of them. We also thank all of our colleagues at the FrameWorks Institute who collaborated in the work summarized here.

1. For most of FrameWorks's existence, we have called these metaphoric devices "simplifying models" to emphasize their function in translating complex expert perspectives to the public in more accessible terms.

2. See FrameWorks Institute (n.d.b).

3. This connection between causal understandings and perceptions of solutions has been widely studied in anthropology (Hurwicz 1995; Kendall-Taylor 2009; Mathews and Hill 1990; Young and Garro 1994). In addition, past FrameWorks research has shown that improved understandings of how issues like child development "work" is important in creating support for policy solutions (Erard et al. 2009).

Editors' Note: The FrameWorks Institute research reports identified in the References Cited can be accessed via the organization's website (FrameWorks Institute n.d.b).

REFERENCES CITED

Aubrun, Axel, and Joseph Grady
    2004 Mind and Monolith: Findings from Cognitive Interviews about Government. Washington, DC: FrameWorks Institute.
Bales, Susan N., and Frank D. Gilliam, Jr.
    2004 Communications for Social Good. Washington, DC: Foundation Center.
Benedict, Ruth
    1922 The Vision in Plains Culture. American Anthropologist 24(1):1–23.
Bennardo, Giovanni
    2011 A Foundational Cultural Model in Polynesia: Monarchy, Democracy, and the Architecture of the Mind. *In* A Companion to Cognitive Anthropology. David B. Kronenfeld, Giovanni Bennardo, Michael D. Fischer, and Victor C. de Munck, eds. Pp. 489–512. Malden, MA: Blackwell.

Boas, Franz

    1902 The Ethnological Significance of Esoteric Doctrines. Science 16(413):872–874.

Bruner, Jerome

    1990 Acts of Meaning. Cambridge, MA: Harvard University Press.

Carey, James W.

    1988 Communications as Culture: Essays on Media and Society. New York: HarperCollins.

Collins, Allan, and Dedre Gentner

    1987 How People Construct Mental Models. *In* Cultural Models in Language and Thought. Dorothy C. Holland and Naomi Quinn, eds. Pp. 243–265. Cambridge: Cambridge University Press.

D'Andrade, Roy

    1984 Cultural Meaning Systems. *In* Culture Theory: Essays on Mind, Self, and Emotion. Richard A. Shweder and Robert A. LeVine, eds. Pp. 88–119. Cambridge: Cambridge University Press.

    1995 Moral Models in Anthropology. Current Anthropology 36(3):399–408.

Davey, Lynn F., and Susan N. Bales

    2010 How to Talk About Budgets and Taxes: A FrameWorks Message Memo. Washington, DC: Frame-Works Institute.

Erard, Michael, Adam Simon, Lynn Davey, and Nat Kendall-Taylor.

    2009 Framing Early Child Development: A FrameWorks Message Brief. Washington, DC: FrameWorks Institute.

    2010a Planning for Our Future: The Contribution of Simplifying Models to Budgets and Taxes. Washington, DC: FrameWorks Institute.

    2010b The Power of Levelness: Making Child Mental Health Visible and Concrete Through a Simplifying Model. Washington, DC: FrameWorks Institute.

Ewing, Katherine

    1990 The Illusion of Wholeness: Culture, Self, and the Experience of Inconsistency. Ethos 18(3):251–278.

FrameWorks Institute

    N.d.a Budgets and Taxes. FrameWorks Institute. http://frameworksinstitute.org/budgetsandtaxes.html, accessed July 10, 2012.

    N.d.b Frameworks Issues. FrameWorks Institute. http://frameworksinstitute.org/allissues.html, accessed July 10, 2012.

Gamson, William A., and Andre Modigliani

    1989 Media Discourse and Public Opinion on Nuclear Power: A Constructionist Approach. American Journal of Sociology 95(1):1–37.

Gilliam, Frank D., Jr.

    2007 Telling the Science Story: An Exploration of Frame Effects on Public Understanding and Support for Early Child Development: A FrameWorks Research Report. Washington, DC: FrameWorks Institute.

Goffman, Erving

    1974 Frame Analysis: An Essay on the Organization of Experience. New York: Harper and Row.

Hastie, Reid, and Bernadette Park

    1986 The Relationship Between Memory and Judgment Depends on Whether the Task is Memory-Based or On-Line. Psychological Review 93:258–268.

Hurwicz, Margo-Lea

    1995 Physicians' Norms and Health Care Decisions of Elderly Medicare Recipients. Medical Anthropology Quarterly 9(2):211–235.

Iyengar, Shanto

    1991 Is Anyone Responsible? How Television Frames Political Issues. Chicago: University of Chicago Press.

Iyengar, Shanto, and Donald R. Kinder

    1987 News That Matters: Television and American Opinion. Chicago: University of Chicago Press.

Jennings, M. Kent

    1991 Thinking about Social Injustice. Political Psychology 12(2):187–204.

Keesing, Roger

    1987 Models, "Folk" and "Cultural": Paradigms Regained? *In* Cultural Models in Language and Thought. Dorothy Holland and Naomi Quinn, eds. Pp. 369–393. Cambridge: Cambridge University Press.

Kempton, Willett

    1987 Two Theories of Home Heat Control. *In* Cultural Models in Language and Thought. Dorothy Holland and Naomi Quinn, eds. Pp. 222–242. Cambridge: Cambridge University Press.

Kendall-Taylor, Nathaniel

    2009 Treatment Seeking for a Chronic Disorder: How Families in Coastal Kenya Make Epilepsy Treatment Decisions. Human Organization 68(2):141–153.

Kendall-Taylor, Nathaniel, and Susan Bales

    2009 Like Mars to Venus: The Separate and Sketchy Worlds of Budgets and Taxes. Washington, DC: FrameWorks Institute.

Kendall-Taylor, Nathaniel, and Anna Mikulak

    2009 Child Mental Health: A Review of the Scientific Discourse. Washington, DC: FrameWorks Institute.

Kendall-Taylor, Nathaniel, and Moira O'Neil

    2009 Priority, Transparency and Agency: Results from Peer Discourse Analysis. Washington, DC: FrameWorks Institute.

Kronenfeld, David B., Giovanni Bennardo, Michael D. Fischer, and Victor C. de Munck, eds.

    2011 A Companion to Cognitive Anthropology. Malden, MA: Blackwell Publishing.

Lakoff, George, and Michael Johnson

    1980 Metaphors We Live by. Chicago: University of Chicago Press.

Lévi-Strauss, Claude

    1963 The Sorcerer and His Magic. *In* Structural Anthropology, vol. 1. Pp. 167–187. New York: Basic.

LeVine, Robert

    1984 Properties of Culture: An Ethnographic View. *In* Cultural Theory: Essays on Mind, Self and Emotion. Richard Shweder and Robert LeVine, eds. Pp. 67–87. New York: Cambridge University Press.

Levy, Robert I.

    1984 Emotion, Knowing, and Culture. *In* Culture Theory: Essays on Mind, Self, and Emotion. Richard A. Shweder and Robert A. LeVine, eds. Pp. 214–237. Cambridge: Cambridge University Press.

Linde, Charlotte

    1987 Explanatory Systems in Oral Life Histories. *In* Cultural Models in Language and Thought. Dorothy Holland and Naomi Quinn, eds. Pp. 343–366. New York: Cambridge University Press.

Lindland, Eric, and Nat Kendall-Taylor

    2011 People, Polar Bears, and the Potato Salad: Mapping the Gap between Expert and Public Thinking about Environmental Health. Washington, DC: FrameWorks Institute.

Mathews, Holly, and Carole E. Hill

    1990 Applying Cognitive Decision Theory to the Study of Regional Patterns of Illness Treatment Choice. American Anthropologist 92(1):155–170.

Mauss, Marcel

    1990 The Gift: The Form and Reason for Exchange in Archaic Societies. W. D. Halls, trans. New York: W. W. Norton.

McCloskey, Michael

    1983 Naïve Theories of Motion. *In* Mental Models. Dedre Gentner and Albert L. Stevens eds. Pp. 299–324. Hillsdale, NJ: Erlbaum.

Ortony, Andrew

    1993 Metaphor and Thought. Cambridge: Cambridge University Press.

Quinn, Naomi

    2005 How to Reconstruct Schemas People Share, From What They Say. *In* Finding Culture in Talk: A Collection of Methods. Naomi Quinn, ed. Pp. 35–81. New York: Palgrave Macmillan.

Quinn, Naomi, and Dorothy Holland

    1987 Culture and Cognition. *In* Cultural Models in Language and Thought. Dorothy Holland and Naomi Quinn, eds. Pp. 3–40. Cambridge: Cambridge University Press.

Rokeach, Milton

    1973 The Nature of Human Values. New York: Free Press.

Sayre, Kenneth M.

    1997 Belief and Knowledge: Mapping the Cognitive Landscape. Lanham, MD: Rowman and Littlefield.

Schank, Roger C.

    1995 Tell Me a Story: Narrative and Intelligence. Evanston, IL: Northwestern University Press.

Schwartz, Shalom H.

    1994 Are There Universal Aspects in the Structure and Content of Human Values? Journal of Social Issues 50(4):19–45.

Sherman, Steven J., Charles M. Judd, and Bernadette Park

    1989 Social Cognition. Annual Review of Psychology 40:281–326.

Shore, Bradd

    1991 Twice-Born, Once Conceived: Meaning Construction and Cultural Cognition. American Anthropologist 93(1):9–27.

    1996 Culture in Mind: Cognition, Culture, and the Problem of Meaning. New York: Oxford University Press.

Simon, Adam F.

    2010a Refining the Options for Advancing Support for Child Mental Health Policies. Washington, DC: FrameWorks Institute.

    2010b An Ounce of Prevention: Experimental Research in Strategic Frame Analysis[TM] to Identify Effective Issue Frames for Public Budgeting and Taxation Systems. Washington, DC: FrameWorks Institute.

Simon, Adam F., and Lynn F. Davey

    2010 College Bound: The Effects of Values Frames on Attitudes Toward Higher Education Reform. Washington, DC: FrameWorks Institute.

Society for Research on Child Development   2009 Healthy Development: A Summit on Young Children's Mental Health—Partnering with Communication Scientists, Collaborating across Disciplines and Leveraging Impact to Promote Children's Mental Health Report. http://www.apa.org/pi/families/summit-report.pdf, accessed November 15, 2011.

Strauss, Anselm L., and Juliet M. Corbin

    1990 Basics of Qualitative Research: Grounded Theory Procedures and Techniques. Newbury Park, CA: Sage.

Strauss, Claudia, and Naomi Quinn

    1997 A Cognitive Theory of Cultural Meaning. Cambridge: Cambridge University Press.

Young, James Clay, and Linda C. Garro

    1994 Medical Choice in a Mexican Village. Prospect Heights, IL: Waveland Press.

EMPATHY AND THE ROBOT:
A NEUROANTHROPOLOGICAL ANALYSIS

KATIE GLASKIN
University of Western Australia

Roboticists developing socially interactive robots seek to design them in such a way that humans will readily anthropomorphize them. For this anthropomorphizing to occur, robots need to display emotion-like responses to elicit empathy from the person, so as to enable social interaction. This article focuses on roboticists' efforts to create emotion-like responses in humanoid robots. In particular, I investigate the extent to which the cultural dimensions of emotion and empathy are factored into these endeavors. Recent research suggests that mirror neurons or other brain structures may have a role to play in empathy and imitation. Notwithstanding this, the effect of sociocultural experience in shaping appropriate empathic responses and expectations is also crucial. More broadly, this article highlights how we are literally anthropomorphizing technology, even as the complexity of technology and the role it plays in our lives grows. Both the actual design process and the understanding of how technology shapes our daily lives are core applied dimensions of this work, from carrying out the research to capturing the critical implications of these technological innovations. [human–robot interaction, empathy, emotion, neuroscience, technology, anthropomorphism]

INTERACTIVE ROBOTS

When Nao is sad, he hunches his shoulders forward and looks down. When he's happy, he raises his arms, angling for a hug. When frightened, Nao cowers, and he stays like that until he is soothed with some gentle strokes on his head.

Nothing out of the ordinary, perhaps, except that Nao is a robot—the world's first that can develop and display emotions. He can form bonds with the people he meets depending on how he is treated. The more he interacts with someone, the more Nao learns a person's moods and the stronger the bonds become. [Jha 2010]

The small humanoid robot called Nao is fully programmable and autonomous. Developed by French company Aldebaran Robotics, Nao was among the humanoid robots on display at the International Robot Exhibition (IREX) held in Tokyo in November 2011. Walking around the exhibition, one could encounter service robots with a variety of different capabilities: a robot that could speak in several languages, more than one robot that could sing, robots that could walk, and a robot that could climb. Some robots could respond to human touch and react accordingly. Robots had motion detection sensors, could recognize human faces using facial recognition software, understand human speech

ANNALS OF ANTHROPOLOGICAL PRACTICE 36, pp. 68–87. ISSN: 2153-957X. © 2012 by the American Anthropological Association. DOI:10.1111/j.2153-9588.2012.01093.x

using voice recognition software, and could learn from their interactions with humans and adjust their behavior. Many of these robots are designed as personal service robots for therapeutic use, or to work with the elderly or the infirm. Many of these robots could and would respond to the humans who stopped in front of them to try to work out what a particular robot did. What distinguished Nao from the other robots on display is that not only could he "show" emotions but he is also able to "develop" them.

In many countries around the world, robotics is big business, and expectations for future growth are high. Although most robotic development worldwide is concentrated on industrial robots, other robots include professional service robots that are able access domains that people cannot, such as in the space industry, in medicine, in mines, in the ocean, and in contexts involving nuclear waste (Bartneck and Forlizzi 2004). The increasing use of robots in warfare has many ethicists concerned (Singer 2009), and a specialized field of robot ethics is emergent (Asaro 2006). Robots initially developed for use in war zones may also be used in other contexts, such as those robots imported from the United States to Japan to assist with the Fukushima disaster.[1] Professional service robots such as these are distinct from service robots designed for domestic and personal use. The latter include robots that can perform domestic chores (such as vacuum cleaning and lawn-mowing robots), and socially interactive robots designed for entertainment, education and leisure. Socially interactive service robots include companion robots, which may be humanoid or in animal form, such as Yume Neko or Yume Hiyoko ("dream cat" and "dream chick," a robotic pet cat and baby chicken, respectively).[2] In terms of developing robots that can express emotion, development is concentrated on social robots and affective computing for personal services.

For those who are unfamiliar with technological developments in this area, the idea of creating emotions or emotion-like responses in robots may seem like science fiction. In these depictions, humanoid robots have often occupied an ambiguous place: on the one hand, they act as man's creation designed to perform certain kinds of labor on man's behalf; on the other hand, if they are able to acquire humanlike attributes, such as emotion and self-awareness, they blur the boundaries between human and machine. The fact that robots develop something that appears as a kind of sentience, in many of these representations, renders them unwieldy and dangerous, a liability to humans. This theme has been explored in iconic movies such as *Blade Runner* (Scott 1982), based on Philip K. Dick's (2004) novel *Do Androids Dream of Electric Sheep,* and *I, Robot* (Proyas 2004), its title drawn from Isaac Asimov's (1950) collection of science fiction stories of the same name.

Those who are less experientially familiar with humanoid robots, with ideas about robots informed primarily by depictions in science fiction, may find the idea uncomfortable that a humanoid robot should have or display emotions. Indeed, when I have presented work in Australia on humanoid robots, I have often encountered this reaction, and part of this is likely to be because of a lack of exposure to robots. This contrasts with the kind of exposure that people have to robotic technology in some other countries, such as Japan. With its enormous number of industrial robots, its scientific investment in humanoid-robot development, and its "robot-themed manga and anime films," Japan is sometimes described as the "Robot Kingdom" (Schodt 2007:98). A significant impetus for Japan's investment in humanoid robot development is its concern about the nation's graying population and associated labor shortfall. In the postwar context Japan pursued automation rather than migration to satisfy its labor requirements and to rebuild its economy. Its robotics industry continues this preference for automation, and, economically, it has been suggested that in this century its robotics industry will be as successful as its car industry was in the last (Robertson 2007:371, 373).

Notwithstanding Japan's significant investment in robot technology, a large amount of work on emotions and robots also occurs in countries outside Japan. These attempts to create artificial emotion stem from a perspective that robots need to display emotion-like responses to elicit empathy from the person to enable social interaction. If, as robot ethicist Ron Arkin (Ulbrick 2008) has argued, "true robot autonomy is the holy grail," with the ultimate goal being "to package all these things in human form," then this aim must be predicated on also creating credible emotional responses in humanoid robots.

ROBOTS AND EMOTIONS

The term *robot* was coined by Josef Capek, Czech playwright Karel Capek's brother, and derives from the term *robota*, meaning forced labor or slave (Nakamura 2007:172; Robertson 2007:373). Robots may be semiautonomous, partially human directed and controlled; or they may be autonomous (Robertson 2007:373). To say that a robot is autonomous, though, is not to say that it operates outside the programming parameters that have been set for it; rather, that it "has considerable control over its sensory inputs and the ability to choose actions based on an adaptive set of criteria rather than too rigidly predesigned a program" (Arbib 2005:371).

Around the world, an extraordinary amount of research and development is currently going on in relation to the creation of emotion-like responses or actual emotions, in robots (e.g., Becker-Asano 2008; Breazeal 2002; el Kaliouby et al. 2006; Fellous and Arbib 2005). This research and development extends beyond humanoid robotic development to other kinds of nonhumanoid robots; to affective computing, defined as "computing that relates to, arises from, or deliberately influences emotions" (Picard 1997:3); and into computer–robot hybrids, such as Reeti le PCBot expressif, a French PCBot that is a mixture of a multimedia computer and a robot that can express feelings.[3] These attempts are motivated by the understanding that for robots to be integrated into everyday human life, their responses to humans need to appear to be natural and intuitive (Breazeal 2002:xii).

One of the aims of human robot interaction research, then, is to identify the necessary characteristics that robots need to display or to have to facilitate sociability, partnership, and "mutual cooperation" with humans (Vidal 2007:918). One of the findings to emerge from these studies has been a positive reassessment of anthropomorphism, the attribution of human qualities to nonhumans, "as the most efficient and most spontaneous register through which humans establish—consciously or not—a strong relationship with artefacts or other nonhuman living beings" (Vidal 2007:919). An important means of facilitating comfortable interaction with robots, then, is to create robots that humans will respond to "as if" they are human. Consequently, the design of socially interactive robots is predicated, to a large extent, on designing robots that humans will readily anthropomorphize, regardless of whether the robots appear in humanoid, animal, or other forms. The physical appearance of the robot, or the way they respond, or both, may contribute to creating the register that allows humans to respond to them as though they are human or as though they have humanlike attributes and responses. This possibly explains why even some of the industrial robots at the IREX exhibition had "faces." These "faces" no doubt augment the human tendency to "attribute emotion to things that clearly do not have emotion" (Breazeal 2002:15; Dubal et al. 2011; Picard 1997:15) by encouraging those working with the machines to see them as in some way humanlike.

Many roboticists developing social robots, robots that are designed to live with and closely interact with humans, focus not just on designing a shape to which humans will respond, although this is an important consideration in humanoid robot design. Nor do they rely only on creating some kind of "face." To specifically facilitate human–robot interaction, they also are designing robots to display emotion, because of the effect this will have on the humans with whom such robots interact. Some working in this field take this further, making an argument for the creation of "emotion" responses in robots, namely, that emotion is central to "basic rational and intelligent behavior" (Picard 1997:2); that emotions are an essential part of intelligence, and contribute vitally to information processing, learning, and memory, functions that Worthman (1999:42) describes as "essential to intelligent being-in-the-world."

In the field of emotions and technology, then, an important distinction is made between the goal of creating "emotion-like responses" and that of inculcating machines with "emotions." As Fellous and Arbib (2005:v) note, those working on the creation of *emotion-like* responses are "content" with creating behavior that, viewed from outside the technology, replicates credible emotional responses, thus facilitating interaction. Much human–robot interaction research is directed toward this end (e.g., Breazeal 2002). Then there are those who wish to create not just the *appearance* of emotions, but "want to parallel, at some level of abstraction," human emotions within machines (Fellous and Arbib 2005:vi). Among the reasons for doing so is that "emotions" within machines (computers or robots) are desirable because of the important role that emotions play in cognition, intelligence, and social interaction (e.g., Picard 1997).

The creation of emotion-like responses and the creation of emotions both present challenges in terms of the cultural aspects of emotions, and most particularly for empathy. By culture, a concept that has been the subject of much anthropological debate (e.g., see Burbank 2011:22), I am referring to patterns of socially learned and shared sociality and experience that, with some variability, significantly shape a person's ontology, that underlie some of their most basic (conscious and unconscious) premises about what it means to be human, and inform how they interact with others. Culture provides premises that, because they are progressively learned from infancy, appear to be "normal" and "natural," simply the way that things "are." Emotional and empathetic expressions are, in that sense, as influenced by culture as is the way that humans around the world sleep (e.g., see Worthman and Melby 2002), which, although a biological imperative, is culturally learned, shaped and experienced.

In designing robots to closely interact with humans, some roboticists are content to create the appearance of an emotion; others consider whether it is possible to create something in machines that is analogous to emotions in humans. Many integrate understandings gleaned from neuroscientific explanations of emotions, combining extremely complex technology with high-end neuroscience in creations that are truly remarkable. In my discussion below, I primarily rely on the written publications of those who are involved in attempts to create emotions or emotion-like responses in both computers and robots. Their interpretations of contemporary neuroscience and psychology in terms of the logical basis required to inculcate emotions in machines forms the focus of the data I present, and can be understood as cultural models of how emotions function that are neurobiologically inspired.[4] This is a vast field, and I have necessarily had to be selective. This article then should be seen as a preliminary discussion of a much larger body of work from a neuroanthropological perspective, one that draws on anthropological and neuroscientific perspectives on emotion and empathy to identify some of the issues that a consideration of culture may have for these attempts. My argument is that if a central goal of creating emotions or emotion-like responses in robots is to enable social interaction, then culture is necessarily implicated.

WIRED FOR EMOTION

Robots that are designed to express emotion are created to elicit an emotional response from the human with whom they interact. Paro, a baby robot seal developed in Japan for therapeutic purposes as a "healing pet," provides a useful initial basis from which to begin to explore the topic of emotion. Paro's designers say that,

> When we engage physically with an animal type robot, it stimulates our affection. Then we have positive emotions such as happiness and love, or negative emotions such as anger and fear. [Shibata et al. 2001:1053]

Three of Paro's attributes are of particular interest for the discussion of virtual emotion: the robot's many sensors that allow it to *interact* with the environment, the ability to *adapt* its behavior as a result of these interactions, and the capacity of the robot to *express* its "feelings" in response to external stimuli.[5] Having interacted with the robot, I know that it will raise its head and close its eyes with apparent "pleasure" when being gently stroked, but will "scream" loudly if someone strokes it too hard. These responses then seem to reflect its "physical" feeling in response to external stimuli. This pattern is significant to how we might think about what an "emotional" response is, and how emotional responses may be elicited from humans by these kinds of interactions.

If we subscribe to neuroscientist Antonio Damasio's distinction between emotions and feelings, we *might* understand these publicly observable expressions made by the robot as a kind of emotional response (rather than as an expression of feelings). Damasio distinguishes between the private, inward nature of feelings, and the public, outward nature of emotions (1999:36); both are "part of a functional continuum" (1999:43). He suggests that "*feeling* should be reserved for the private, mental experience of an emotion, while the term *emotion* should be used to designate the collection of responses, many of which are publicly observable" (Damasio 1999:42). These observable responses include facial expressions and reactions, qualities of breath (such as breathlessness, expulsion of air, sharp intake of breath), qualities of voice, pulse rate, and posture, among others. Feelings are evolved mechanisms enabling responses to environmental challenges; they are connected to preserving homeostasis, keeping equilibrium in the body by providing it with important feedback (Adolphs 2005:14; Damasio 1994). Thus, for Damasio (1999:42), a person perceives their own emotional state when they are conscious of a feeling within themselves; this means that "no-one can observe your own feelings, but some aspects of the emotions that give rise to your feelings will be patently observable to others."

Damasio's distinction between emotions and feelings is widely drawn on by those writing about the emotions in general, and also by those working on the creation of emotions and emotion-like responses in computers and robots (e.g., Picard 1997; Prinz 2004; Becker-Asano 2008). Prinz (2004:6) describes Damasio's theory as a somatic theory of emotion, one that theorizes that changes to *the body* (the respiratory, endocrine, digestive, circulatory, and musculoskeletal systems) constitute an emotion. Change in facial expressions or heart rates are among such somatic changes (Prinz 2004:7). These bodily changes are neurally mapped in specific structures (Adolphs 2005:14). If an emotion involves bodily change, then we know that we feel this emotion through the pattern of arousal in the brain.

Damasio also distinguishes between primary and secondary emotions. He says that "primary" emotions are "universal," and limits these universal emotions to just six: "happiness, sadness, fear, anger, surprise, or disgust" (1999:50). These are the "basic emotions," emotions that are innate and "not derived from other emotions" (Prinz 2004:88). This is the same set of basic emotions that Ekman and colleagues (1969) identified in their early cross-cultural research among the Fore of Papua New Guinea on universal facial expressions; a list that Ekman (1999) has subsequently expanded. In contrast to primary emotions, seen as innate and universal in this view, secondary emotions are "social emotions." Some roboticists working on emotions take up this distinction between "primary" and "secondary" emotions, factoring these distinctions into their design principles. For example, in his doctoral thesis, Christian Becker-Asano (2008:19) says that "for the aim of this thesis only the six basic emotions . . . are important," these being the six emotions Ekman and colleagues (1969) identified as basic emotions corresponding with particular facial expressions.

Becker-Asano is a German android scientist who deals extensively with the topic of emotions. His work has included postdoctoral research in Japan on people's reactions to robots and "virtual agents" (Iolini 2010:2; see also becker-asano.de), and applying affective computing to humanoid robots and androids in Japan, under the guidance of Japanese roboticist Hiroshi Ishiguro.[6] In his doctoral thesis, Becker-Asano (2008:54) says that he derives certain "assumptions" from Damasio's (1994) distinction between primary and secondary emotions.[7] The "assumptions" he draws are these:

> 1. In contrast to primary emotions, the process resulting in secondary emotions starts with conscious, cognitive evaluation. (A)
> 2. The deliberation process uses and modifies aspects of the past (memories, experiences) and the future (expectations). (A)
> 3. Some kind of higher-order, dispositional representation forms the basis of so-called "mental images" which can be pictorial or linguistical [*sic*] (A)
> 4. The past experiences are crystallized in pairings of situations and (primary) emotions. Nonconscious processes work on these experiences to derive appropriate second-order dispositional representations that are needed for secondary emotions. (B)
> 5. The bodily responses (a), (b), and (c) cause an "emotional body state" (Damasio 1994, p. 138) that is subsequently analyzed in the thought process after having been signaled back "to the limbic *and* somatosensory systems." (italics in the original) (C)
> 6. In parallel, the cognitive state itself (i.e. the brain) is directly modulated during the process. (C) [Becker-Asano 2008:54]

Becker-Asano's discussion illustrates that while the attempt to create virtual emotions relies on neuroscientific understandings of what is occurring in the human brain, these understandings need to be relayed as a series of "processing steps" that "are explicit enough for a computational implementation" (Becker-Asano 2008:54). This approach signals an underlying assumption that such processes are capable of being rendered in computational terms. Keeping in mind the idea of primary and secondary emotions, one of the difficulties that occurs in relation to these computational processing steps (as Becker-Asano himself identifies) lies precisely with the creation of "secondary emotions." Drawing on Damasio, Becker-Asano says that these begin with "conscious, cognitive evaluation" that "uses . . . and modifies aspects of the past (memories, experiences) and the future (expectations)"; are informed by "some kind of higher-order, dispositional representation," and that are effected by "nonconscious processes" (2008:54). Implicit in Becker-Asano's approach, then, is a significant question about the cultural aspects of emotion, because this includes nonconscious processes associated with experience, memory, and expectation, all of which have social dimensions.

Earlier I noted that there was a distinction between two approaches to emotions and robots: those who work to create *emotion-like* responses, and those who work to create emotions (or responses that could be considered their equivalent). In his thesis, Becker-Asano (2008) is primarily interested in the problem of creating *emotion-like* responses: his thesis subtitle, "Affect simulation for agents with believable interactivity," is indicative of this commitment.

EMOTION IN THE MACHINE

In contrast, Rosalind Picard (1997) advocates for the creation of emotions (as distinct from "emotion-like responses") in affective computing. Picard (1997:60) acknowledges the significant difficulty involved in answering a question about whether a machine, such as a computer or robot, could really experience emotions, noting that the question of subjective feelings is inevitably linked to a consideration of consciousness. To address this question, Picard identifies five components that she argues must be present within a system to say that it "has" emotions, although she also says that it is not necessarily a precondition that all five components are always operative at any given time to say this (Picard 1997:61). The first of the five components is what she calls "emergent emotions"; emergent here referring to attributions of emotions to robots or machines, given their "observable behavior" (Picard 1997:61). Machines that "express emotions" are likely to have emotions attributed to them. Attempts to create *emotion-like* responses can be seen as building toward this first condition.

The second component is what Picard (1997:62) calls "fast primary emotions," which involve a rapid physiological response to situations that require it, of which fear (related to survival) is a usual exemplar (e.g., Picard 1997:62). Drawing on Damasio, Picard (1997:62) says that the neural mechanisms involved in primary emotions involve two "communicating systems—a rough pattern recognition system [the limbic system] that acts fast, and can 'hijack' the cortex ... and a finer pattern recognition system [the cortical system] that is slower and more precise." Programming computers or robots so that they always display an appropriate behavior following a specific stimulus accords more with creating emotion-like responses than actual emotions; and Picard (1997:63) argues that this response is unlikely to be the way that humans and other animals operate, because even though "the fear response may be innate," the subsequent behavior has other influences that shape it.

Picard's third component is that of "cognitively generated emotions," involving "explicit reasoning" which then activates "limbic responses and bodily feelings" (Picard 1997:63, 64). In computer technology, most "emotions" are generated through cognitive reasoning, in which specific inputs interact with a set of rules to produce emotional states (Picard 1997:64). In computing, the Ortony, Clore, and Collins structure (OCC) is most often used to generate emotions in this manner, allowing the computer to use cognitive reasoning "to deduce that a sequence of events causes an emotion to rise" (Picard 1997:64; and see Becker-Asano 2008:39, 40–46). Although this sounds, at first blush, quite a bit like creating *the appearance* of emotional responses in robots, Picard argues that the OCC structure allows computers to generate emotions using the same cognitive reasoning applied to its personal events (Picard 1997:64). In other words, the relevant inputs here are those things that the computer (or robot) can be said to have "experienced."

Picard's fourth component, "emotional experience," involves cognitive awareness (recognizing and labeling emotional experience), physiological awareness (of that emotion's "physiological accompaniments") and "internal *subjective feeling* or 'gut feeling'" (Picard 1997:65). This accords with Damasio's distinction between emotion and feeling, in which feeling is the inward, subjective experience of an emotion. Needless to say, the latter is the most difficult to produce in a machine. At the time of writing and subsequently, Picard (1997:65; 1999:137) noted that it was not yet possible to "measure and observe" biochemical substances during "emotional arousal," such as to be able to describe the relationship between the physiological and subjective experience in scientific terms. Yet she argues that one of the reasons for this being an important aspect of emotions for machines to have is precisely because it is "through our emotional experience [that] we gain insight into our own motivations and values" (Picard 1997:66).

Picard's final component of emotion is "body–mind interactions," what we do know of how emotion affects "cognitive and bodily functions" and how emotions in turn are impacted by cognitive thoughts and biochemical processes (Picard 1997:67). In computers or robots, equivalent processes would be those that work with processes that emulate "human cognitive and physical functions," including memory, learning, perception, decision making, motivation, concerns, goals, attention, prioritizing, immune system functions, regulatory mechanisms, and the physical ways emotional states are expressed (Picard 1997:70–71, 135). Once humans can effectively duplicate these, then, Picard (1999:137) argues, the machine will have mechanisms that "are essentially emotions."

In terms of the attempts to create emotions or emotion-like responses in robots, then, a number of issues and questions arise. For the robotics question under consideration here, the development of "secondary" or "social" emotions such as shame, guilt, pride, and jealousy—which have been described as "self-conscious emotions" and as "cognition-dependent" (Tracy and Robins 2007:5)—would arguably require the robot to develop a sense of self (Leary 2007). If emotions are socially expressed and regulated, and these social understandings, expressions and expectations are shaped in patterned ways specific to different cultural contexts, then another question concerns how even an emotionally sophisticated and expressive robot could successfully negotiate cross-cultural situations in which different understandings of what we are calling here emotion, and of appropriate emotional responses, might occur.

EMBODIMENT AND DEVELOPMENT

Given the role of socialization in human development, one argument that could be made is that if the social and cultural aspects of emotion are to be successfully factored into the creation of emotional responses in humanoid robots, it would require, at the very least, that robots have learning and developmental capabilities; it would require an embodied and developmental approach. Indeed, such a developmental approach is one that Vernon et al. (2010) take in their "roadmap" to developing cognition in humanoid robots. Robotic learning can be "embodied" in the sense that robots have mechanical "bodies" that can be covered in "skin" that includes "pain sensors" and "algorithms for learning" (Picard 1997:72). Although many robots have some learning algorithms, some robots, such as "CB2" ("child robot with biomimetic body," which is being developed at Osaka University), have very sophisticated learning capabilities. CB2's human creators explicitly intend that the robot's learning would mimic the embodied development of a child, through which it "learns" how to use particular "muscles" to walk and talk. The robot is being taught to "read" and evaluate facial expressions, which it then "clusters . . . into basic categories, such as happiness and sadness," and that it can "memorise" and "match" with "physical sensations" (Suzuki 2009). The further development of "child" robots such as CB2 that "learn" to walk and to speak by emulating the human developmental process may be a step toward the creation of humanoids that "learn" appropriate emotion-like responses within a particular cultural context. Similarly, the robot Nao is said to be learning emotions "using facial and body language recognition," in which "special Nao prototypes will form attachments to those humans that teach them the most. The robots will then pick up on emotional cues and mimic the way they are used" (Saenz 2010). Notwithstanding such astounding achievements, Arbib (2005:344, 374) points out that robots lack "flesh and blood" evolutionary history, the "biological imperatives [that] have shaped the evolution of motivational and emotional systems for biological creatures." For this reason, he questions whether the term "emotion" is therefore suitably applied in relation to such creations.

EMOTIONS CROSS-CULTURALLY

What is absent from these discussions about emotions, whether about the development of something analogous to human emotion or about believable emotional responses, is a consideration of the relationship between emotions and culture. Questions about the extent to which our emotions are biologically wired and the extent to which they are culturally shaped and learned have elicited considerably different responses, partly stemming from the understanding of "emotion" drawn on by those who have sought to answer this (e.g., see Adolphs 2005; Kitayama and Markus 1994; Milton and Svašek 2005; Prinz 2004:131–159; Tracy and Robins 2007). A consideration of the role of empathy in human interaction, and the influence of culture in empathetic interactions, complicates things even further (Hollan and Throop 2008).

The ways in which humans anthropomorphize cross-culturally varies, and is connected to the ways in which humans perceive and impute emotions, intentionality, and sentience. By way of example, I consider here, briefly, the case of Japan where, as mentioned earlier, there is an enormous amount of robotic development. The place of humanoid robots in contemporary Japan clearly arises from a complex interrelationship between aspects of Japanese history and culture. Although it is not possible to explore this fully here, I briefly discuss some factors that can be understood as contributing to the comfort that many Japanese people have with robots.

Historically, the robot in Japan was preceded by *karakuri*, or *karakuri ningyo*, a Japanese term used to describe mechanical or wind-up dolls. The technological connection between *karakuri* and robots in Japan is one that has been explicitly made, with many commentators considering *karakuri*, which flourished during the Tokugawa period (between 1603 and 1868) to have been Japan's first robots, a kind of "prototype" for those proliferating today (Plath 1990:241; Masao 2001:78). Nakamura (2007:172, 173) argues that the performance of the play R.U.R. ("Rossum's Universal Robots") in Japan in 1924 prompted a large shift in the way that the automaton in Japan was conceptualized, and that it was instrumental in bringing about a "robot boom in modern Japan." Nakamura

(2007) describes the enormous interest generated in making robots (*jinzo ningen*, artificial humans) that followed, their depictions in popular *manga* (a kind of illustrated story), and in *anime* (Japanese animations), particularly in the postwar era of the 1950s, when the commercial production of *anime* really took hold. The airing of Tetsuwan Atom in 1963 ("Mighty Atom," known as "Astro Boy" in the West), had an extraordinary impact in Japan, and was the first among many animations about humanoid robots that would subsequently follow. Tezuka Osada first created the character of Atom for manga in 1951, at a time in which, Tezuka said, Japan had "an inferiority complex about science," because "Japan lost the war because of science and technology" (Schodt 2007:98, 99). Schodt (2007:114) argues that in Japan, Mighty Atom came to symbolize advanced technology, in part because of the balance struck between Atom's human qualities and his "artificial intelligence and superhuman abilities."

The connection between Japanese robotics research and manga and anime characters, particularly that of Mighty Atom, does not appear to be incidental (e.g., see Schodt 2007:117). When talking about the place of robots in contemporary Japan, many commentators, and Japanese people themselves, talk about the ways in which robots have been popularized through the mediums of manga and anime. Robotics researcher Eiji Nakano's book, titled *Atomu no ashiato* (*Footsteps of Mighty Atom*) and published in 2003, discussed why it is that humanoid robotic research has the popularity in Japan that it does, suggesting that along with "religious, cultural and historical differences between Japan and the West," there is what he called "the 'Atom Effect'" (Schodt 2007:118). The "Atom Effect," along with a burgeoning robotics industry that reflects Japan's pursuit of a policy of automation rather than migration to meet the country's labor requirements (see Robertson 2007), has undoubtedly made a significant contribution to Japanese perceptions of robots today.

For many Japanese people, too, there is an additional dimension to their comfort with robots. Japanese roboticist Minoru Osada has said that because of animism in Japan, Japanese people have a different attitude toward robots—"everything has a soul therefore a robot has a soul"—and that this makes companion robots easier to accept in Japan (Ulbrick 2008). Shinto, the oldest religion in Japan, is animistic, and understands *kami* (a hidden, "vital" energy), to be present in "all aspects of the world and universe": this includes natural phenomena, but also, "human creations" such as dolls and robots (Robertson 2007:377). The analogy between dolls, humans, and robots is one that the well-known Japanese animation movie *Ghost in the Shell 2: Innocence* (Oshii 2004) explicitly shows, drawing all of them as kinds of animate persons.

The Japanese language distinguishes between animate and inanimate things. The verb *to be*, or *to exist*, has two forms: *imas* [iru] (for animate things) and *arimas* [aru] (for inanimate things). In his discussion concerning early conceptualizations of whether things were considered animate or inanimate among two–three-year-old Japanese- and English-speaking children, psychologist Rakison (2003:295) found that English- and Japanese-speaking children tended to divide things up in much the same way, except when it came to "ambiguous entities that lie near the [animate-object] boundary," in which case Japanese-speaking children were more likely to class these as animate than their

English-speaking counterparts. Thus, this argument is that the distinction in Japanese, concerning the verb *to be*, as applied to animate or inanimate objects, is likely to have an effect on how children think about "things." One of his conclusions is that there is a strong connection between cognition, language, and ontology: that how we are in the world, how we perceive and think about the world, is strongly correlated with the language that we learn to describe it (Rakison 2003:300). Cultural ontologies are strongly embedded in language, and this impacts on cognition and thus on perception. Demography and history provide part of the reason for the proliferation of robots and their acceptance in Japan, as discussed earlier, and are connected to political, economic, and industrial developments, especially in the post-WWII period. In addition, though, it is apparent that the extent to which humans anthropomorphize nonhuman entities have inflections that are cultural as well as historical, and that this will also affect how people might empathize with or attribute emotion to nonhuman things, and hence, impact on their acceptance of them.

Damasio does not hold that all emotions are biologically based: he takes the view that some (the primary emotions) are wholly biological, while others (secondary emotions) have "biologically based parts" (Prinz 2004:134; see also Damasio 1999:50). Prinz (2004:10) describes this approach as a "hybrid theory," one that recognizes the somatic basis of emotion along with conscious experiences ("feelings"). The theory is "hybrid" in that it accommodates aspects of two opposing perspectives on emotions: an evolutionary psychological perspective that sees emotions as evolutionary adaptations that are purely biological, and social or cultural constructionist perspectives that argue that emotions are cognitive appraisals derived from our socialization and enculturation, some of which may have embodied correlates and some of which may not (Prinz 2004:10–14). In this regard, Damasio's distinction between the "primary" and "secondary" emotions reflects aspects of evolutionary and constructionist perspectives.[8]

Although Adolphs (2005:15) argues for the importance of understanding the role of culture in the social emotions (such as shame, guilt, and embarrassment), suggesting that interpretation, categorization and the naming of emotions is culturally varied, he also suggests the likelihood that "emotional states themselves" are "quite invariant across cultures." These emotional states may be "modified" in specific cultural contexts, but he maintains that the primary emotions are part of "a basic, culturally universal emotion set that is sculpted by evolution and implemented in the brain" (Adolphs 2005:15). This reflects a hybrid theory of emotions as described above. Prinz (2004) has advanced a more dialectical view about how culture contributes to the somatic experience of emotion, and I return to this later. What is important to note at this point is how hybrid theories, which pose a distinction between primary and secondary emotions (biologically innate emotions, and those that are "social"), are clearly reflected in approaches taken to the emotions by some roboticists and those involved in affective computing.

For Adolphs (2005:11), creating *emotion-like* responses is a behaviorist approach that, especially if credibly inculcated in a humanoid robot that is otherwise indistinguishable from a human, is destined to "violate" our "background assumptions about the robot," which would create cognitive and emotional confusion for humans who interact with it (something that accords with Mori's 1970 theory of the "uncanny valley"). Background assumptions about a humanoid robot that can "pass" as human include expectations about the emotional and empathic aspects of its interaction. Adolphs identifies a further problem with an approach that equates behavior with emotion. Our behavior and our emotions are linked, he argues, but "only dispositionally," such that any attempt to comprehensively match emotions with particular behaviors in specific circumstances, to program robots accordingly, is unlikely to be successful (Adolphs 2005:12).

It may be that those working on the creation of emotion-like responses in robots or computing programs are content to have these work within particular sets of parameters (that might include a specific cultural context) rather than to try to anticipate all the contingencies as Adolphs has noted. If the goal is to facilitate human–robot interaction, and a limited set of emotion-like responses is sufficient for this within that certain context, then issues such as that of cross-cultural variability in emotion-like responses may not be an issue. Given globalization and commodity reach, however, it would seem likely that ultimately many of the products developed will need to reach across cultural markets.

EMPATHY IN THE MACHINE

Another element of significance to the consideration of the anthropomorphization of robots is the interesting role of empathy in human interaction, and how this might operate in human and humanoid–robot interaction. Notwithstanding some of the extraordinary developments discussed above, just how a robot would come to "learn" the social and cultural dimensions of empathic responses, even if it can be programmed to adjust its behavior "with respect to both its own as well as the interlocutor's emotional state," to be experienced by the human interlocutor as "a more sensible and trustworthy interaction partner" (Becker-Asano et al. 2005), remains a challenging design problem.

Given the significance of empathy in communication, the creation of empathic-like responses is important for those who seek to inculcate machines with believable emotional interactivity, yet it also poses particular challenges. Unlike the "basic" emotions, empathy involves a specifically other-directed focus, one that both involves and transcends one's own "feeling," by feeling "*into* the emotions of others," such that one way of describing empathy is "feeling with/for someone" (Gieser 2008:308). Empathy involves a "subject-subject" relationship, and thus highlights intersubjectivity (Gieser 2008:308, 311). Hollan summarizes empathy as "a first-person-like, *experiential* understanding of another person's perspective"; an understanding that involves cognition and imagination, as well as emotion (2008:475).

Experiments that have used positron emission topography (PET scans) and functional magnetic resonance imaging (fMRI) to observe the effect on the brain of thinking about acting, such as one might experience when one observes someone else executing that action, have shown that there is a significant relationship between how various parts of the brain respond when performing an action and how they respond when observing that action performed (Jeannerod 2005:158). This is relevant to the question of empathy insofar as it suggests that, neurologically speaking, the same mechanisms are involved in experiencing an action or feeling and in understanding what we see when we observe another person doing or experiencing something similar. Recent research on mirror neurons, "those that become activated merely by observing another's actions or behaviors" (Hollan 2008:480), suggest that these have a role to play in empathy and in imitation (Downey 2010; Hrdy 2009:48).

Jeannerod (2005:160) has argued that whether mirror neurons specifically simulate emotion is not specifically supported by existing scientific data, but do reveal that the amygdala is one of the main neural structures involved in recognizing, processing, and appraising emotional stimuli, in "inferring emotion from all relevant cues." On the question of the role of mirror neurons in empathy, Hrdy (2009:52) has argued that "by themselves mirror-neurons could scarcely be sufficient to explain the development of human-caliber empathy, since other primates possess mirror neurons as well." Nevertheless, the important fact remains that we can make a connection between "this incredible, unintentional capacity of the brain to literally 'participate in' or reflect and embody the experience of the other" and "the work of understanding" that we call empathy (Hollan 2008:480). The capacity to put oneself in the position of another relies not just on a shared human biology, but also on experience and imagination; and on how one understands "one's self" vis-à-vis others.

"Systemization" is one method described by el Kaliouby and colleagues (2006:232) for creating empathic responses in computers or robots. Systemization "involves sensing, pattern recognition, learning, inference, generalization, and prediction" (el Kaliouby et al. 2006:231). They note, though, that this approach poses a considerable challenge, because of the complexities and variation in the social world. Given the same situation and context, people's empathic responses may differ, they may rely on nonverbal communication, and they may not really reflect "their true feelings and thoughts" (el Kaliouby et al. 2006 :232).

For those who are interested in creating emotions in robots or computers, the experiential dimension of empathy poses particular difficulty that some acknowledge may be insurmountable. In discussing this challenge, Picard (1997:80) notes that what allows humans insight into the emotional experience of others is that "we have similar brains and bodies," whereas humans and machine have different "physiology," a different "conscious awareness," and hence their "emotional experiences" will not be the same. As a result, even if a machine "has" emotions, "we cannot expect a machine to really *feel* what we feel" (Picard 1997:80). Indeed, in a discussion about attempts to inculcate emotion with a robotics developer at the International Robotics Exhibition in Tokyo, the developer expressed the view that a robot's emotions would be different from human emotions, because of its embodiment. The logical corollary of this perspective is that if the robot had its own emotions, or something that we understand as analogous to an emotion, then it would also come to have its own "feelings," or something that we might consider analogous to feelings.

Should it be possible to create a robot with believable human interactivity that appears to "have" emotions, or that indeed does "have" emotions, what are the implications if in fact it had no empathy?

Like emotions, empathy has social and cultural dimensions that may "inhibit" or "amplify" both the expression and the experience (Hollan 2008:480). The cultural conventions of empathic expression are likely to be dynamic and regionally variable. When is it appropriate to empathize, in what social contexts, how empathy should be expressed, and with whom or what, will necessarily involve different social and cultural expectations and understanding, linked with questions of morality and value. Indeed, researchers have made the case that empathy is integral to moral development, moral thought, and moral behavior (e.g., Eisenberg 2000; Hoffman 1991). Moral values necessarily depend on specific cultural ontologies and epistemologies, as in a Shinto ontology that extends animacy to entities that might not be considered animate in other cultural contexts. In Japan, then, getting humans to feel empathy for robots is likely to prove less difficult than it might in some other contexts. Throop (2008) has identified temporality, intentionality, discernability, and appropriateness as four dimensions that shape empathic processes and that are likely to vary cross-culturally. Among many remote-dwelling Indigenous Australians, for example, close kinship relationships, structural equivalences between siblings, and conceptual equivalences between other relational categories of person means that empathy is a significant factor in interactions and relationships between particular people but not, as necessarily, between others (see Glaskin 2012). When is empathizing with someone inappropriate, because it creates equivalences between your experience and theirs that may not be reciprocally felt? When does a failure to empathize constitute a denial of relationship? What if overt behavior is not where the embodied dimensions of empathy can really be found but, rather, in the health effects of stress created by an empathically shared sense of loss or disempowerment (Burbank 2011)? What if the rules of empathic engagement with others are not the kinds of things that can be easily articulated, let alone codified, depending on many intersecting variables? These are just some of the questions around empathy and culture that arise. These questions return us to more fundamental issues about how culture may literally be "embodied" in our emotions (as well as our feelings).

In Damasio's model of the relationship between primary and secondary emotions, which is drawn on by many robotics developers, secondary emotions are "informed" by such things as memory, perception and experience, all of which have cultural dimensions (Glaskin 2011). Like Prinz (2004), I would argue, too, that the role of culture in emotion is not confined to the so-called "secondary" or social emotions. Prinz (2004:158) argues that while "all emotions are ... neural responses to patterned bodily states," culture influences these patterned body states and hence our experience of the emotion. Culture (and experience) shape the "habits of the body," "blends" basic emotions together and "calibrates" these in response to "sets of eliciting conditions" into specific cultural configurations that in turn influence how our body patterns detect "new classes of exter-nal elicitors" (Prinz 2004:158). In this way, what constitutes a "class" of "external elicitors" will be culturally variable. In arguing this, I do not mean to suggest that I see emotions in purely cognitive or constructionist terms. Rather, along with Prinz (2004:20), I would argue for an approach to emotion that recognizes the embodied dimensions of emotion as a "form of perception" that is "not merely perceptions of the body but also perceptions of our relations to the world." This approach recognizes the somatic nature of emotion and the influence of culture in shaping and elaborating our embodied responses. Given that the oft-stated goal of creating emotion-like responses in robots, or even emotions, is to facilitate social interaction between humans and robots, the contribution that I hope to make in an applied sense is to raise the important issue of the relationship between culture and emotion, and culture and empathy, in social interaction.

The philosopher Gunderson (1968:109) once posed a question: "might we after all be a kind of robot? Or might certain sorts of robots after all be a kind of us?" Endeavors to replicate human attributes such as emotion and empathy in robots continue to raise questions about the boundaries between human and machine, between nature and artifice, and, as we have seen here, about the relationship between biology and culture. Brooks has argued that "we, all of us, overanthropomorphize humans, who are after all, mere machines" (Vidal 2007:917). Haraway offers another perspective: that humans in the late 20th century could already be thought of as cyborgs, "theorized and fabricated hybrids of machine and organism" (1991:149, 151, 152). One of the critical implications of these technological innovations, then, include that even as we literally anthropomorphize technology, we are also interrogating what it means to be human, and investing in a future in which interactions with such technologies may also come to shape how we think about this. Roboticists' reliance on Damasio's distinction between emotion and feeling, and between primary and secondary emotions, means that particular understandings of emotions, and indeed of empathy, are being advanced. In this sense, these robotic endeavors might be understood as "culture producing" in this area of thinking about emotion.[9] A neuroanthropological approach to these issues reminds us that the "social" in human–robot social interaction will inevitably have a cultural component, whether this is explicitly factored into robotic development, or not.

NOTES

1. Japan has an enormous investment in robotic technology, but its postwar constitution prevents it from developing a military, and this has also prevented it from developing robots to use in combat. Following the tsunami in Japan in 2011 and the subsequent crisis at the Fukushima nuclear power plant, robots developed for use in combat zones were used to assist in efforts to bring the situation under control. See McPherson (2011). Unfortunately, the lack of "communications infrastructure, combining wired and wireless capabilities" meant that although these robots were remote-controlled, those controlling them still worked in dangerous proximity to the radioactive and unstable reactors (Guizzo 2011).

2. See Japan Trend Shop n.d.a.

3. See Reeti n.d.

4. I am grateful to an anonymous peer reviewer for this observation.

5. These attributes included that it "has a diurnal rhythm of morning, afternoon, and night"; that it has "five kinds of sensors: tactile, light, audition, temperature, and posture"; "can recognize light and dark"; "can feel being stroked and the amount of pressure"; "understands when it is being held"; "can recognize the direction of sound"; "recognizes its name, greetings, and praise"; "remembers interactions and adapts"; "imitates the voice of a real baby seal," and "expresses feelings through noises, body movements, and facial expressions." See Japan Trend Shop n.d.b.

6. Ishiguro is a well-known Japanese roboticist who famously created a robot that is almost identical to himself, called a geminoid.

7. Although Damasio also talks about "background emotions . . . such as well-being, malaise, calm or tension" (1999:51), Becker-Asano does not refer to these.

8. The view that facial expressions correlate with a basic emotion set, and the idea that there are six basic (innate, universal) emotions has been subject to much debate (e.g., see Kitayama and Markus 1994:7; Prinz 2004:150), with one of the criticisms being that these reflect a Western cultural and linguistic bias that does not adequately capture identifications and experiences of emotion in different cultural contexts.

9. I am indebted to Greg Downey for this observation.

REFERENCES CITED

Adolphs, Ralph
  2005 Could a Robot Have Emotions? Theoretical Perspectives from Social Cognitive Neuroscience. *In* Who Needs Emotions? The Brain Meets the Robot. Jean-Marc Fellous and Michael A. Arbib, eds. Pp. 9–25. Oxford: Oxford University Press.
Arbib, Michael A.
  2005 Beware the Passionate Robot. *In* Who Needs Emotions? The Brain Meets the Robot. Jean-Marc Fellous and Michael A. Arbib, eds. Pp. 333–383. Oxford: Oxford University Press.
Asaro, Peter M.
  2006 What Should We Want From a Robot Ethic? International Review of Information Ethics 6(12):9–16.
Asimov, Isaac
  1950 I, Robot. New York: Gnome.
Bartneck, Christoph, and Jodi Forlizzi
  2004 Shaping Human-Robot Interaction: Understanding the Social Aspects of Intelligent Robotic Products. April. Pp. 1731–1732. Vienna: CHI2004 Extended Abstracts.
Becker-Asano, Christian
  2008 WASABI: Affect Simulation for Agents with Believable Interactivity. Dissertation zur Erlangung des Grades eines Doktors der Naturwissenschaften (Dr. rer. nat.) [Ph.D. dissertation], Universität Bielefeld.
Becker-Asano, Christian, Helmut Prendinger, Mitsuru Ishizuka, and Ipke Wachsmuth
  2005 Empathy for Max. Preliminary Project Report. *In* Proceedings of the 2005 International Conference on Active Media Technology, AMT-05. Pp. 541–545. Piscataway, NJ: IEEE Conference.
Breazeal, Cynthia L.
  2002 Designing Sociable Robots. Cambridge, MA: MIT Press.
Burbank, Victoria K.
  2011 An Ethnography of Stress: The Social Determinants of Health in Aboriginal Australia. New York: Palgrave Macmillan.
Damasio, Antonio R.
  1994 Descartes' Error: Emotion, Reason, and the Human Brain. New York: Putnam.
  1999 The Feeling of What Happens: Body and Emotion in the Making of Consciousness. New York: Harcourt Brace.
Dick, Philip K.
  2004 [1968] Do Androids Dream of Electric Sheep? *In* Five Great Novels. Philip K. Dick. Pp. 351–494. London: Gollancz.

Downey, Greg

2010 Practice Without Theory: A Neuroanthropological Perspective on Embodied Learning. Journal of the Royal Anthropological Institute 16:S22–S40.

Dubal, Stéphanie, Aurélie Foucher, Roland Jouvent, and Jacqueline Nadel

2011 Human Brain Spots Emotion in Non Humanoid Robots. Social Cognitive and Affective Neuroscience 6(1):90–97.

Eisenberg, Nancy

2000 Emotion, Regulation and Moral Development. Annual Review of Psychology 51:665–697.

Ekman, Paul

1999 Basic Emotions. *In* The Handbook of Cognition and Emotion. Tim Dalgleish and Mick J. Power, eds. Pp. 45–60. New York: John Wiley and Sons.

Ekman, Paul, E. Richard Sorenson, and Wallace V. Friesen

1969 Pan-Cultural Elements in Facial Displays of Emotions. Science 164(3875):86–88.

el Kaliouby, Rana, Rosalind Picard, and Simon Baron-Cohen

2006 Affective Computing and Autism. Annals of the New York Academy of Sciences 1093:228–248.

Fellous, Jean-Marc, and Michael A. Arbib, eds.

2005 Who Needs Emotions? The Brain Meets the Robot. Oxford: Oxford University Press.

Gieser, Thorsten

2008 Embodiment, Emotion and Empathy: A Phenomenological Approach to Apprenticeship Learning. Anthropological Theory 8(3):299–318.

Glaskin, Katie

2011 Dreams, Memory and the Ancestors: Creativity, Culture and the Science of Sleep. Journal of the Royal Anthropological Institute 17(1):44–62.

2012 Anatomies of Relatedness: Considering Personhood in Aboriginal Australia. American Anthropologist 114(2):297–308.

Guizzo, Erico

2011 Fukushima Robot Operator Writes Tell-All Blog. IEEE Spectrum. http://spectrum.ieee.org/automaton/robotics/industrial-robots/fukushima-robot-operator-diaries, accessed October 12, 2011.

Gunderson, Keith

1968 Robots, Consciousness, and Programmed Behaviour. British Journal of Philosophical Science 19(2):109–122.

Haraway, Donna J.

1991 Simians, Cyborgs, and Women: The Reinvention of Nature. New York: Routledge.

Hoffman, Martin L.

1991 Empathy, Social Cognition, and Moral Action. *In* Handbook of Moral Behavior and Development, vol. 1: Theory. William M. Kurtines and Jacob L. Gewirtz, eds. Pp. 275–301. Hillsdale, NJ: Erlbaum.

Hollan, Douglas

2008 Being There: On the Imaginative Aspects of Understanding Others and Being Understood. Ethos 36(4):475–489.

Hollan, Douglas, and C. Jason Throop

2008 Whatever Happened to Empathy? Ethos 36(4):385–401.

Hrdy, Sarah Blaffer

2009 Mothers and Others: The Evolutionary Origins of Mutual Understanding. Cambridge, MA: Belknap Press of Harvard University Press.

Iolini, Robert

2010 Post Human. Program transcript 360 Documentaries. Australian Broadcasting Commission, Radio National. October 23. http://www.abc.net.au/radionational/programs/360/post-human/2971136, accessed February 1, 2012.

Japan Trend Shop

N.d.a Dream Cat Venus. Japan Trend Shop. http://www.japantrendshop.com/dream-cat-venus-yume-neko-robotic-cat-p-681.html, accessed October 12, 2011.

N.d.b Paro Robot Seal Healing Pet: World's Most Therapeutic Robot. http://www.japantrendshop.com/paro-robotic-healing-seal-p-144.html, accessed October 12, 2011.

Jeannerod, Marc

2005 How do we Decipher Others' Minds? *In* Who Needs Emotions? The Brain Meets the Robot. Jean-Marc Fellous and Michael A. Arbib, eds. Pp. 147–169. Oxford: Oxford University Press.

Jha, Alok

2010 First Robot Able to Develop and Show Emotions is Unveiled. *Guardian*, August, 9. http://www.guardian.co.uk/technology/2010/aug/09/nao-robot-develop-display-emotions, accessed January 25, 2012.

Kitayama, Shinobu, and Hazel Rose Markus, eds.

1994 Emotion and Culture: Empirical Studies of Mutual Influence. Washington, DC: American Psychological Association.

Leary, Mark R.

2007 How the Self Became Involved in Affective Experience: Three Sources of Self-Reflective Emotions. *In* The Self-Conscious Emotions: Theory and Research. Jessica L. Tracy, Richard W. Robins and June Price Tangney, eds. Pp. 38–52. New York: Guilford.

Masao, Yamaguchi

2001 Karakuri: The Ludic Relationship between Man and Machine in Tokugawa Japan. *In* Japan at Play: The Ludic and Logic of Power. Joy Hendry and Massimo Raveri, eds. Pp. 72–83. New York: Routledge.

McPherson, Stephanie M.

2011 How Battle-Tested Robots are Helping out at Fukushima. Popular Mechanics, April 18. http://www.popularmechanics.com/technology/military/robots/how-battle-tested-robots-are-helping-out-at-fukushima-5586925, accessed October 12, 2011.

Milton, Kay, and Maruška Svašek, eds.

2005 Mixed Emotions: Anthropological Studies of Feeling. Oxford: Berg.

Mori, Masahiro

1970 Bukimi no Tani: The Uncanny Valley. Karl F. MacDorman and Minato Takashi, trans. Energy 7(4):33–35.

Nakamura, Miri

2007 Marking Bodily Differences: Mechanized Bodies in Hirabayashi Hatsunosuke's "Robot" and Early Showa Robot Literature. Japan Forum 19(2):169–190.

Nakano, Eiji

2003 Atomu no Ashi Ato [Footsteps of Mighty Atom]. Tokyo: Suken Shuppansha.

Oshii, Mamoru

2004 Ghost in the Shell 2: Innocence. 100 min. Animation. TM and Go Fish Pictures. Glendale, CA.

Picard, Rosalind W.

1997 Affective Computing. Cambridge, MA: MIT Press.

1999 Response to Sloman's review of Affective Computing. AI Magazine 20(1):134–137.

Plath, David W.

1990 My-Car-Isma: Motorizing the Showa Self. Daedalus 119(3):229–244.

Prinz, Jesse J.

2004 Gut Reactions: A Perceptual Theory of Emotion. Oxford: Oxford University Press.

Proyas, Alex

2004 I, Robot. 115 min. Twentieth Century Fox Film Corporation. Hollywood.

Rakison, David H.

2003 Parts, Motion, and the Development of the Animate-Inanimate Distinction in Infancy. *In* Early Category and Concept Development: Making Sense of the Blooming, Buzzing Confusion. David H. Rakison and Lisa M. Oakes, eds. Pp. 159–192. Oxford: Oxford University Press.

Reeti

N.d. Reeti: An Expressive and Communication Robot! http://reeti.fr/fr, accessed October 2011.

Robertson, Jennifer

2007 Robo Sapiens Japanicus: Posthuman Robots and the Posthuman Family. Critical Asian Studies 39(3):369–398.

Saenz, Aaron

    2010 Nao Robot Develops Emotions, Learns to Interact With Humans. Singularity Hub. http://singularityhub.com/2010/08/17/nao-robot-develops-emotions-learns-how-to-interact-with-humans-video/ accessed February 9, 2012.

Schodt, Frederik L.

    2007 The Astro Boy Essays: Osamu Tezuka, Mighty Atom, and the Manga/Anime Revolution. Berkeley: Stone Bridge Press.

Scott, Ridley

    1982 Blade Runner. 117 min. Warner Brothers Pictures. Hollywood.

Shibata, Takanori, Teruaki Mitsui, Kazuyoshi Wada, Akihiro Touda, Takayuki Kumasaka, Kazumi Tagami and Kazuo Tanie

    2001 Mental Commit Robot and its Application to Therapy of Children. Proceedings of the IEEE/ASME International Conference on Advanced Intelligent Mechatronics, July 8–12, 2001. Como, Italy. Pp. 1053–1058. Piscataway, NJ: IEEE Conference.

Singer, Peter W.

    2009 Wired for War: The Robotics Revolution and Conflict in the 21st Century. New York: Penguin.

Suzuki, Miwa

    2009 Japan Child Robot Mimicks [sic] Infant Learning. Phys.org. http://www.physorg.com/news158151870.html, accessed February 9, 2012.

Throop, C. Jason

    2008 On the Problem of Empathy: The Case of Yap, Federated States of Micronesia. Ethos 36(4):402–426.

Tracy, Jessica L., and Richard W. Robins

    2007 The Self in Self-conscious Emotions: A Cognitive Appraisal Approach. In The Self-Conscious Emotions: Theory and Research. Jessica L. Tracy, Richard W. Robins and June Price Tangney, eds. Pp. 3–20. New York: Guilford.

Ulbrick, Andrea

    2008 Rodney's Robot Revolution. Documentary. 53 min. Essential Media and Entertainment. Sydney.

Vernon, David, Claes von Hoftsen, and Luciano Fadiga

    2010 A Roadmap for Cognitive Development in Humanoid Robots. Cognitive Systems Monographs, vol. 11. Berlin: Springer-Verlag.

Vidal, Denis

    2007 Anthropomorphism or Sub-Anthropomorphism? An Anthropological Approach to Gods and Robots. Journal of the Royal Anthropological Institute 13(4):917–933.

Worthman, Carol

    1999 Emotions: You Can Feel the Difference. In Biocultural Approaches to the Emotions. Alexander Laban Hinton, ed. Pp. 41–74. Cambridge: Cambridge University Press.

Worthman, Carol, and Melissa K. Melby

    2002 Toward a Comparative Developmental Ecology of Human Sleep. In Adolescent Sleep Patterns: Biological, Social, and Psychological Influences, Mary A. Carskadon, ed. Pp. 69–117. New York: Cambridge University Press.

APPLYING NEPALI ETHNOPSYCHOLOGY TO PSYCHOTHERAPY FOR THE TREATMENT OF MENTAL ILLNESS AND PREVENTION OF SUICIDE AMONG BHUTANESE REFUGEES

Brandon A. Kohrt
The George Washington University School of Medicine, Washington, D.C.

Sujen M. Maharjan
Tribhuvan University, Kirtipur, Nepal

Damber Timsina
Grady Memorial Hospital, Atlanta, Georgia

James L. Griffith
The George Washington University School of Medicine, Washington, D.C

Addressing mental health needs of 100,000 ethnic Nepali Bhutanese refugees relocated from Nepal is a new challenge for mental health clinicians in the receiving countries. A limitation of current services is the lack of knowledge about cultural understandings of mental health. Ethnopsychology is the study of emotions, suffering, the self, and social relationships from a cultural perspective. Nepali ethnopsychology can be used to develop and adapt mental health interventions for refugees. We discuss applying ethnopsychology to provide safe and effective mental healthcare for Bhutanese refugees, including cultural adaptation of cognitive behavior therapy, interpersonal therapy, and dialectical behavior therapy. Psychological interventions are proposed for the high rates of suicide among Bhutanese refugees. The contribution of ethnopsychology to applied anthropology and the growing field of neuroanthropology are discussed. [ethnopsychology, Bhutanese refugees, culture, psychotherapy, suicide, somatization, Nepal]

In the late 1980s, the Bhutanese government enacted legislation restricting the civil, political, and economic rights of ethnic Nepali Bhutanese, also known as Lhotshampa (Hutt 2003). They accompanied this legislation with state-sponsored confiscation of land, expulsion from professional and government posts, abduction of activists, and rape of Nepali Bhutanese women. This led to the exodus of Nepali Bhutanese into adjacent India and nearby Nepal. Since the early 1990s, over 100,000 Nepali Bhutanese have been living in refugee camps in southeastern Nepal. After nearly two decades of confinement to refugee camps, the United Nation High Commission on Refugees (UNHCR), the International Organization for Migration (IOM), and myriad resettlement agencies have been relocating Nepali Bhutanese to the United States, Australia, and Western Europe.

ANNALS OF ANTHROPOLOGICAL PRACTICE 36, pp. 88–112. ISSN: 2153-957X. © 2012 by the American Anthropological Association. DOI:10.1111/j.2153-9588.2012.01094.x

Thousands of these refugees have resettled in the United States. Ultimately, over two-thirds of the Nepali Bhutanese refugees will be resettled in the United States (Schininà et al. 2011).

Unfortunately, resettlement, often in impoverished and crime-afflicted areas of the United States and amid a nationwide shortage in employment opportunities, has not been an anodyne for a population that suffered persecution in their home country and a generation living in refugee camps. In the United States, many Nepali Bhutanese have been exploited in high risk employment settings or have been forced to travel long distances for work (Dahal 2011). Lack of healthcare has been a major challenge in the United States. In refugee camps the Bhutanese had medical care provided through UNHCR and IOM. In the United States refugees typically are limited to only a few months of healthcare, and this policy varies by state. Unfortunately, Nepali Bhutanese are being resettled in states in the South and Southeast United States that have the most limited access to healthcare.

Although resettlement is rarely an easy process, the current environment for resettlement in the United States may be exacerbating mental health problems. One of the most concerning health issues has been the rate of suicide among the Nepali Bhutanese in the United States. One estimation of the current rate is 35 in 100,000 (Schininà et al. 2011). This is more than three times the national average in the United States, which is 11 in 100,000 (WHO 2011). The rate is a significant increase from the rate in the refugee camps, which was estimated to be 21 in 100,000 (Schininà et al. 2011). The United States has the highest rate of suicide among countries where Nepali Bhutanese refugees have been resettled according to one estimate: the U.S. rate is almost 30 percent greater than other resettlement countries (Schininà et al. 2011).

Given the high suicide rates and other psychological sequelae of resettlement and trauma, one area of needed intervention is improved mental health services. Although mental health services in isolation will not address the underlying economic, social, and other structural processes that contribute to impaired functioning and health, improving mental health services can foster better coping and adjustment in the face of resettlement problems (Porter 2007; Porter and Haslam 2005). Mental health services can be tailored to promote assertive coping, strengthen social networks, and improve problem solving related to economic and other acculturation stressors (Kira et al. 2012).

The goal of this article is to discuss the application of ethnography with Nepalis to therapeutic work with Nepali Bhutanese refugees using ethnopsychology and neuroanthropology as heuristics for clinical interactions. This article provides a framework to increase awareness among health professionals and resettlement agencies about Nepali Bhutanese experiences and interpretations of distress. We outline Nepali ethnopsychological concepts of the mind, body, and mental illness, which we then apply to psychotherapy. We reflect on how Nepali ethnopsychology can be mapped onto neuroscience models of mental disorders to facilitate both theoretical and applied work. Moreover, we address the issue of suicide and propose approaches for reducing suicide risk. To illustrate therapeutic application, we employ examples from clinical experiences with Nepali Bhutanese patients treated in a refugee mental health clinic in the United States. This information is intended to improve mental health and psychosocial functioning and help augment protective mental health factors to reduce the risk of suicide.

PART ONE: NEUROANTHROPOLOGY AND PSYCHOTHERAPY

Neuroanthropology is a maturing discipline with a mission to examine "the enculturation of the nervous system" (Lende and Downey 2012:56). Researchers interested in neuroanthropology take advantage of the growing field of cultural neuroscience, which uses neuroimaging to examine group and cultural differences in processing of experience (Lende and Downey 2012:64–65). Neuroanthropology provides a framework for transitioning anthropological theory into practice, such as our application of ethnography for mental healthcare. The underlying schema in this endeavor is that culture shapes experience, which shapes neural processes, which in turn produce behaviors that replicate and transform culture (Lende and Downey 2012). Psychotherapy is a microcosm of this process. Relationships and personal experience, shaped by neurobiological attentional and categorizing processes, produce individual differences in reactions to trauma, experiences of distress, and trajectories of recovery (Levine 2010):

> Attachment styles shape how personal narratives are constructed. Social hierarchy selects which stories of one's people are told and retold or ignored. Social exchange guides which interactions in one's life teach moral lessons that are remembered in storied form. Neurobiology opens and closes shutters to the world—opening awareness of one person's pain, closing awareness of another, marking certain scenes or interactions as alarm buttons for entering survival mode. [Griffith 2010:242–243]

Three mechanisms can be distinguished in enculturation from a neuroanthropological perspective: (1) behavioral reaction and reinforcement, (2) language and framing, and (3) defining of in-group versus out-group categories. These processes are most salient in child development. A child's behavior and language are shaped by the reaction and reinforcement behaviors of others in his or her social world (Vygotsky 2006). Language helps frame and label behaviors, groups of people, and types of experiences. Enculturation leads to categorization of in-groups and out-groups based on behavioral patterns, language use, and other group symbols (Cozolino 2010; Goffman 1963).

Psychotherapy operates along these three neuroanthropological domains of enculturation as well (Cozolino 2010). The therapist is trained to react to and reinforce specific behaviors, which will vary based on the therapist's school of practice and training (Sparks et al. 2008). The therapist uses certain language and encourages reflection on language by the client or patient, and shifts in language and interpretation occur alongside changes in framing of experience (Epston et al. 1992; White 2004; White and Denborough 2011). Both shamanic healing and psychotherapy use manipulation of languages and symbols to produce change in emotional states (Dow 1986). The therapist also works with the client or patient to examine group association. People may arrive in therapy because of a lack of felt association with an individual, family, or group (Klerman et al. 1984). Others may define themselves as part of group characterized by a certain emotional or behavioral impairment. The therapist's model of the patient also should change from seeing the client in his or her group role to seeing him or her as a unique individual (Griffith 2010).

The neuroscience of enculturation during child development is echoed by the neuro-processing changes observed during therapy (Cozolino 2010). The frontal lobes, which are involved in planning, inhibition, social regulation, and an array of executive functions, develop over the longest period of time and are the last to reach their mature and functional state. During psychotherapy, the frontal lobes are the main site of change, with increased frontal lobe activity observed during and after cognitive behavior therapy (DeRubeis et al. 2008).

The major components of psychotherapy are (1) hope and expectancy of change, (2) extratherapeutic and contextual factors, (3) therapeutic alliance, and (4) specific psychotherapeutic technique (e.g., cognitive behavior therapy vs. interpersonal therapy; see Miller et al. 1997). Mobilizing hope is a therapeutic process in which the client or patient sees him or herself as having the agency to affect change and the ability to identify pathways for change (Griffith and D'Souza 2012; Snyder et al. 2002). This process draws on the neuroanatomical circuits for motivation and planning, which are influenced by development and enculturation (Cozolino 2010). Contextual factors refer to those processes outside the therapy session ranging from amount of social support to availability of employment (White 2004). The cultural contexts that reinforce or discourage certain frames of self-appraisal are important contextual factors that influence if and how therapy will work. The therapeutic relationship refers to the bond and trust that develop between therapist and client or patient (Winston and Muran 1996). Cultural differences in appraisal of authority, models for self-disclosure, and the shared language between therapist and patient all influence therapeutic relationships (Jordans et al. 2007; Tol et al. 2005). Below, we discuss using ethnography to build ethnopsychological models for psychotherapy grounded in neuroanthropology.

PART TWO: FROM ETHNOGRAPHY TO ETHNOPSYCHOLOGY

Ethnopsychology refers to cultural models of understanding emotions, the self, social connections, perception, and cognition (Bock 1999; Kirmayer 1989; Kohrt and Harper 2008; Kohrt and Maharjan 2009; Shweder and Sullivan 1993; Westermeyer 1976; White 1992). Historically, Western culture's ethnopsychology has been characterized by a split between mind and body, often referred to as Cartesian duality (Scheper-Hughes and Lock 1987), as well as an associated split between thoughts–rationality and feelings–emotions (Damasio 1994). Another division is between the soul and the body, which was instantiated in Christian religious doctrine (Lindland 2005). Individualism is a hallmark of Western ethnopsychology, with the assumption that individuals are separable from their familial and social relationships (Carrithers et al. 1985; Markus and Kitayama 1991). These cultural beliefs are reflected in aspects of Western healing systems such as the division of physical and mental health, therapies that focus on emotions and cognitions as separable phenomena, and individualized approaches to mental health care (Kleinman 1988). However, neuroscience and psychology research are modifying Western ethnopsychology into a system that challenges many of the earlier divisions of emotion versus rationality, the body versus the mind, and the self versus the collective (Damasio 1994, 1999, 2003).

An overly simplistic division of Western from non-Western ethnopsychology holds that while dualism characterizes the former, holism is the trademark of the latter (Scheper-Hughes and Lock 1987). However, when non-Western ethnopsychologies have been studied by anthropologists and psychologists, this does not bear out (Fox 2003; Keys et al. 2012; Kohrt and Harper 2008; Kohrt et al. 2004). In reality, there is tremendous heterogeneity in ethnopsychologies, and some aspects considered hallmarks of Western ethnopsychology are common in other cultures. For example, mind–body divisions have been observed from West Africa to the Indian subcontinent (Desjarlais 1992; Fox 2003). Gendered frameworks of emotions are present from Pacific islands to Himalayan mountains (Lutz 1988; McHugh 1989, 2004). Other aspects of ethnopsychology, such as the role of the spirit or soul, are important in both Western psychotherapy (Griffith 2010; Griffith and Griffith 2002) and in other cultural healing practices (Desjarlais 1992; Wikan 1989).

In Nepal and among the Nepali diaspora, including Nepali Bhutanese, it would be misleading to claim that there is a single ethnopsychology. Nepal is home to greater than 40 ethnic groups and 100 languages (Bhattachan 2008). This diversity also is represented within Nepali Bhutanese. That said, through our ethnographic work, we have been able to cull core components of the self that should be incorporated into mental health treatment for Nepali Bhutanese refugees ranging from Sanskrit-language speakers to Tibeto-Burman language speakers. Both Sanskrit languages and Tibeto-Burman languages have terms referring to heart–mind, brain–mind, and souls (Desjarlais 1992; McHugh 1989, 2001). Thus, for the purposes of this article, we will refer to "Nepali ethnopsychology" while being cognizant that this is an oversimplified heuristic to function as an entry point into mental health dialogues, which can then allow for further exploration and nuance related to one's linguistic, religious, educational, and geographic background.

In Nepal, over a decade of ethnography was used to develop an ethnopsychological model that captures Nepali ways of understanding the self and emotions (Kohrt and Harper 2008). Our ethnographic work included participant-observation with traditional healers, biomedical mental health professionals, and psychosocial NGO workers. The types of complaints, ways of framing illness and healing, and myriad practices for restoration of well-being were documented. This work revealed the importance of bodily complaints in expression of distress, as well as the realization that both physical pathology and psychological distress contribute to the somatic presentation of suffering (Kohrt and Schreiber 1999; Kohrt et al. 2005, 2007). Ethnography of the biomedical clinical encounter revealed commonalities with traditional healing in regard to self and emotion terminology. These commonalities helped establish a foundation for understanding a generalized ethnopsychological model (Kohrt and Harper 2008). The next phase of research was an examination of psychological trauma, which was addressed not only with traditional healers and psychiatrists but also with NGOs that viewed suffering through the lens of human rights violations (Kohrt and Hruschka 2010; Kohrt and Maharjan

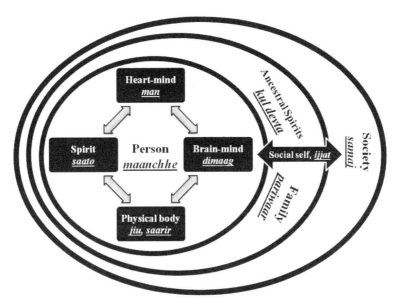

FIGURE 1. Nepali ethnopsychological model of the self.

2009). These ethnographic experiences, taken together, are integral to understanding the experience and narrative surrounding ethnic Nepali Bhutanese refugees' interpretation of mental health services. Since the arrival of Bhutanese refugees in the United States, further observations have evolved out of clinical endeavors with recently relocated individuals and families.

Nepali ethnopsychology, not dissimilar to Western ethnopsychology, includes multiple divisions of the self (see Figure 1). The main components are the physical body (Nepali: *jiu* or *saarir*), the heart–mind (*man*), the brain–mind (*dimaag*), the spirit (*saato*), the soul (*atma*), and one's social status (*ijjat*) (Kohrt and Harper 2008; Kohrt and Hruschka 2010). Other important divisions are the family (*pariwaar*), which includes the extended family, and the spiritual world, especially connections with one's ancestral deities (*kul devta*). For mental health treatment, the heart–mind and brain–mind are crucial topics. The heart–mind is the locus of memory and emotions. When one desires something, it is felt in his or her heart–mind. A bad or good memory arises from the heart–mind. Traumatic or intrusive memories often are identified as wounds or sores on the heart mind (*manko gaau*). Worries and anxiety are located in the heart–mind (e.g., *manmaa kura khelne* [thoughts playing in the heart–mind]). The heart–mind is what makes every person unique through their personal desires and wishes. In contrast, the brain–mind is the organ of cognition, attention, and social regulation. The brain–mind, when working correctly, will monitor thoughts and desires from the heart–mind, then inhibit socially inappropriate desires or actions. When someone acts in a socially inappropriate manner, such as when drunk, he or she is considered to have problems in the brain–mind. Someone who does not follow appropriate gender or caste norms is considered to have brain–mind problems. In some context, a woman who is not subservient to a man may be accused of having a brain–mind problem. Violence and uncontrolled anger are also problems of the brain–mind. Lastly, psychosis and severe mental illness are brain–mind problems that are highly feared and stigmatized.

Not surprisingly, social implications of heart–mind and brain–mind problems vary considerably. Heart–mind problems are considered commonplace. Individuals often will share openly about "thoughts playing in the heart–mind" or "worries in the heart–mind." However, to discuss a brain–mind problem invokes a heavy social stigma. Because of the social unpredictability of brain–mind problems, people with these symptoms and behavior are shunned. Many who have brain–mind problems are imprisoned within their homes and have severely constrained social lives. A family in which one person has a brain–mind problem will find that other family members have difficulty with arranged marriages. Having a family member with a brain–mind problem also can lead to job loss, exclusion from cooperative work or investment activity, or rejection from public festivals. Moreover, some brain–mind problems, such as psychosis, are considered communicable by sharing a cup or a plate.

Based on our experience working within Nepal and with Nepali Bhutanese patients in the United States, there is an important liminal state at the intersection of heart–mind and brain–mind problems. Although heart–mind problems are socially acceptable, there is also a concern that a prolonged intense heart–mind problem eventually can lead to a brain–mind problem. Child soldiers, in a multiday workshop in which they gradually developed rapport with facilitators, eventually disclosed that they were concerned that they may be going crazy (*paagal*) and that their brain–mind was going "out" (*dimaag out bhayo*) because of chronic heart–mind problems (Karki et al. 2009; Kohrt et al. 2010). Nepali Bhutanese patients similarly stated that they thought their brain–minds were becoming impaired and could no longer socially regulate the emotions and desires in their heart–minds. Love and lust are powerful emotions in the heart–mind that need to be controlled through the brain–mind. Overwhelming love is thought to make one irrational and thus impair his or her brain–mind making him or her do "crazy" things. Lust must be controlled by the brain–mind to prevent engaging in socially inappropriate acts. There is a traditional healing practice in Nepal conducted by shamans (*dhami-jhankri*) in which the heart–mind is ritualistically bound (*man baadne*) to calm its desires and intense emotions, ranging from jealousy to sadness to love, so that the brain–mind is not overpowered and socially acceptable behavior can be maintained (Kohrt in press).

The other parts of the self and society are associated with the heart–mind and brain–mind. The *ijjat* or social self is maintained by appropriate functioning of the brain–mind. If the brain–mind is not operating properly one suffers *bejjat* (loss of *ijjat*, or social status), which is associated with social marginalization and in extreme cases "social death." Historically, certain socially inappropriate acts, especially those where caste or gender norms were violated, resulted in social death in the form of banishment from a village or town (Höfer 2004). Because of the importance of the social unit, *bejjat* (loss of status) also is experienced by family members of the person with a brain–mind problem.

The *saato* is the spirit. It is a supernatural part of oneself connected to the supernatural world of ancestors and spirits of places and animals. In most Nepali ethnopsychologies, people are thought to have multiple spirits. The *saato* is crucial for vitality and physical health. When one becomes frightened or possibly cursed, the spirit may be lost (*saato jaane*, spirit goes) (Desjarlais 1992; McHugh 2001). As in many cultures with the concept of "soul loss," the loss of spirit leads to vulnerability to other supernatural and physical maladies (Rubel et al. 1984; Simons 1985; Wikan 1989). A child who has lost his or her spirit may then develop a life threatening diarrheal disease, respiratory infection, or fever. Although adults do not lose their *saato* as easily as children do, they also become vulnerable to disease and generalized weakness when the *saato* is gone. Losing one's spirit has important mental health implications. A trauma or sudden fright, which intensely activates the heart–mind, can dislodge the *saato* resulting in its loss. Therefore, after a traumatic or frightening event, individuals are vulnerable to physical maladies and may be overcome with generalized weakness. Healing by *dhami-jhankri* shamans is used in these instances to call the *saato* back to restore health and vitality. The *atma*, often translated as soul, has some overlap with *saato*. *Atma* is referred to by persons who have learned to read Sanskrit religious text and is thus an aspect of the self more salient to religious scholars.

The physical body (*jiu, saarir*) is the site of physical suffering and pain. For physical problems, individuals may seek home remedies, the care of a *dhami-jhankri* shaman, or go to a health clinic. When the physical body is sick or in pain, this leads to worries in the heart–mind. It is not unexpected to have worries in the heart–mind translate into bodily pain, headaches, stomach upset (*gyastrik*), and numbness and tingling sensations (*jham-jham*; see Kohrt et al. 2005; Kohrt et al. 2007). Within the physical body, the *dimaag* is located in the head. The location of the *heart–mind* may be in the region of the chest. However, interpretations of its location vary. The *saato* and *atma* do not have specific locations in the body.

A study of suicide and ethnopsychology among Bhutanese refugees found that 55 percent of family members of suicide completers felt that the suicide victim had problems in the brain–mind, 25 percent felt that the suicide victim had problems in the heart–mind, and 10 percent felt the suicide victim had *ijjat* problems (Schininà et al. 2011). These family perceptions focusing on behavioral control (brain–mind problems) more than sadness and depression (heart–mind problems) parallel epidemiological data about suicide studies in Asia (Hendin et al. 2008). In China and India, suicide shows only a weak association with depression and other mood disorders (Hendin et al. 2008). Mood disorders are especially rare among women in South Asia who have attempted suicide (Maselko and Patel 2008; Zhang et al. 2010). The disorders commonly associated with suicide in Asia and in low-income countries in general are impulse control disorders (Nock et al. 2008), which would be considered *dimaag* or brain–mind dysfunctions in ethnopsychological terms. In contrast, in the United States three-fifths of suicides are associated with mood disorders (Nock et al. 2010), which would be heart–mind problems.

Nepali ethnopsychology overlaps with neuroscience partitions of functioning. In mental disorders ranging from posttraumatic stress disorder (PTSD) to depression, there is increasing emphasis on the division between the prefrontal cortex and the limbic system, especially the amygdala (Canli 2005; Kemp et al. 2007; Ressler and Nemeroff

2000). In both depression and PTSD, the amygdala may have increased activity (Bryant et al. 2008; Siegle et al. 2007). Conversely, the prefrontal cortex is considered hypoactive (Goldapple et al. 2004; Putnam and McSweeney 2008). The interaction of the prefrontal cortex and the amygdala parallel the ethnopsychological divisions of the *dimaag* and the *man*. The heart–mind is the locus of fear similar to the amygdala. The prefrontal cortex is the center of planning and social appropriate behavior comparable to the brain–mind. In the famous case of Phineaus Gage, it was damage to the prefrontal cortex that led to impaired social behavior and recklessness (Damasio 1994). In Nepali ethnopsychological terms, Gage undoubtedly would have been suffering from a brain–mind dysfunction. Mental health workers providing care for Bhutanese refugees could choose to include a psychoeducation component that gives credence to a neurological basis for the brain–mind and heart–mind division. This may be fruitful for some patients, but more work is required to determine if a biomedical interpretation of Nepali ethnopsychology would impact patient–doctor alliances or treatment adherence behavior. Instead, we feel that a key application of ethnopsychology is for psychotherapy.

PART THREE: PSYCHOTHERAPY FOR NEPALI AND BHUTANESE PATIENTS

Nepali ethnopsychology can be applied to psychotherapies such as cognitive behavior therapy, interpersonal therapy, and dialectical behavior therapy. One indispensible element with any of these approaches is that an effective therapist also acts as an ethnographer. Taking on the role of Other, rather than seeing the patient or client as Other, leads to elicitation of individual ethnopsychologies, rather than imposing biomedical models: "From a position as Other, a clinician can ask questions that might never be addressed to a patient from within his or her world. These questions can be asked with authenticity, concern, and respect, but their unique value lies in their otherness" (Griffith 2010:251).

Cognitive Behavior Therapy

Aaron T. Beck developed cognitive behavior therapy (CBT) as an approach to treat depression, which he conceptualized as a disorder in *thinking* that resulted in the negative *feelings* associated with depression (Beck et al. 1979; Rush et al. 1977). CBT is based on the model that activating events lead to behaviors that result in negative consequences (Beck 2011; Trinidad et al. 2011). The activating events trigger automatic thoughts that lead to the specific behavioral responses. In CBT, automatic thoughts are one of three types of cognitions, the others being conditional beliefs and underlying schemas. Treatment is based on short-term weekly therapy combined with homework to build insight for associations among thoughts, feelings, and behavior. CBT has been tested in numerous randomized control trials for multiple types of mental illness (DeRubeis et al. 2008; Harvey et al. 2003; Mehta et al. 2011). CBT consistently outperforms treatment as usual, and CBT has performed equally well to psychiatric medication in some trials (DeRubeis et al. 2008).

Kamal is a middle-aged Nepali Bhutanese refugee man who was brought to a mental health clinic in the United States because of intractable seizures.[1] Kamal had seizures since his late teens first starting around the time of his marriage then again in his mid-twenties when his mother had a stroke. Despite treatment with numerous antiepileptic medications in refugee camps, these seizures did not abate. However, they did improve with the amount of time elapsed from major life events: his marriage and his mother's stroke. In the United States, Kamal's seizure frequency increased again. He was prescribed myriad antiepileptic medications without improvement. The pattern of Kamal's seizures raised concerns for conversion disorder, a type of mental disorder in which an individual will display neurological symptoms, but in which no neurological etiology can be identified (Couprie et al. 1995). Pseudoseizures, a common manifestation of conversion disorder, are observable in most populations around the world from high income to low income settings (Bowman and Markand 1996; Guinness 1992).

CBT is a possible treatment for pseudoseizures. In CBT, the first goal would be to highlight the connection among automatic thoughts, feelings, and the seizure behaviors. For example, Kamal's seizures often were precipitated by major life changes. Kamal revealed that he thought his mother had her stroke because he did not properly care for her and because he had not become a *pujari* (priest) like his father.

Kamal revealed that not living with his parents in the United States was another sign of his failure as a son. Kamal is the eldest son in his family. Kamal lived with his parents in the refugee camp in Nepal. Often, it is the expectation that the eldest son will look after his elderly parents. However, when the family was resettled not all of the sons were relocated in the same region of the United States, and the elderly parents were resettled with Kamal's younger brother in a different state from Kamal. Kamal was worried that problems would befall his parents in the United States, and he would not be able to fulfill his responsibility as the eldest son, which entailed caring for their well-being. The thoughts of being a failure as a son typically preceded his seizures. For example, Kamal had one seizure when his father called and said that there was no longer health insurance to pay for his mother's blood pressure medication. Pseudoseizures are often associated with unspoken dilemmas within families (Griffith et al. 1998).

An essential element of CBT is psychoeducation. Psychoeducation for CBT, as well as other forms of psychotherapy can be explained in terms of Nepali ethnopsychology to facilitate understanding (see Table 1). For Kamal and his family, the explanatory model for Kamal's seizures was that he had a brain–mind problem that was manifest as epilepsy. Epilepsy typically is considered a brain–mind disease in Nepal and is treated by psychiatrists. This was the starting point for ethnopsychological grounding of CBT. Kamal was asked to identify what could affect the brain–mind. He pointed out that alcohol affects the brain–mind, not getting enough sleep affects the brain–mind, and too many thoughts in his heart–mind affect his brain–mind. Kamal identified worries of being separated from his parents as a major anxiety in his heart–mind that affected his brain–mind.

Eventually, Kamal discovered that his automatic thought, which preceded seizures, was "I am the main person responsible for taking care of my parents. If anything bad happens to them and they do not get help, it will be my fault." His conditional belief was "as long as I am sick with epilepsy, it is not my responsibility to take care of my parents. If I am sick, then someone else needs to take care of them." When these

TABLE 1. Components of Nepali ethnopsychology in therapy modalities

Ethno-psychology Component	Description	Cognitive Behavior Therapy (CBT)	Interpersonal Therapy (IPT)	Dialectical Behavior Therapy (DBT)
Heart-mind (*man*)	Organ of emotions, memories, and desires	'Feelings' in CBT should reference heart-mind processes	Heart-mind processes are examined in the context of social relationships; IPT grief theme relates to the heart-mind	Radical acceptance and change framed in heart-mind and brain-mind conflicts
Brain-mind (*dimaag*)	Organ of social responsibility and behavioral control	'Thoughts' and 'appraisals' in CBT should reference brain-mind processes	Behavioral control through the brain-mind is examined in the context of social relationships	Brain-mind and heart-mind conflicts are reduced; the brain-mind is responsible for regulating "opposite actions" and "response prevention"
Physical body (*jiu, saarir*)	Physical sense organ, topography of pain	Somatic complaints in CBT may be consequence of heart-mind and brain-mind processes	The connection between physical suffering and relationships is explored through the social world, heart-mind, and physical body	"Opposite actions" and "response prevention" are used to prevent self-injury to the body
Spirit (*saato*)	Vitality, energy, immunity to illness	Lost vitality in CBT can be associated with strong emotions in heart-mind (anger, fear)	Loss of vitality can be tied to difficulties in interpersonal relationships with both family and ancestral spirits	Preventing soul loss (*saato jaane*) is addressed through reducing intensity of emotions in heart-mind
Social status (*ijjat*)	Personal and family social standing and respect	Social status can be maintained through better insight into thoughts and feelings in CBT	Social status is explored by considering network of relationships; interpersonal deficits related to perceived social status can be challenged	Distress from perceived social status loss (*bejjat*) is managed through heart-mind emotional acceptance
Family and community relationships	Social support and social burden	The brain-mind processes related to relationships are explored for their effect on heart-mind processes	IPT themes of interpersonal disputes and role transitions examine social relationships	The group therapy component of DBT is used to discuss and model appropriate social relationships

issues were discovered, Kamal examined the ways that he could help his parents even if they were resettled in another state. He also recognized that it was not his fault that his parents were separated from him in the resettlement process. The treatment goal moving forward was to help Kamal reduce the worry in his heart–mind arising from perceived powerless to help his parents. In therapy, Kamal examined the evidence regarding his power to help his parents while they lived with his brother. Kamal identified one solution: to help his mother identify affordable generic medications, which he could send her money to buy. The family, patient, and therapist worked to create an atmosphere in which Kamal's pseudoseizures could improve by examining the damaging worries in his heart–mind that led to dysfunction of his brain–mind. This treatment goal was framed as minimizing worries in the heart–mind by changing thoughts and behaviors related to his perceived powerlessness, which then reduced brain–mind distress that caused pseudoseizures.

In neuroimaging studies of CBT, increased prefrontal cortical activity and decreased amygdala activity have been observed (DeRubeis et al. 2008). Depending on the academic background of the patient or the investment in biomedical explanatory models, a mental health worker could add that CBT treatment is associated with improved brain–mind activity (i.e., the prefrontal cortex) and decreased heart–mind activity (i.e., the amygdala). Interestingly, this resembles the traditional practice of *man baadne*, heart–mind binding, in *dhami-jhankri* shamanic treatments in Nepal (Kohrt in press).

In some cases, reality testing may not be therapeutic because of real threats to well-being. For many Nepali and Nepali Bhutanese female clients, triggering events are related to interpersonal interactions with their husbands. For example, a triggering event may be giving birth to a girl instead of a boy. The *automatic thought* would be "my husband is going to get a second wife" or "my husband is going to abandon me." This automatic thought leads to feelings of panic, distress, fear, and hopelessness. The *conditional belief* that underlies this automatic thought is "If I do not produce a son, my husband will leave me," or, "I am not a real woman until I have been given birth to a son." These conditional beliefs may be grounded in variants of universal schemas such as "I am helpless" or "I am unlovable." Unfortunately, the issue of abandonment may be a real threat. Therefore in these cases, alternative therapies such as Interpersonal Therapy may be more appropriate.

Interpersonal Therapy

Interpersonal Therapy (IPT) evolved from the work of Harry Stack Sullivan who emphasized the importance of culture in psychiatry and the need to address interpersonal, and not just intrapsychic, phenomenon (Klerman et al. 1984). For Harry Stack Sullivan, the contexts in which relationships form, evolve, and deteriorate were crucial to determine the appropriate treatment. IPT was established as a short-term psychotherapy by Gerald Klerman and colleagues (1984). IPT often occurs over approximately 16 weekly sessions. Regarding cross-cultural applicability, group IPT has shown efficacy in the reduction of depression symptoms among women in Uganda (Bolton et al. 2003, 2007; Verdeli et al. 2003, 2008). IPT produces changes in the limbic system, specifically in the limbic right posterior cingulate and right basal ganglia activation (Martin et al. 2001).

The first trimester of treatment is devoted to the diagnostic assessment and review of current social functioning. Sessions in this section include (1) dealing with depression, giving the syndrome a name, and giving the patient the "sick role," (2) relating depression to interpersonal context, (3) identifying major problem areas, and (4) explaining the IPT concepts and contract (Klerman et al. 1984). In Nepali, the syndrome being treated by IPT can best be described as *manosamajik samasya* (Kohrt and Harper 2008). This term is used by many NGOs working with trauma survivors and refugees in Nepal. The common translation is "psychosocial problem." The literal translation is "heart-mind—society problem." *Manosamajik* highlights the problem neither as intrapsychic nor as exclusively external to the self. Rather, the root of distress is at the intersection of one's heart–mind and the experience of social interactions. This captures the ethos of IPT. Therefore, although one could use the psychiatric term *depression*, we feel that framing treatment around *manosamajik samasya* better captures the framing and treatment within IPT. This framing also avoids the stigmatization of a brain–mind problem (Kohrt and Harper 2008). Once the person's problem has been defined as *manosamajik samasya*, then the treatment plan will highlight both goals for modifying one's social relations and for changes in one's emotional appraisal of those relations.

In the first trimester of IPT, the concept of "sick role" is introduced (Klerman et al. 1984). When one treats their psychological distress as a disease, he or she is more likely to take time to recover, modify his or her current behavior to achieve recovery, and prioritize medical care such as psychotherapy or psychopharmacology. Moreover, identifying psychological distress as an illness shifts attention from explanatory models that attribute the distress to personal weakness or inadequacy. We still are struggling with how best to address this with Nepali and Nepali Bhutanese patients. One option is to tell someone that they have a *maanasik rog* (mental sickness). However, this has the potential to greatly stigmatize a patient (Kohrt and Harper 2008). The term *mental illness* is viewed as psychotic or schizophrenic in Nepali ethnopsychology. Concepts such as depression and anxiety are framed differently from psychotic mental illness. Instead of using the label *maanasik rog*, we advocate for emphasizing the goals of the "sick role" framing (e.g., greater investment in self-care, reduction in self-blame, and adherence to treatment) without labeling someone as mentally ill. This is an area that will require greater exploration.

The second trimester of treatment identifies the main problem areas: (1) grief, (2) interpersonal disputes, (3) role transitions, or (4) interpersonal deficits (Klerman et al. 1984). Among refugees, interpersonal disputes and role transitions are common sources of distress (Miller et al. 2002; Porter 2007; Weine et al. 2004). Gender roles may be altered as a woman gets a job and her husband remains at home (Westermeyer et al. 1984). Age-based stratification of roles is inverted as children become parentified because of their greater aptitude with English (Ajdukovic and Ajdukovic 1993). It is not uncommon for a teenage boy or girl to be attending school, working nights and weekends for the family income, and then driving and translating for healthcare and social service visits for their parents. This can lead to interpersonal disputes when parents and children conflict about disciplinary action and behavior expectation. In the final trimester, therapeutic goals are consolidated. IPT has shown comparable efficacy to medication in the treatment of major depression (de Mello et al. 2005; Fournier et al. 2009).

Phulmaya is an elderly woman who presented with problems sleeping, poor concentration, low mood, inability to enjoy activities, feelings of guilt, and pain in her abdomen and scalp. She met criteria for major depressive disorder. Phulmaya is from a low caste Hindu group known as Dalit and historically referred to as "untouchable." In Nepal, Dalit groups have significantly greater levels of depression and anxiety compared to high caste groups (Kohrt 2009; Kohrt et al. 2009). After multiple sessions, Phulmaya revealed that her heart–mind problems of negative feelings, her brain–mind problems of poor concentration, and her physical pain all began when her adult children, with whom she lives, converted to Christianity. Her adult children told her that she could longer practice Hindu *puja* (prayer) in the home and she had to dismantle her small prayer shrine with pictures of Hindu deities. Phulmaya became increasingly distressed about the family's *karma* and the consequences that the Christian conversion would have on suffering in this life and the next for her and her family. She was worried that misfortune would befall her and her children. Phulmaya was referred to us because of her depressed mood as well as visualizations of demons when she was going to sleep. Phulmaya explained that it was acceptable for her that her children converted, but that she still wanted to be able to perform *puja* to pray for them.

Within an IPT framework, the first phase of treatment was to develop a shared therapist and patient understanding of the problem. The ethnopsychological approach to IPT emphasized the connection between the distress in Phulmaya's heart–mind and her social life, that is, her family relationships, which together resulted in a *manosamajik samasya*. Phulmaya framed her distress as occurring at that intersection of her feelings and her relationship with her adult children. Phulmaya then traced her symptoms progression to being forced to remove her *puja* shrine. Once this framing was established, it opened an opportunity to employ components of IPT to address the interpersonal difficulties. Phulmaya developed strategies for negotiating with family regarding continuing to perform *puja*. Because of Phulmaya's self-perceived powerlessness in the household, the plan involved enlisting others in the community to communicate the psychosocial issues with her family. Church members were enlisted to speak with the therapist about the impact of the *puja* prohibition on the Phulmaya's health. In a meeting facilitated by the therapist, the church members explained to Phulmaya's adult children that conversion to Christianity was a choice and not forced on everyone in the household. The church members explained to Phulmaya's adult children that they could pray for Phulmaya. Similarly, Phulmaya could perform *puja* for her adult children and grandchildren. This allowed each party to engage in the practice that was meaningful for them and allowed them to express their concerns for other family members in a religiously consonant fashion. Moreover, using IPT, Phulmaya focused on her role in the relationships with her adult children. Although improving assertiveness was limited because of the expectations of hierarchy in the household, Phulmaya and the therapist discussed strategies for disclosing what was in her heart–mind. Ultimately, by focusing on Phulmaya's relationship, rather than individual pathology, we were able to work in collaboration to reduce inter- and intrapersonal dimensions of distress.

Dialectal Behavior Therapy

A third type of manualized psychotherapy that has been tested with randomized control trials is dialectal behavior therapy (DBT; Kliem et al. 2010; Linehan et al. 2006; McMain et al. 2009; Soler et al. 2005). DBT was developed by Marsha Linehan to work with individuals who engage in self-injurious and suicidal behavior (Linehan 1987). Given the high rate of suicide among Nepalis and Nepali Bhutanese, DBT is an important therapy to consider for these patients. Although we have not directly applied DBT to a Nepali patient at this time, we will review the basic tenets and make suggestions for how Nepali ethnopsychology could be employed, especially in relation to reducing the risk of suicide. Moreover, DBT is ideal for persons with borderline personality disorder (Lynch et al. 2007), which often overlaps significantly with complex posttraumatic stress disorder (PTSD; Eichelman 2010; Southwick et al. 2003).

The goal of DBT is "the reduction of ineffective action tendencies linked with dysregulated emotions" (Lynch et al. 2006:459). The targets are to reduce suicidal behavior, behaviors that interfere with treatment delivery, and other dangerous or destabilizing behaviors (Linehan et al. 2006). DBT does this by improving five functions: increasing behavioral capabilities, improving motivation for skillful behavior, assuring generalization of gains to the natural environment, structuring the treatment environment to reinforce functional behavior, and enhancing therapist capabilities. DBT is intended to be delivered via weekly individual psychotherapy, weekly group sessions, occasional skill trainings, telephone consultations on an "as needed" basis, and weekly therapist team meetings.

DBT was designed with elements of Buddhist and Hindu philosophy such as mindfulness and the connection between radical acceptance and change (Lynch et al. 2006). In DBT, patients are supported as they employ mindfulness to improve their awareness about their own emotional tenor and its association with interpersonal experiences. In radical acceptance, behaviors and feelings are not given a valence of "good" or "bad" but, rather, are to be seen as "just is." Moreover, after developing increased awareness of one's emotional and bodily states, patients are taught to engage in "opposite actions" or "response prevention." A key emotion–behavior cycle to break in DBT is the experience of shame and concomitant shameful behavior such as hiding, withdrawing, or disappearing, of which suicide can be the extreme example.

Within Nepali ethnopsychology, mindfulness is built on the concept of meditation and attentiveness. *Dyan garne* refers to meditation and *dyan dine* refers to giving one's attention, focusing, or concentrating. *Dyan dine* is a brain–mind function, whereas *dyan garne* involves the brain–mind but with the ultimate goal of facilitating peace in the heart–mind. Patients can be supported in efforts to attend to their inner states to help facilitate affect stability. DBT also relies on divisions among perception, affect, and behaviors with the goal of separating these so that a person does not see self-harm as an inevitable consequence of negative feelings (Lynch et al. 2006). DBT works to increase awareness about one's sensations and emotions so that individuals are better able to see associations among the body, the heart–mind, the brain–mind, and the social self. Ultimately, DBT holds promise as an important intervention that can be adapted within Nepali ethnopsychology and can be used to reduce suicide risk.

PART FOUR: CAN ETHNOPSYCHOLOGY USEFULLY INFORM MENTAL HEALTH INTERVENTIONS IN OTHER POPULATIONS?

In Nepali culture, an ethnopsychological perspective has effectively aligned clinical concepts and actions of Western psychotherapies with Nepali understandings of self and emotions so that their therapeutic benefits can be realized with a reduction in stigma.

One can consider whether this approach may be generalizable to other refugee populations with similar benefits.

A fortuitous goodness of fit could appear to exist in Nepali culture between a neuroscience model of regulation of amygdala emotion-processing by the prefrontal cortex and Nepali regulation of heart–mind emotion processing by the brain–mind. In most cultures, however, some form of cognition (e.g., brain-mind) generates pathways toward goals and regulates emotions (e.g., heart-mind; see Damasio 1994; Fox 2003; Keys et al. 2012). Mental health thus requires balance and coordination between brain-mind and heart-mind, and disruptions in this balance result in mental illnesses (c.f. Clifford 1990; Kohrt et al. 2004). As in Nepali culture, stigma often travels most closely with disruptions owing to brain-mind problems because of their greater risk for damaging family relationships and social structures. Perhaps life is so sorrow-laden that a wounded heart is easy to normalize in most cultures.

To the extent that such a regulatory model can be perceived within the ethnopsychology of a culture, a Western model of psychotherapy may be refitted within the categories of the culture. This suggests that an ethnopsychological refitting of a Western psychotherapy should assess the following:

1 How is cognitive regulation of emotion processing formulated within the psychological categories of the local culture?
2 In what ways can dysregulation generate suffering that threatens the individual?
3 In what ways can dysregulation disrupt the functioning of families and extended kin (clan) relationships?
4 In what ways can dysregulation disrupt the function of relationships with the numinous or spirit world?
5 Which of the above forms of disruption are most stigmatized?

This inquiry can be used to guide reformulation of Western psychotherapy concepts and interventions within categories of the local culture. It also can give guidance for what type of psychotherapy might best fit the greater concerns of the culture and whether to prioritize cognitive, emotional, or relational interventions to best reduce stigma.

Decades of psychotherapy outcome research have established that most of the effectiveness of any specific psychotherapy depends on its capabilities for activating the "common factors" of psychotherapy—making good use of a patient's unique strengths and competencies, mobilizing hope and expectancy of change, and facilitating a robust therapeutic alliance (Frank and Frank 1991; Miller et al. 1997). An ethnopsychological approach holds promise for maximizing these common factors by rendering psychotherapy sensible and usable within the assumptive world and categories of meaning of a local culture.

There are examples where ethnopsychology effectively has been incorporated into psychotherapy for other refugee groups. Hinton and colleagues have detailed various ways that conceptions of the self and conceptions of the body vary across cultures (Hinton and Hinton 2002; Hinton and Otto 2006). Although we have used the term *ethnopsychology* throughout this article, Hinton and colleagues refer to ethnophysiology as the cultural model of how the body works including experience and regulation of distress (Hinton and Hinton 2002). Hinton and colleagues have developed versions of CBT that draw on ethnophysiologies of Cambodian refugees (Hinton and Otto 2006), Vietnamese refugees (Hinton et al. 2006), and Latinas (Hinton et al. 2011). These culturally adapted therapies emphasize the somatic-looping of how the body is experienced, the meanings attributed to sensations, and the cycle of distress exacerbating both somatic sensations and emotional distress (Hinton and Hinton 2002). Culturally adapted CBT is an ideal therapy to interrupt these cycles of distress (Hinton et al. 2009, 2012). In Haiti, we have found that ethnopsychological differences in interpretation among biomedical health workers, Vodou *hougan*-s (priests), and laypersons leads to avoidance of biomedical practitioners because of their perceived failure to present a coherent ethnopsychological explanation and treatment for mental illness (Keys et al. 2012; Khoury et al. 2012). Ethnopsychology, thus, can be a key element in developing culturally appropriate and compelling psychological treatments.

CONCLUSION

Neuroanthropology provides a framework for considering the cocreation of experience and neural pathways of perception, processing, and behavior (Lende and Downey 2012). The process of enculturation studied in neuroanthropology is recapitulated in the therapeutic process. One product of culture is ethnopsychology—the cultural framing of the self, emotions, and suffering. Ethnopsychology is the outcome of as well as the progenitor of perception, language, and behavior. Understanding ethnopsychology can help achieve therapeutic goals of promotion of hope and expectancy of change. Moreover, using ethnopsychology can aid adaptation of specific schools of psychotherapy, such as CBT, IPT, and DBT. Ethnopsychology can complement other types of adaptation of psychotherapy for Bhutanese, such as adaptations that focus on augmenting community resources and social networks (Kira et al. 2012).

There is a dearth of mental health care in Nepal (Regmi et al. 2004) and among the Nepali diaspora including ethnic Nepali Bhutanese refugees. Despite misconceptions that so-called non-Western psychologies are characterized by holism, Nepali ethnopsychology involves complex divisions of the self. Nepali ethnopsychological terms fit well with the growing body of neuroscience literature on mental illness. The heart–mind and brain–mind divisions capture the division between the amygdala's and the prefrontal cortex's roles in psychopathology. Furthermore, drawing on Nepali ethnopsychology will prevent unnecessary stigmatization through use of inappropriate terms for mental disorders (Kohrt and Harper 2008; Kohrt and Hruschka 2010). Nepali ethnopsychology is compatible with three of the major evidence-based psychotherapies: CBT, IPT, and DBT. DBT may be a key in addressing the epidemic of suicide among Bhutanese refugees.

The goal of using neuroanthropology and ethnopsychology is not simply to be a "culturally competent" therapist or researcher for a specific group. Griffith cautions, "A person is not a person if known only as a category" (Griffith 2010:251). Rather these are tools to be used so that identity categories, such as "refugee" or "Bhutanese," are no longer the defining feature of the individual. Ultimately, these conceptual frameworks are means to establish a conversation not between cultures but among human beings.

NOTE

Acknowledgments. Research in Nepal was supported by an NIMH Pre-Doctoral National Research Service Award (F31 MH075584) and a Wenner-Gren Dissertation Research Grant. Thanks to Liana Chase, Daniel Lende, and Greg Downey for their comments on this manuscript. Thanks to Ian Harper for original discussions that led to the Nepali ethnopsychology framework. Special thanks to Michael Saenger for his clinical dedication to the Bhutanese community. Portions of this article were presented for the John Spiegel Fellowship at the Society for the Study of Psychiatry and Culture, June 2011, Seattle, Washington.

1. All names of patients are pseudonyms. Cases represent amalgamations of different patients, narratives, and treatment regimens to protect anonymity.

REFERENCES CITED

Ajdukovic, M., and D. Ajdukovic
    1993 Psychological Well-Being of Refugee Children. Child Abuse and Neglect 17(6):843–854.
Beck, Aaron T., A. John Rush, Brian F. Shaw, and Gary Emery
    1979 Cognitive Therapy of Depression. New York: Guilford.
Beck, Judith
    2011 Cognitive Behavior Therapy: Basics and Beyond. New York: Guilford.
Bhattachan, Krishna B
    2008 Indigenous Peoples and Minorities of Nepal. Nepal Indigenous Federation of Minorities Peoples (NEFIN). http://www.nefin.org.np/hppics/42562_MRG-Nepal-Final%20Report%20by%20Bhattachan.doc, accessed November 9, 2011.
Bock, Philip K.
    1999 Rethinking Psychological Anthropology: Continuity and Change in the Study of Human Action. Prospect Heights, IL: Waveland Press.
Bolton, Paul, Judith Bass, Theresa Betancourt, Liesbeth Speelman, Grace Onyango, Kathleen F. Clougherty, Richard Neugebauer, Laura Murray, and Helen Verdeli
    2007 Interventions for Depression Symptoms Among Adolescent Survivors of War and Displacement in Northern Uganda: A Randomized Controlled Trial. JAMA 298(5):519–527.
Bolton, Paul, Judith Bass, Richard Neugebauer, Helen Verdeli, Kathleen F. Clougherty, Priya Wickramaratne, Liesbeth Speelman, Lincoln Ndogoni, and Myrna Weissman
    2003 Group Interpersonal Psychotherapy for Depression in Rural Uganda: A Randomized Controlled Trial. JAMA 289(23):3117–3124.
Bowman, E. S., and O. N. Markand
    1996 Psychodynamics and Psychiatric Diagnoses of Pseudoseizure Subjects. American Journal of Psychiatry 153(1):57–63.
Bryant, Richard A., Andrew H. Kemp, Kim L. Felmingham, Belinda Liddell, Gloria Olivieri, Anthony Peduto, Evian G., and Leanne M. Williams
    2008 Enhanced Amygdala and Medial Prefrontal Activation During Nonconscious Processing of Fear in Posttraumatic Stress Disorder: An fMRI Study. Human Brain Mapping 29(5):517–523.
Canli, Turhan
    2005 Amygdala Reactivity to Emotional Faces Predicts Improvement in Major Depression. Neuroreport 16:1267–1270.
Carrithers, Michael, Steven Collins, and Steven Lukes
    1985 The Category of the Person: Anthropology, Philosophy, History. New York: Cambridge University Press.

Clifford, Terry

1990 Tibetan Buddhist Medicine and Psychiatry. York Beach, Maine: Samuel Weiser, Inc.

Couprie, W., E. F. M. Wijdicks, H. G. M. Rooijmans, and J. Vangijn

1995 Outcome in Conversion Disorder—Acx Follow-up-Study. Journal of Neurology, Neurosurgery and Psychiatry 58(6):750–752.

Cozolino, Louis

2010 The Neuroscience of Psychotherapy: Healing the Social Brain. New York: W. W. Norton.

Dahal, Kamal

2011 Funeral Rites of Deceased Over; One Injured Still Reported to be Critical. Bhutan News Service. March 25. http://www.bhutannewsservice.com/main-news/funeral-rites-of-deceased-completes-one-injured-still-under-critical-condition/, accessed February 1, 2012.

Damasio, Antonio R.

1994 Descartes' Error: Emotion, Reason, and the Human Brain. New York: G. P. Putnam.

1999 The Feeling of What Happens: Body and Emotion in the Making of Consciousness. New York: Harcourt Brace.

2003 Looking for Spinoza: Joy, Sorrow, and the Feeling Brain. Orlando, Fla.: Harcourt.

de Mello, Marcelo Feijo, Jair de Jesus Mari, Josue Bacaltchuk, Helen Verdeli, and Richard Neugebauer

2005 A Systematic Review of Research Findings on the Efficacy of Interpersonal Therapy for Depressive Disorders. European Archives of Psychiatry and Clinical Neuroscience 255(2):75–82.

DeRubeis, Robert J., Greg J. Siegle, and Steven D. Hollon

2008 Cognitive Therapy versus Medication for Depression: Treatment Outcomes and Neural Mechanisms. Nature Reviews Neuroscience 9(10):788–796.

Desjarlais, Robert R.

1992 Body and Emotion: The Aesthetics of Illness and Healing in the Nepal Himalayas. Philadelphia: University of Pennsylvania Press.

Dow, J.

1986 Universal Aspects of Symbolic Healing—A Theoretical Synthesis. American Anthropologist 88(1): 56–69.

Eichelman, Burr

2010 Borderline Personality Disorder, PTSD, and Suicide. American Journal of Psychiatry 167(10):1152–1154.

Epston, David, Michael White, and Kevin Murray

1992 A Proposal for a Re-Authoring Therapy: Rose's Revisioning of Her Life and a Commentary. In Therapy as Social Construction. S. McNamee and K. J. Gergen, eds. Pp. 96–115. Thousand Oaks, CA: Sage.

Fournier, Jay C., Robert J. DeRubeis, Richard C. Shelton, Steven D. Hollon, Jay D. Amsterdam, and Robert Gallop

2009 Prediction of Response to Medication and Cognitive Therapy in the Treatment of Moderate to Severe Depression. Journal of Consulting and Clinical Psychology 77(4):775–787.

Fox, Steven H.

2003 The Mandinka Nosological System in the Context of Post-Trauma Syndromes. Transcultural Psychiatry 40(4):488–506.

Frank, Jerome D., and Julia B. Frank

1991 Persuasion and Healing: A Comparative Study of Psychotherapy. Baltimore: Johns Hopkins Press.

Goffman, Erving

1963 Stigma: Notes on the Management of Spoiled Identity. Englewood Cliffs, NJ: Prentice-Hall.

Goldapple, Kimberly, Zindel Segal, Carol Garson, Mark Lau, Peter Bieling, Sidney Kennedy, and Helen Mayberg

2004 Modulation of Cortical-Limbic Pathways in Major Depression: Treatment-specific Effects of Cognitive Behavior Therapy. Archives of General Psychiatry 61(1):34–41.

Griffith, James L.

2010 Religion that Heals, Religion that Harms: A Guide for Clinical Practice. New York: Guilford.

Griffith, James L., and Anjali D'Souza

2012 Demoralization and Hope in Clinical Psychiatry and Psychotherapy. *In* The Psychotherapy of Hope: The Legacy of Persuasion and Healing. R. D. Alarcon and J. B. Frank, eds. Pp. 158–177. Baltimore: Johns Hopkins University Press.

Griffith, James L., and Melissa Elliott Griffith

2002 Encountering the Sacred in Psychotherapy: How to Talk with People about Their Spiritual Lives. New York: Guilford.

Griffith, James L., Alexis Polles, and Melissa E. Griffith

1998 Pseudoseizures, Families, and Unspeakable Dilemmas. Psychosomatics: Journal of Consultation Liaison Psychiatry 39(2):144–153.

Guinness, E. A.

1992 Relationship between the Neuroses and Brief Reactive Psychosis: Descriptive Case Studies in Africa. British Journal of Psychiatry—Supplement 16:12–23.

Harvey, Allison G., Richard A. Bryant, and Nicholas Tarrier

2003 Cognitive Behaviour Therapy for Posttraumatic Stress Disorder. Clinical Psychology Review 23(3): 501–522.

Hendin, Herbert, Michael R. Phillips, Lakshmi Vijayakumar, Jane Pirkis, Hong Wang, Paul Yip, Danuta Wasserman, Jose Bertolote, and Alexandra Fleischmann, eds.

2008 Suicide and Suicide Prevention in Asia. Geneva: Department of Mental Health and Substance Abuse, WHO.

Hinton, Devon, and Susan Hinton

2002 Panic Disorder, Somatization, and the New Cross-Cultural Psychiatry: The Seven Bodies of a Medical Anthropology of Panic. Culture, Medicine and Psychiatry 26(2):155–178.

Hinton, Devon E., Stefan G. Hofmann, Mark H. Pollack, and Michael W. Otto

2009 Mechanisms of Efficacy of CBT for Cambodian Refugees with PTSD: Improvement in Emotion Regulation and Orthostatic Blood Pressure Response. CNS Neuroscience and Therapeutics 15(3): 255–263.

Hinton, Devon E., Stefan G. Hofmann, Edwin I. Rivera, Michael W. Otto, and Michael H. Pollack

2011 Culturally Adapted CBT (CA-CBT) for Latino Women with Treatment-resistant PTSD: A Pilot Study Comparing CA-CBT to Applied Muscle Relaxation. Behaviour Research and Therapy 49(4):275–280.

Hinton, Devon E., and Mark W. Otto

2006 Symptom Presentation and Symptom Meaning among Traumatized Cambodian Refugees: Relevance to a Somatically focused Cognitive-Behavior Therapy. Cognitive and Behavioral Practice 13(4): 249–260.

Hinton, Devon E., Edwin I. Rivera, Stefan G. Hofmann, David H. Barlow, and Michael W. Otto

2012 Adapting CBT for Traumatized Refugees and Ethnic Minority Patients: Examples from Culturally Adapted CBT (CA-CBT). Transcultural Psychiatry 49(2):340–365.

Hinton, Devon E., Steven A. Safren, Mark H. Pollack, and Minh Tran

2006 Cognitive-Behavior Therapy for Vietnamese Refugees with PTSD and Comorbid Panic Attacks. Cognitive and Behavioral Practice 13(4):271–281.

Höfer, András

2004 The Caste Hierarchy and the State in Nepal: A Study of the Muluki Ain of 1854. Lalitpur: Himal.

Hutt, Michael

2003 Unbecoming Citizens: Culture, Nationhood, and the Flight of Refugees from Bhutan. New Delhi: Oxford University Press.

Jordans, Mark J., Annalise S. Keen, Hima Pradhan, and Wietse A. Tol

2007 Psychosocial Counselling in Nepal: Perspectives of Counsellors and Beneficiaries. International Journal for the Advancement of Counselling 29(1):57–68.

Karki, Rohit, Brandon A. Kohrt, and Mark J. D. Jordans

2009 Child Led Indicators: Pilot Testing a Child Participation Tool for Psychosocial Support Programmes for Former Child Soldiers in Nepal. Intervention: International Journal of Mental Health, Psychosocial Work and Counselling in Areas of Armed Conflict 7(2):92–109.

Kemp, Andrew H., Kim Felmingham, Pritha Das, Gerard Hughes, Anthony S. Peduto, Richard A. Bryant, and Leanne M. Williams
  2007 Influence of Comorbid Depression on Fear in Posttraumatic Stress Disorder: An fMRI Study. Psychiatry Research 155(3):265–269.
Keys, Hunter M., Bonnie N. Kaiser, Brandon A. Kohrt, Nayla M. Khoury, and Aimee-Rika T. Brewster
  2012 Idioms of Distress, Ethnopsychology, and the Clinical Encounter in Haiti's Central Plateau. Social Science and Medicine 75(3):555–564.
Khoury, Nayla M., Bonnie N. Kaiser, Hunter M. Keys, Aimee-Rika T. Brewster, and Brandon A. Kohrt
  2012 Explanatory Models and Mental Health Treatment: Is Vodou an Obstacle to Psychiatric Treatment in Rural Haiti? Culture, Medicine and Psychiatry 36(3):514–534.
Kira, Ibrahim A., Asha Ahmed, Fatima Wasim, Vanessa Mahmoud, Joanna Colrain, and Dhan Rai
  2012 Group Therapy for Refugees and Torture Survivors: Treatment Model Innovations. International Journal of Group Psychotherapy 62(1):69–88.
Kirmayer, Laurence J.
  1989 Cultural Variations in the Response to Psychiatric Disorders and Emotional Distress. Social Science and Medicine 29(3):327–339.
Kleinman, Arthur
  1988 Rethinking Psychiatry: From Cultural Category to Personal Experience. New York: Free Press–Collier Macmillan.
Klerman, Gerald L., Myrna M. Weissman, Bruce J. Rounsaville, and Eve S. Chevron
  1984 Interpersonal Psychotherapy of Depression. New York: Basic.
Kliem, Soren, Christoph Kroger, and Joachim Kosfelder
  2010 Dialectical Behavior Therapy for Borderline Personality Disorder: A Meta-Analysis Using Mixed-Effects Modeling. Journal of Consulting and Clinical Psychology 78(6):936–951.
Kohrt, Brandon A.
  2009 Vulnerable Social Groups in Post-Conflict Settings: A Mixed-Methods Policy Analysis and Epidemiology Study of Caste and Psychological Morbidity in Nepal. Intervention: International Journal of Mental Health, Psychosocial Work and Counselling in Areas of Armed Conflict 7(3):239–264.
  In press The Role of Traditional Rituals for Reintegration and Psychosocial Wellbeing of Child Soldiers in Nepal. In Legacies of Mass Violence. Alex L. Hinton and Devon E. Hinton, eds. Durham, NC: Duke University Press.
Kohrt, Brandon A., and Ian Harper
  2008 Navigating Diagnoses: Understanding Mind-Body Relations, Mental Health, and Stigma in Nepal. Culture, Medicine and Psychiatry 32(4):462–491.
Kohrt, Brandon A., and Daniel J. Hruschka
  2010 Nepali Concepts of Psychological Trauma: The Role of Idioms of Distress, Ethnopsychology and Ethnophysiology in Alleviating Suffering and Preventing Stigma. Culture, Medicine and Psychiatry 34(2):322–352.
Kohrt, Brandon A., Daniel J. Hruschka, Holbrook E. Kohrt, Nova L. Panebianco, and G. Tsagaankhuu
  2004 Distribution of Distress in Post-Socialist Mongolia: A Cultural Epidemiology of Yadargaa. Social Science and Medicine 58(3):471–485.
Kohrt, Brandon A., Mark J. D. Jordans, and Chrisopher A. Morley
  2010 Four Principles of Mental Health Research and Psychosocial Intervention for Child Soldiers: Lessons Learned in Nepal. International Psychiatry 7(3):58–60.
Kohrt, Brandon A., Richard D. Kunz, Jennifer L. Baldwin, Naba R. Koirala, Vidya D. Sharma, and Mahendra K. Nepal
  2005 "Somatization" and "Comorbidity": A Study of Jhum-Jhum and Depression in Rural Nepal. Ethos 33(1):125–147.
Kohrt, Brandon A., and Sujen M. Maharjan
  2009 When a Child Is No Longer a Child: Nepali Ethnopsychology of Child Development and Violence. Studies in Nepali History and Society 14(1):107–142.

Kohrt, Brandon A., and Steven S. Schreiber

    1999 Jhum-Jhum: Neuropsychiatric Symptoms in a Nepali Village. Lancet 353(9158):1070.

Kohrt, Brandon A., Rebecca A. Speckman, Richard D. Kunz, Jennifer L. Baldwin, Nawaraj Upadhaya, Nanda Raj Acharya, Vidya Dev Sharma, Mahendra K. Nepal, and Carol M. Worthman

    2009 Culture in Psychiatric Epidemiology: Using Ethnography and Multiple Mediator Models to Assess the Relationship of Caste with Depression and Anxiety in Nepal. Annals of Human Biology 36(3): 261–280.

Kohrt, Brandon A., Wietse A. Tol, and Ian Harper

    2007 Reconsidering Somatic Presentation in Nepal. Journal of Nervous and Mental Disease 195(6):544.

Lende, Daniel H., and Greg Downey, eds.

    2012 The Encultured Brain: An Introduction to Neuroanthropology. Cambridge, MA: MIT Press.

Levine, Peter A.

    2010 In an Unspoken Voice: How the Body Releases Trauma and Restores Goodness. Berkeley, California: North Atlantic.

Lindland, Eric H.

    2005 Crossroads of Culture: Religion, Therapy, and Personhood in Northern Malawi. Atlanta: Emory University.

Linehan, Marsha M.

    1987 Dialectical Behavior Therapy for Borderline Personality Disorder. Theory and Method. Bulletin of the Menninger Clinic 51(3):261–276.

Linehan, Marsha M., Katherine Anne Comtois, Angela M. Murray, Milton Z. Brown, Robert J. Gallop, Heidi L. Heard, Kathryn E. Korslund, Darren A. Tutek, Sarah K. Reynolds, and Noam Lindenboim

    2006 Two-Year Randomized Controlled Trial and Follow-Up of Dialectical Behavior Therapy vs Therapy by Experts for Suicidal Behaviors and Borderline Personality disorder. [Erratum appears in Arch Gen Psychiatry. 2007 Dec;64(12):1401]. Archives of General Psychiatry 63(7):757–766.

Lutz, Catherine

    1988 Unnatural Emotions: Everyday Sentiments on a Micronesian Atoll and Their Challenge to Western theory. Chicago: University of Chicago Press.

Lynch, Thomas R., Alexander L. Chapman, M. Zachary Rosenthal, Janice R. Kuo, and Marsha M. Linehan

    2006 Mechanisms of Change in Dialectical Behavior Therapy: Theoretical and Empirical Observations. Journal of Clinical Psychology 62(4):459–480.

Lynch, Thomas R., William T. Trost, Nicholas Salsman, and Marsha M. Linehan

    2007 Dialectical Behavior Therapy for Borderline Personality Disorder. Annual Review of Clinical Psychology 3:181–205.

Markus, Hazel R., and Shinobu Kitayama

    1991 Culture and the Self—Implications for Cognition, Emotion, and Motivation. Psychological Review 98(2):224–253.

Martin, Stephen D., Elizabeth Martin, Santoch S. Rai, Mark A. Richardson, and Robert Royall

    2001 Brain Blood Flow Changes in Depressed Patients Treated with Interpersonal Psychotherapy or Venlafaxine Hydrochloride: Preliminary Findings. Archives of General Psychiatry 58(7):641–648.

Maselko, Joanna, and Vikram Patel

    2008 Why Women Attempt Suicide: The Role of Mental Illness and Social Disadvantage in a Community Cohort Study in India. Journal of Epidemiology and Community Health 62(9):817–822.

McHugh, Ernestine L.

    1989 Concepts of the Person among the Gurungs of Nepal. American Ethnologist 16(1):75–86.

    2001 Love and Honor in the Himalayas: Coming to Know Another Culture. Philadelphia: University of Pennsylvania Press.

    2004 Moral Choices and Global Desires: Feminine Identity in a Transnational Realm. Ethos 32(4):575–597.

McMain, Shelley F., Paul S. Links, William H. Gnam, Tim Guimond, Robert J. Cardish, Lorne Korman, and David L. Streiner

2009 A Randomized Trial of Dialectical Behavior Therapy versus General Psychiatric Management for Borderline Personality Disorder. [Erratum appears in American Journal of Psychiatry (2010) 167(10):1283]. American Journal of Psychiatry 166(12):1365–1374.

Mehta, Swati, Steven Orenczuk, Kevin T. Hansen, Jo-Anne L. Aubut, Sander L. Hitzig, Matthew Legassic, Robert W. Teasell, and Team Spinal Cord Injury Rehabilitation Evidence Research Team.
2011 An Evidence-Based Review of the Effectiveness of Cognitive Behavioral Therapy for Psychosocial Issues Post-Spinal Cord Injury. Rehabilitation Psychology 56(1):15–25.

Miller, Kenneth E., Gregory J. Worthington, Jasmina Muzurovic, Susannah Tipping, and Allison Goldman
2002 Bosnian Refugees and the Stressors of Exile: A Narrative Study. American Journal of Orthopsychiatry 72(3):341–354.

Miller, Scott D., Barry L. Duncan, and Mark A. Hubble
1997 Escape from Babel: Toward a Unifying Language for Psychotherapy Practice. New York: W. W. Norton.

Nock, Matthew K., Guilherme Borges, Evelyn J. Bromet, Jordi Alonso, Matthias Angermeyer, Annette Beautrais, Ronny Bruffaerts, Wai Tat Chiu, Giovanni de Girolamo, Semyon Gluzman, Ron de Graaf, Oye Gureje, Josep Maria Haro, Yueqin Huang, Elie Karam, Ronald C. Kessler, Jean Pierre Lepine, Daphna Levinson, Maria Elena Medina-Mora, Yutaka Ono, Jose Posada-Villa, and David Williams
2008 Cross-National Prevalence and Risk Factors for Suicidal Ideation, Plans and Attempts. British Journal of Psychiatry 192(2):98–105.

Nock, Matthew K., Irving Hwang, Nancy A. Sampson, and Ronald C. Kessler
2010 Mental Disorders, Comorbidity and Suicidal Behavior: Results from the National Comorbidity Survey Replication. Molecular Psychiatry 15(8):868–876.

Porter, Matthew
2007 Global Evidence for a Biopsychosocial Understanding of Refugee Adaptation. Transcultural Psychiatry 44(3):418–439.

Porter, Matthew, and Nick Haslam
2005 Predisplacement and Postdisplacement Factors Associated with Mental Health of Refugees and Internally Displaced Persons: A Meta-Analysis. JAMA Journal of the American Medical Association 294(5):602–612.

Putnam, Katherine M., and Lauren B. McSweeney
2008 Depressive Symptoms and Baseline Prefrontal EEG Alpha Activity: A Study Utilizing Ecological Momentary Assessment. Biological Psychology 77(2):237–240.

Regmi, S., A. Pokharel, S. Ojha, S. Pradhan, and G. Chapagain
2004 Nepal Mental Health Country Profile. International Review of Psychiatry 16(1–2):142–149.

Ressler, Kerry J., and Charles B. Nemeroff
2000 Role of Serotonergic and Noradrenergic Systems in the Pathophysiology of Depression and Anxiety Disorders. Depression and Anxiety 12 Suppl 1:2–19.

Rubel, Arthur J., C. W. O'Nell, and R. Collado
1984 Susto: A Folk Illness. Berkeley and Los Angeles: University of California Press.

Rush, Augustus J., Aaron T. Beck, Maria Kovacs, and Steven D. Hollon
1977 Comparative Efficacy of Cognitive Therapy and Pharmacotherapy in the Treatment of Depressed Outpatients. Cognitive Therapy and Research 1(1):17–38.

Scheper-Hughes, Nancy, and Margaret M. Lock
1987 The Mindful Body: A Prolegmenon to Future Work in Medical Anthropology. Medical Anthropology Quarterly 1(1):6–41.

Schininà, Guglielmo, Sonali Sharma, Olga Gorbacheva, and Anit Kumar Mishra
2011 Who Am I? Assessment of Psychosocial Needs and Suicide Risk Factors among Bhutanese Refugees in Nepal and after Third Country Resettlement. International Organization for Migration. http://www.iom.int/jahia/webdav/shared/shared/mainsite/published_docs/studies_and_reports/Bhutanese-Mental-Health-Assessment-Nepal-23-March.pdf, accessed January 12, 2012.

Shweder, Richard A., and Maria A. Sullivan
  1993 Cultural Psychology: Who Needs It. Annual Review of Psychology 44:497–523.
Siegle, Gary J., Wesley Thompson, Cameron S. Carter, Stuart R. Steinhauer, and Michael E. Thase
  2007 Increased Amygdala and Decreased Dorsolateral Prefrontal BOLD Responses in Unipolar Depression:
        Related and Independent Deatures. Biological Psychiatry 61:198–209.
Simons, Ronald C.
  1985 The Fright Illness Taxon: Introduction. In The Culture-Bound Syndromes: Folk Illnesses of Psychiatric
        and Anthropological interest. Ronald C. Simons and Charles C. Hughes, eds. Pp. 329–332. Boston:
        D. Reidel.
Snyder, C. R., Stacy C. Parenteau, Hal S. Shorey, Kristin E. Kahle, and Carla Berg
  2002 Hope as the Underlying Process in the Psychotherapeutic Change Process. International Gestalt
        Journal 25(2):11–29.
Soler, Joaquim, Juan Carlos Pascual, Josefa Campins, Judith Barrachina, Dolors Puigdemont, Enrique Alvarez,
        and Victor Perez
  2005 Double-Blind, Placebo-Controlled Study of Dialectical Behavior Therapy plus Olanzapine for
        Borderline Personality Disorder. [Erratum appears in American Journal of Psychiatry (2008)
        165(6):777]. American Journal of Psychiatry 162(6):1221–1224.
Southwick, Steven M., Seth R. Axelrod, Sheila Wang, Rachel Yehuda, C. A. Morgan III, Dennis Charney,
        Robert Rosenheck, and John W. Mason
  2003 Twenty-Four-Hour Urine Cortisol in Combat Veterans with PTSD and Comorbid Borderline
        Personality Disorder. Journal of Nervous and Mental Disease 191(4):261–262.
Sparks, Jacqueline A., Barry L. Duncan, and Scott D. Miller
  2008 Common Factors in Psychotherapy. In Twenty-First Century Psychotherapies: Contemporary Ap-
        proaches to Theory and Practice. J. L. Lebow, ed. Pp. 453–497. Hoboken, NJ: John Wiley and
        Sons.
Tol, Wietse A., Mark J. Jordans, Sushama Regmi, and Bhogendra Sharma
  2005 Cultural Challenges to Psychosocial Counselling in Nepal. Transcultural Psychiatry 42(2):317–333.
Trinidad, Anton C., Brandon A. Kohrt, and Lorenzo Norris
  2011 Cognitive Behavioral Therapy and Cancer. Psychiatric Annals 41(9):439–442.
Verdeli, H., K. Clougherty, P. Bolton, L. Speelman, N. Lincoln, J. Bass, R. Neugebauer, and M. M. Weissman
  2003 Adapting Group Interpersonal Psychotherapy for a Developing Country: Experience in Rural Uganda.
        World Psychiatry 2(2):114–120.
Verdeli, Helen, Kathleen Clougherty, Grace Onyango, Eric Lewandowski, Liesbeth Speelman, Teresa S.
        Betancourt, Richard Neugebauer, Traci R. Stein, and Paul Bolton
  2008 Group Interpersonal Psychotherapy for Depressed Youth in IDP Camps in Northern Uganda:
        Adaptation and Training. Child and Adolescent Psychiatric Clinics of North America 17(3):605–
        624.
Vygotsky, Lev
  2006 Thought and Word. In Knowledge and Learning in the Firm, vol. 1: The Fundamentals of Embodied
        Cognition. B. Nooteboom, ed. Pp. 80–131. Cheltenham, UK: Elgar.
Weine, Stevan, Nerina Muzurovic, Yasmina Kulauzovic, Sanela Besic, Alma Lezic, Aida Mujagic, Jasmina
        Muzurovic, Dzemila Spahovic, Suzanne Feetham, Norma Ware, Kathleen Knafl, and Ivan Pavkovic
  2004 Family Consequences of Refugee Trauma. Family Process 43(2):147–160.
Westermeyer, Joseph
  1976 Anthropology and Mental Health: Setting a New Course. Chicago: Mouton.
Westermeyer, Joseph, Mayka Bouafuely, and Tou Fu Vang
  1984 Hmong Refugees in Minnesota: Sex Roles and Mental Health. Medical Anthropology 8(4):229–
        245.
White, Geoffrey M.
  1992 Ethnopsychology. In New Directions in Psychological Anthropology. Theodore Schwartz, Geoffrey
        M. White, and Catherine Lutz, eds. Pp. 21–46. New York: Cambridge University Press.

White, Michael

    2004 Folk Psychology and Narrative Practices. *In* The Handbook of Narrative and Psychotherapy: Practice, Theory, and Research. L. E. Angus and J. McLeod, eds. Pp. 15–51. Thousand Oaks, CA: Sage.

White, Michael, and David Denborough

    2011 Narrative Practice: Continuing the Conversations. New York: W. W. Norton.

WHO

    2011 Suicide Prevention and Special Programmes. http://www.who.int/mental_health/prevention/suicide/country_reports/en/index.html, accessed November 16, 2011.

Wikan, Unni

    1989 Illness from Fright or Soul Loss: A North Balinese Culture-Bound Syndrome? Culture, Medicine and Psychiatry 13(1):25–50.

Winston, Arnold, and J. Christopher Muran

    1996 Common Factors in the Time-Limited Psychotherapies. American Psychiatric Press Review of Psychiatry 15:43–68.

Zhang, Jie, Shuiyuan Xiao, and Liang Zhou

    2010 Mental Disorders and Suicide among Young Rural Chinese: A Case-Control SPsychological Autopsy Study. American Journal of Psychiatry 167(7):773–781.

TOWARD AN APPLIED NEUROANTHROPOLOGY OF PSYCHOSIS: THE INTERPLAY OF CULTURE, BRAINS, AND EXPERIENCE

Neely Anne Laurenzo Myers
The George Washington University

Psychotic disorders emerge from the interplay between culture, brains, and experience. Understanding psychotic disorders and intervening effectively to prevent them or alleviate their effects requires a rich understanding of all three, which may best be captured by the transdisciplinary methods and theory of an applied neuroanthropology. Neuroanthropology investigates the ways that cultural context interacts with vulnerable people's brains to both encourage and inhibit the neurodevelopmental processes that lead to a psychotic disorder like schizophrenia. Culturally grounded investigations enable us to investigate the ways a person's lived experiences perpetuate neural changes in the brain that may shape the onset and course of psychotic disorders. This article presents an ethnographic case study of a young man diagnosed with a psychotic disorder after spending 80 days in solitary confinement. Building on his narrative, this article explores his development of a psychotic disorder from an ethnographic and neuroscience perspective. Future transdisciplinary, neuroanthropological studies could rigorously investigate issues that his narrative highlights, including the seemingly inhumane use of solitary confinement and the paucity of meaning-making efforts in biomedical treatment for psychotic disorders. Applied neuroanthropological research on the interplay of culture, brains, and experience in psychotic disorders can contribute to clinical and policy recommendations that improve the lives of people diagnosed with a psychotic disorder around the globe in ways that are locally meaningful for them. [neuroanthropology, culture, schizophrenia, psychosis, psychotic disorder, solitary confinement, stress]

INTRODUCING PSYCHOSIS

"It is so puzzling," a clinical psychologist with over 40 years of experience working with young, psychotic patients—mostly diagnosed with schizophrenia—told me. "How is it that a perfectly lovely young person with all the promise in the world can go off to college or out on their own, get overwhelmed by life, and end up completely dilapidated sitting in a back ward somewhere chain smoking and watching TV? So much investment and potential lost, just at the moment when the child was supposed to thrive on their own."

Over the past decade, I have conducted ethnographic research in the urban United States on the lived experiences of people who have severe psychiatric disabilities, many of whom have been diagnosed with schizophrenia. Eugene Bleuler (1911) first used the word *schizophrenia* to reference a splitting (*schiz*, Latin) of the heart, diaphragm, or

ANNALS OF ANTHROPOLOGICAL PRACTICE 36, pp. 113–130. ISSN: 2153-957X. © 2012 by the American Anthropological Association. DOI:10.1111/j.2153-9588.2012.01095.x

mind (*phren*, Latin). Schizophrenia may affect around 1 percent of the global population, although research suggests its prevalence varies considerably across contexts (Bauer et al. 2010; Gecici et al. 2010). The personal, social, and financial consequences of psychotic symptomatology make psychotic disorders like schizophrenia one of the top five global health burdens of our time (Collins et al. 2011).

Psychosis is a complete break with reality (Compton and Broussard 2009). Experiencing psychosis means that one may believe that something is true that no one else believes, which is known as a delusion. Or one may have a sensory hallucination, such as hearing voices talking in one's head that others do not hear, or smelling smoke when there is no fire. People with a psychotic disorder experience delusions and hallucinations lasting at least one month (American Psychiatric Association 2000). These "positive" symptoms may generate a great deal of fear and anxiety—both in the person experiencing them and in the people around them who do not understand what is happening to their loved one (Neugeboren 1997; Nudel 2009). Also present are "negative symptoms," which include a seemingly flat affect, low motivation, and social withdrawal (American Psychiatry Association 2000). Cognitive symptoms of a psychotic disorder, such as memory loss or difficulty paying attention may also be present.

In her wonderful memoir, Dr. Elyn Saks describes the creep of psychosis as "disorganization":

> Consciousness gradually loses its coherence. One's center gives away. The center cannot hold. The "me" becomes a haze, and the solid center from which one experiences reality breaks up like a bad radio signal. There is no longer a sturdy vantage point from which to look out, take things in, assess what's happening. No core holds things together, providing the lens through which to see the world, to make judgments and comprehend risk. Random moments of time follow one another. Sights, sounds, thoughts and feelings don't go together. No organizing principle takes successive moments in time and puts them together in a coherent way from which sense can be made. And it's all taking place in slow motion [Saks 2007:13].

These experiences tend to be quite disruptive. In 2004, Maison, a 65-year-old Creole man, told me about his experiences with psychosis. "It's just like when you're on acid, you know, LSD . . . But you have no control over it," he said as tears began to trail down his withered cheeks. "You didn't choose it and it won't go away." Maison's psychotic disorder led him from being a respected veteran, nurse, homeowner, husband, and father to eating out of a dumpster behind Kentucky Fried Chicken before he found the help he needed.

This article will discuss emergent findings in the neurosciences and the social sciences that point to the promise of an applied neuroanthropology for furthering our understanding of psychotic disorders. Epidemiological studies suggest that outcomes for schizophrenia vary cross-culturally, with people in non-Western countries often having better outcomes than people in the West (Hopper 2007). Studying culture and using neuroscience techniques enables the exploration of the nuanced ways that a person's lived experiences may shape the onset and course of neurodevelopmental psychotic disorders.

As described in more detail elsewhere, culture can be a source of both risk and protection for people diagnosed with psychotic disorders (Myers 2011). Analyzing the role of culture can account for the importance of the social order (e.g., institutional hierarchies, relationships of regard) and social context (e.g., urban vs. rural) in the course and outcome of psychotic disorders while also capturing the ways people enlist culturally available resources to make sense of and adapt to psychotic symptoms (Tranulis et al. 2009). Cultural analyses heed the key moral commitments people must meet to thrive in local moral worlds. A Bedouin diagnosed with schizophrenia, for example, will receive support from his family when he can claim his experiences are spiritual attacks but may not if he tells them he has a biological illness (Sartorius and Schultze 2005). Moreover, an Indian daughter's family may tolerate her psychiatric disability more once she has married, and especially if she has children (Thara and Srinivasan 1997). These local, moral features may change the trajectory of the disorder.

Once one has developed working hypotheses about what is culturally helpful or harmful for people experiencing psychotic disorder, a neuroanthropological study might expand the scope of these claims to either address or prevent psychosis. Neuroscience methods present valuable tools for assessing a core interest of anthropology—the study of human adaptation—to ask how culture might get "under the skin." This is especially interesting in the context of psychosis, which is thought to have a neurodevelopmental course. If a psychotic disorder develops over time, specific events and the neural changes they induce may lead to the development of the disorder in vulnerable people.

Collaborations between neuroscientists and anthropologists to create targeted neuroanthropological studies can move the field toward understanding what pushes people over the edge of shared, social reality into a state of psychosis, and how to better prevent or at least cushion that fall. This article proposes ideas for such studies, grounded in ethnographic findings and building on some of the latest neuroscience research about psychotic disorders. The article opens with a case study of a young man who participated in a recent ethnographic study conducted in New York. The article then shifts to look at this case from a neuroscience perspective. Blending the two perspectives, the article speculates on how these perspectives might inform each other in future research projects to advance an applied neuroanthropology of psychotic disorders.

PSYCHOTIC DISORDERS: AN ETHNOGRAPHIC PERSPECTIVE

For eight months in 2011, I rode the great artery of train track connecting our nation's capital to New York's Penn Station one day each week. After another subway ride, and a half mile walk up a broad and bustling avenue, I arrived at my destination: an unassuming, seven-story, brick building. On the sixth floor, a fledgling clinic offered services to people with psychiatric disabilities. At this clinic, I conducted mixed methods research using ethnographic participant-observation, semistructured interviews, and psychometric assessments to ask how clients learned to take charge of their own lives.

The clinic was sunny, and painted a cheery shade of lime. Bamboo-colored paneling and frosted glass partitions carved up the space. Most of the clinic's clients, who called themselves "participants," thought of this place as "program." For some, "program" was court mandated or a requirement to establish or maintain a meager government stipend for their psychiatric disability. Many also thought of program as a place to work on self-improvement projects. Administrators organized this unusual program "like a university," and offered "classes" that ran from 9 a.m. until 4 p.m. on a variety of topics. Psychosocial education classes, for example, included lessons on how to live by one's self in the community, prepare for employment, apply for continuing education, and practice coping skills.

Leroy was a bright, 32-year-old African American male that I met the first day I attended the program. During my more than 25 visits to this clinic in 2011, I conducted two hourlong interviews with him. We also spent time together as we attended the program's classes, mingled with others in the dining area, used the computers, strolled to the library, and lingered with the smokers in front of the building.

Leroy lived nearby in an apartment with his parents and siblings. He was tall and broad, and kept the hood of his sweatshirt pulled up over his black football cap with silver insignia. He also wore a black backpack at all times. One day at the library, I asked him for a pen. He removed the backpack and sat down in a chair. I sat across from him, and he placed the bag between us. As he searched for a pen, he showed me the contents. Inside were well-drawn designs for Yu-Gi-Oh!–themed T-shirts based on the Japanese anime series and various informative social services brochures. He liked to be ready to help other people, he explained, when they had questions about where to go for help.

Over time, I came to think of Leroy as a wise observer. He watched everything carefully and rarely interjected unless he could help. He was an excellent informant, and seemed to know about everyone's daily lives. In joyous moments, he had a striking smile and booming laugh. Everyone liked him, but Leroy seemed shy. Whenever we talked, he slouched so low in his chair that he peered cautiously up at me from the shadow of his hat.

Leroy "presents really well," the staff would say, indicating that they found him to be smart and sociable. "I would hire him," they told each other—a standard benchmark in U.S. clinics for assessing one's mental health. Leroy was well-loved, thoughtful, resourceful, smart, and easy to be around most of the time. People gravitated to him.

On paper, Leroy was an alcoholic and a felon on parole with a diagnosis of schizoaffective disorder. I wanted to know how Leroy reconciled these titles and the institutional treatment they prescribed for him (regardless of whether or not he deserved them) with his self-perception, and how the paradoxical elements of how he viewed himself and who he was thought to be affected his ability to "take charge of his own life," a task the clinic prescribed for him. As my fieldwork proceeded, I was struck by the multiple ways that the trajectory of his psychiatric disability seemed to be, in part, shaped by the social context of the institutions in which Leroy participated. To understand more, I collected a detailed history of his psychotic experiences during his short life, paying close attention to the ways his experiences unfolded and were explained and managed across contexts.

During our audio taped interviews, Leroy told me about his early experiences of psychosis. He recalled a frightening female zombie reaching for him from his sister's lower bunk bed during the night when he was about ten years old. Then, as a teenager, Leroy stepped off of a bus and was struck by a car. He lost consciousness for a few hours. The doctors, he claimed, told him he was lucky to be alive.

Recovering at his aunt's house, he experienced vivid hallucinations of women trying to seduce him as he lay in bed. Frightened, he called for his aunt who tried to calm him. She also told him a story. When he was born, his grandmother yelled at his mother because he was "born with a veil over his face." His grandmother predicted that he would see things that other people could not see. When I asked where his grandmother came from, Leroy told me "the South. A Southerner." When I asked what this story meant to him, Leroy told me that he thought the story came from the "folklore" of his ancestors. When he tried to explain his aunt's theory that he might be hearing spirits to his doctors, he said, they told him it was nonsense. So, he speculated, the veil was probably just his hair flattened across his face at birth. He was born with a lot of hair, his mother had told him.

When I asked him if anyone else in his family saw spirits, he said no, but that his aunt had taken his problem very seriously. She lit candles in his room and performed an exorcism to drive out the spirits. After that, she made sure he had what he called a "white cube in water" next to his bed at night. He did not know what the cube was, but his aunt told him the spirits would eat the cube instead of him. He did not have any visions after that for a long time.

Always intelligent, Leroy did well in school. He also grew up poor in a tough neighborhood. As a young teen, a prostitute from the crack house next door asked him to help her regain her wallet from a thieving customer. She still had the customer's car keys, and so she expected him to return. Would Leroy trade the keys for her wallet when he did? Leroy told me that he recognized her as a classmate and felt sorry for her. A heated exchange between Leroy and the customer for the wallet ensued as a policeman looked on. This altercation led to Leroy's first arrest for carrying a concealed weapon. Leroy said all of the kids carried weapons for safety.

After graduating from high school, Leroy's best friend David began to work at a bank. Leroy commuted to a "white neighborhood" for work. But then, a female coworker told him that he did not fit in there. He told me "'why not?' I asked her, and she said, 'Oh, cuz you're black.'"

Embarrassed, Leroy quit and began to work security in his own neighborhood. Then David lost his job at the bank. David, Leroy explained, still had to support his mom and sisters, so he asked Leroy to help him sell marijuana. "I did not want to ruin people's lives," Leroy claimed, "I just saw it as a service. People wanted something so I got it for them." But while they made enough to buy new shoes or cool jeans, they never made enough to pay rent. "We could never get ahead," Leroy noted.

Then David came to visit one night. "'Why can't we get ahead? Why?' David asked me," Leroy said quietly. "He [David] had tears running down his face and I had never seen him cry. I was, like, whoa-" Leroy leaned back in his chair as he said this to accentuate his point.

The next day, David came over with a new product to sell. They could make more money, he insisted, if they sold crack. Leroy wanted to say no, he claimed, but he had never seen David so depressed. He agreed to help. And then they started to use the crack, too. And they still could not get ahead.

One night, Leroy was hanging out with some girls who were high on crack. He told me that he was sober. They asked him to help them rob a cab. He had robbed a cabbie successfully before without getting caught, and wanted to keep everyone safe—the to-be-robbed cabbie and the girls—so he decided to go along. He brought along a cap gun to expedite the whole operation. At some point, though, the cabbie resisted and one of the girls pressed a knifepoint into the back of his neck. Leroy feared she would kill him. "People who want crack," he told me, "will do just about anything to get their fix." Leroy told the driver to get out of the car. As he did so, the other girl jumped in the driver's seat and drove off.

This time, Leroy was charged with armed robbery and grand theft auto. At his sentencing, the judge, he said, told him that he was a good kid and she liked him, but he had that first offense—the concealed weapons charge. "The best I can do is eight years," she told him, and the gavel fell.

Leroy served six of his eight years well. He did everything right. "But," he told me, licking his lips nervously, "I did them too right." The jail hired him to work, and he sent money home. "Good money, but this was too good," he said. The other inmates began to "pay too much attention" and ask for favors. At first he did them, but then he stopped. He did not want get caught and penalized. "I just wanted to get home," he said in a desperate tone. "And then," he told me, "the real trouble began."

People walked away from him in the yard. They refused to talk to him, and made aggressive remarks. He began to sense patterns in their movements, to perceive threatening behaviors in every gesture, to fear the gaze and attention of everyone. He quit his job as a clerk hoping they would leave him alone, but they did not.

"One brother is a snitch, and the other brother is a gangsta," he heard two people walking by say one afternoon. His brother, a real gangster, was also incarcerated at another penitentiary. Leroy was sure they were talking about him. And now, he thought in terror, they thought he was a snitch. "Really strange stuff started happening," Leroy recalled. He stopped talking to others and looked forward to calling home, but he could only make one call each month.

At one point, Leroy lit a cigarette to calm down, and a sergeant saw him. The sergeant shouted, "Hey! Put that out!"

"No," he told me he said angrily, "I am not putting shit out. I'll just go up to my cube [the term he used for his prison cell]." He started to head for his cube. A few puffs later, the sergeant caught up to him. Leroy flicked his cigarette on the ground in anger, watching as it landed near the sergeant's foot.

For this offense, the sergeant charged Leroy with inciting a riot and disobeying a direct command. He received a sentence: 80 days in "the box." "The box" is a prisoner's term for solitary confinement. It is illegal to sentence someone to more than 40 days in solitary confinement, so Leroy would be transferred between prisons to serve 40 days each in two locations.

"The box"—a seamless, metal, cubic space with a toilet, a shower, and a metal bed—was aptly named. A narrow, vertical slit high on one wall gave Leroy a view of other inmates walking in "the yard" about 200 yards away. The C.O. (correctional officer) used a thin, horizontal slot in the door to unlock or put on handcuffs, and pass him meals, a book, or a pen and paper. The C.O. also peered through the slot, Leroy said, to "make sure you don't hang yourself or something," but "you can't see nobody." Leroy could read, write, and listen to music, but he had no human interaction. Each day, he spent one hour outside (alone) to pace a concrete space about the size of his room.

This experience, Leroy claimed, "was messing with my head." One day he heard a voice that said, "Satan is coming." At first, he thought the guards were "messing with me," but when he asked if they had said anything, they answered with the only word permitted to be spoken to people in the box: "no."

One of the guards brought him the book *Roots* and he asked for a Christian Bible. He read them both. Over time, Leroy found, patterns and connections emerged from the text. The voices came more frequently. At first, Leroy thought he might be conversing with the people outside the window despite the distance and the glass. When he tried to yell back through the vertical slit, the C.O. opened the door slot and yelled, "no!"

Leroy realized he was "being tested." He knew then that he had to prove himself worthy. He "had to pass the test."

They transferred Leroy to another prison after 40 days to bypass the legal limits of 40 days. This time he had a roommate. The voices in Leroy's head often clamored. He found his roommate to be bizarre, dominating, and at times revolting. He said this man often used the bathroom without being decent about the process (there was no door or curtain on the toilet or shower), had several pornographic magazines, and spoke freely of sexual topics that made Leroy uncomfortable. When his 40 days in that room were up, the administration transferred Leroy into the general population of the new prison.

Leroy carried the Bible everywhere with him "for protection." One man that Leroy thought was a friend mocked him. "Man, the Bible is for church," he told Leroy one afternoon while bouncing in a seated position on Leroy's bed. "He knew that's like a prison sign," Leroy explained, "a very negative sign for him to be doing that on my bed." Leroy avoided him. Staff decided he was "too religiously occupied. That's what they told me later."

One afternoon, a man and woman asked him to whom he was talking, and Leroy said he could not remember. They laughed and told Leroy he failed the test. This statement resonated with all of his beliefs about being tested by "demons." "I was so scared going back to my cube," he told me later. "I thought it was going to rain fire and brimstone because I failed. I was holding the Bible up to protect my head."

Without explanation, the guards chained Leroy, put him into a van, and drove him up a long hill in the rain. "It was the longest ride I ever took," he said softly. He was terrified; he had no idea where he was going and the dense fog reminded him of purgatory. Along the way, one of the two guards leaned back over the seat and offered him a cup of juice. Then the overwhelming visual hallucinations began. Leroy realized in terror that the guard was the devil. He had long fingernails and a wicked smile. The guard, he felt sure, had poisoned his juice. Then, he told me, "I really started seeing stuff." More than he had ever seen before.

On arrival at the new location, he was taken into an empty room, stripped down, hosed off by a man larger than himself, and put into "a skirt." The guard commented that the skirt was never going to fit him. Leroy watched in horror as the skirt magically grew larger to fit his body. Then, they put him alone in another room—a room in which all of the lights were on. He did not know the time, and there were no windows.

Leroy told me that he did not understand until later that the medical staff were observing him around the clock through a one-way mirror to determine whether or not he was sane. But at the moment, he only knew that he was alone in another strange, bright box. At some point, he recalled, the staff swarmed around him, telling him, "you're not the only one being tested. We're being tested, too."

When the doctors offered him medication, he told me, the "demons" became very distressed. They mocked him. "Oh, so you don't want to play the game?" they shrieked. He tried to refuse the medication, and was put into physical restraints and administered a shot of Haldol, an antipsychotic drug that has a strong sedative effect.

The medication made the demons go away, Leroy said, but he also felt resentful. "They just wanted to medicate me to keep me quiet. And now, because I took the medication I can't hear the directions anymore. And I am going to be stuck on medication for the rest of my life."

Leroy was transferred to a psychiatric hospital and diagnosed with a psychotic disorder, schizoaffective disorder. In 2008, he made parole one year early and transferred to community mental health services—first one program and then another. He received a Social Security Disability Income for his new psychiatric disability that left him living well below the poverty level. Because he needs health insurance to afford his expensive antipsychotic medications that silence the "demons," Leroy is unlikely to work full time for fear he will lose the Medicaid coverage that comes with his disability.

As his story ended, Leroy shuddered and slouched further in his chair. "I failed the test," he said huskily, shaking his head, his eyes moist with wonder. "It's the only explanation for why we are sitting here. I failed the test."

PSYCHOTIC DISORDERS: A NEUROSCIENCE PERSPECTIVE

Neuroscientists have long been investigating what happens in the brains of people like Leroy to trigger psychotic episodes, but the etiology of psychotic disorders such as schizophrenia remain unclear. In a recent *Nature* article, neuroscientist David Lewis stated that the knowledge we have about schizophrenia is best understood through the old parable of blind men trying to collectively describe the nature of an elephant. At the moment, researchers are gaining "a bit more synchrony" in their findings so that they can agree, perhaps, on the description of one part (Dobbs 2010).

For example, there is no known gene for schizophrenia. Even in identical twins, there is only a 50 percent chance of the other twin developing schizophrenia if one twin has the condition (Owen et al. 2002). The partial concordance between identical twins suggests that epigenetic effects, or alterations in gene expression during a person's lifetime in response to lived experiences, are involved. Epigenetic effects, some argue, may have a more potent effect on the development of psychotic disorder than the influence of genes or environment alone (Oh and Petronis 2008; Van Winkel et al. 2010). Epigenetic changes also fit into the long-accepted diathesis-stress model of schizophrenia (Howes and Kapur 2009), which posits that a person with schizophrenia has a biological vulnerability to overreact to normal stressors that eventually leads to the development of psychotic symptoms under duress (Walker et al. 2008). Did Leroy have such a vulnerability? And is it possible that the intense duress he experienced, authorized by institutions charged with his rehabilitation no less, nudged his vulnerability into a full-blown psychotic disorder?

The new "psychosis–proneness–persistence continuum" model of schizophrenia suggests that stressful and persistent events (e.g., childhood trauma) may well lead to psychosis in vulnerable people. The model places people who experience nonclinical, "psychotic-like experiences" (PLEs) that are shorter in duration and do not disrupt everyday life (about 5–7 percent of the general population) at one end of the continuum, and people who experience a psychotic disorder at the other end of the continuum (Kelleher and Cannon 2011; Van Os et al. 2009). In this model, psychotic symptoms may be part of a common neurodevelopmental process that becomes pathological when a person has biological traits (e.g., genetic markers, neurological soft signs) that render them "prone" to the effects of adversity. Depending on a person's "prone-ness," a mounting accumulation of social stressors may lead to a psychotic disorder. Many initial psychotic episodes occur as young people transition to adulthood, for example, a developmental period involving a high volume of stressors in a young person's life (McGorry 2011).

Epidemiological research also suggests that stressors prevalent in specific contexts can increase a person's risk of developing schizophrenia. Incidence, or a person's risk of developing schizophrenia over time, varies substantially according to seemingly stress-related social factors. Urbanicity, migration, seeming different among one's peer group, poverty, adverse life events, cumulative social disadvantage, and knock-on effects (the increasing impact of social factors as they accumulate) can each raise a person's risk of developing psychotic symptoms (Kirkbride and Jones 2011; Myers 2011). In urban Tanzania, for example, the experience of two or more stressful life events in the past year led to increased psychotic symptoms (Jenkins et al. 2010). Physical abuse in childhood among British women made them twice as likely as controls to report psychotic symptoms (Fisher et al. 2009). Exposure to trauma in South Africa (Burns et al. 2011) and exposure to trauma with intention to harm (e.g., bullying) as a child, even with controlled genetic liability for psychosis, also led to an increased incidence of psychosis in Britain (Arseneault et al. 2010). In a recent case-control study, cumulative social disadvantage (e.g., the adding-up of instances of unemployment, discrimination, adverse life events, parental separation before the age of 16, and childhood trauma across the life course) had a linear correlation with higher rates of PLEs in the Black Caribbean ethnic population (Morgan et al. 2009).

The evidence all points to the idea that contextual stress pushes vulnerable people toward a psychotic disorder. What neuroscience lacks is a strong sense of what kinds of life experiences, during what neurodevelopmental phases, and with what effects, may lead to the onset of psychotic symptoms. In other words, what is the interplay between culture, brains, and experience over time for people who develop a psychotic disorder?

One theory suggests that neural changes in psychotic disorder may result from long-term "allostatic overload," which also plays a role in cardiovascular disease and abdominal obesity (McEwen 1998; Pedrini et al. 2012). Allostasis is a "balance" sought by the body as it seeks to adapt to new and stressful circumstances (McEwen 1998). Allostatic load is the energy expended by the body to maintain this neurophysiological balance in moments of distress. When an animal is under great duress, the energy demanded exceeds supply—known as allostatic overload. At this point, the body enters "survival mode" and releases inflammatory cytokines (such as IL-1 and IL-6) and other glucocorticoids (of which cortisol is one) to decrease the allostatic overload. After the difficult circumstances recede, the body exits survival mode. If the difficult circumstances do not recede and social conflict and other types of social dysfunction continue—for example, as happens with animals in captivity—the allostatic load remains high.

Conditions of increased oxidative stress that occur in allostatic overload—such as the continued surge of glucocorticoids and inflammatory cytokines—detectably alter inflammation-related pathways, which are common in people diagnosed with psychiatric disorders (Dean 2011; Kaur and Cadenhead 2010; McEwen 1998; Pedrini et al. 2012). Altered inflammation-related pathways are also strongly implicated in the neurophysiological mechanisms of schizophrenia (Miller et al. 2011; Pedrini et al. 2012). Because schizophrenia has a specific developmental trajectory, with onset typically occurring in late adolescence or early adulthood, it is reasonable to hypothesize that culture, as defined above, contributes to elevated oxidative stress during sensitive periods of neurodevelopment that engenders neural changes related to psychosis in the brains of young adults (McGorry 2011; Pedrini et al. 2012).

Neuroscientists, however, have yet to determine how oxidative stress—such as elevated levels of inflammatory cytokines—correlates with specific, neurophysiological changes relevant to psychotic disorders that stem from specific, contextualized life events. If this connection were made, we may begin to understand how and when stress gets "under the skin" to trigger upstream neurophysiological events that contribute to one's downstream development of psychotic symptoms. With careful, longitudinal research, we may be able to better unpack, for example, what pushes a prone person along the psychotic continuum from having "PLEs" to experiencing a psychotic episode. Moreover, in experiments with mice, allostatic overloads can only be reduced by "learning and changes in the social structure" (McEwen 1998). Culture may also be protective, or capable of teaching vulnerable people how to better handle distress.

Psychotic disorder may well be a neurodevelopmental adaptation of one's brain to lived experience that has gone awry. The lived experience of psychosis, anthropology teaches us, is also embedded in the webs of significance that men have both spun for themselves, and in which they are also suspended (Geertz 1973). Understanding psychotic symptoms as a phenomenon that emerges from a continual interplay between culture, brains, and experience will require the methods and theory of an applied neuroanthropology, which can push the limits of both disciplines to ask—how does culture interact with vulnerable people's brains over time to both generate and inhibit neurodevelopmental processes that lead to psychosis?

TOWARD AN APPLIED NEUROANTHROPOLOGY OF PSYCHOSIS

Applied anthropology asks that we pragmatically engage with the problems of our contemporary worlds to be part of the solution (Rylko-Bauer et al. 2006). I am an anthropologist, not a neuroscientist. The ideas I present below are meant to plant seeds for collaboration and imagine ways forward, but do not reflect rigorously planned studies. Leroy's narrative presents us with strong examples of the ways the life histories of people with psychiatric disabilities often contain accumulating adversity; in his case, violence, incarceration, unemployment, powerlessness in the clinical encounter, and discrimination. Experiences such as these often rigidify one's social position as a helpless and hopeless person in a situation that some refer to as "structural violence" (Farmer 2004; Kelly 2005). An applied neuroanthropology of psychosis could work to identify how one's experience of culture (e.g., structural violence) alters the neural architecture of the brain in ways that may exacerbate or alleviate one's progression along the psychosis continuum.

Anthropologists could produce, for example, prospective, contextualized histories of developmental experiences in high risk populations who possess relevant genetic and neurological vulnerabilities. Developmental insults may amount to the emergence of a disease state, even in the context of what appears to be minor or transient events, as they lead to subtle alterations in developing circuitry and neurochemistry (Niwa et al. 2010). Targeted early intervention during sensitive periods, prior to the onset of a psychotic disorder, may "reroute" the neurodevelopmental trajectory away from pathological functioning (Thompson and Levitt 2010). Through nuanced, prospective studies of adolescents at-risk, anthropologists can help identify the social processes and sensitive periods that matter, and possibly even the culturally available resources needed for protective neural rerouting (as with the mice whose allostatic overload could only be overcome with learning and changes in social structure [McEwen 1998]).

One application of neuroanthropology going forward, then, is to inform clinical interventions. If vulnerable people encountering social adversity experience neurodevelopmental alterations that move them from being prone to PLEs (like hearing voices on occasion or feeling psychic) toward "first-episode psychosis," and then multiple psychotic episodes, can we correlate relevant life events (e.g., juvenile incarceration, trauma) with neural effects in specific developmental periods that may push sensitive people toward psychotic illness (Van Os et al. 2009)? And if we can, might it be possible to intervene in ways that prevent or counteract those neural events in high risk youth? An applied neuroanthropology could work to pinpoint what aspects of culture and experience drive the neurodevelopment of a psychotic disorder for some, and locally relevant ways culture may protect others.

Leroy's story provides an excellent example with which to speculate on how such studies could be useful to researchers, clinicians, and public policymakers. Leroy's early experiences with zombies and spirits in dark rooms sound similar to the PLEs described on the nonpathological side of the psychosis continuum. PLEs include magical thinking, hearing voices, and having visions, but these occur for less than one day and do not lead to a complete break with reality. Although PLEs share the same continuum with psychotic disorder, the vast majority of people never transition from experiencing PLEs to experiencing psychosis (Kelleher and Cannon 2011). Even among a group of people considered to be at "ultrahigh risk" of developing a psychotic disorder (owing to specific genetic markers and neurological soft signs), only 19 percent transitioned to having a psychotic disorder (Ruhrmann et al. 2010). What happened to the young people who transitioned from experiencing PLEs to having psychotic disorder? Was Leroy like them? Did he share the ultrahigh risk profile? Or, to articulate these questions in context, would his childhood propensity to see spirits in a dark room have progressed to a psychotic disorder if he had not been incarcerated and sentenced to spend an *illegal* number of days—through willful institutional jockeying no less—in solitary confinement?

Rhodes's (2004:32–34) blistering ethnography of prison life makes plain that solitary confinement may be psychotogenic. And by Rhodes's account, the guards were fully aware of this possibility—almost ashamed of it—but the entire institution was complicit in this form of "rehabilitation." Rhodes is not the first to make this claim (Ignatieff 1978:9). Additionally, prison rules limit the amount of mental health services a person can receive in solitary confinement (Metzner and Fellner 2010). Given the negative impacts of solitary confinement on people's minds, should this practice not be changed? A neuroanthropological study might conclusively establish that people who experience PLEs are inclined to develop a psychotic disorder when placed in solitary confinement. If we could, for example, recruit people in prison who meet criteria for being "ultrahigh risk" for psychotic disorder, take extensive life histories, and then track both their development (if any) of psychiatric symptoms (perhaps asking them to use a mini video recorder to report their status each day) and their neurophysiological status (perhaps collecting a daily saliva or blood sample), we might learn more about the effects of incarceration on mental health. Moreover, if we compared ultrahigh risk people who remained in the general population to ultrahigh risk people experiencing solitary confinement, we could learn more about how this specific practice affects the bodies and minds of vulnerable people, and potentially move society toward ending an inhumane practice.

As with Leroy, people experiencing psychosis in the West also have few opportunities to mitigate or make sense of their highly disorienting psychotic experiences, such as "voices" that are often dismissed as unreal and therefore not part of one's actual self

(Estroff 2004). As Leroy so poignantly stated, this led him to believe that he "failed the test." Leroy felt that the "demons" would eventually make clear to him what his instructions should be, but the powerful antipsychotic medication, Haldol, involuntarily administered to him, silenced his "demons" before he understood how to "pass the test." From then on, he fantasized about what it would be like to stop taking his medications and interact with the demons again so that he might find out what they wanted and how to not fail the test. This is not to say that the demons were real (how can we know) nor that Leroy needed to follow their instructions to relieve his psychosis, but the involuntary silencing of this deeply personal and meaningful experience generated distress. He had no chance to integrate these confusing experiences with his own life narrative.

The idea of "biochemical imbalance" that informed Leroy's treatment with medications, anthropologist Jenkins (2010) argues, is grounded in what she calls the "pharmaceutical imaginary," or the conception that pharmaceutical drugs will bring us closer to our imagined potentials. The notion of "chemical imbalance" and the kinds of treatment it produces in the clinic (namely, the prescription of antipsychotic drugs), Jenkins continues, does little to address what mattered most to patients—namely, their concerns with the impact of their diagnosis and its treatment on their sense of agency, kinship relations and moral worth. Jenkins' arguments reveal much about Leroy's own plight. Although many people describe psychopharmaceuticals as a critical aspect of their ability to maintain well-being, they also need more than psychopharmaceuticals to thrive.

Western people experiencing psychotic symptoms often long to make sense of their experiences in a socially acceptable way, but lack opportunities to do so in Western countries. Anthropologists Corin and colleagues (2004) and Lucas (2004) both described how Western people with schizophrenia turn to marginalized religious sects or parapsychology groups because these groups sometimes received their experiences as real. Anthropologist McGruder (2004) also described how, in Zanzibar, some people accepted that hostile spirits, which may be responding to the action of any relative or ancestor, explained psychotic behavior. In this case, the onus was not on the individual—they were likely neither the source of the problem nor the solution—so the family sacrificed to insure their comfort. Similarly, one of Robert Lemelson's ethnographic films on schizophrenia in Bali, *Shadows and Illuminations*, enables us to witness the acceptance of one man diagnosed with schizophrenia's interactions with the spirit world by his family. The presence of spirits is generally accepted in Bali, and traditional rituals offered means with which to assign meaning to their presence and ways to encourage them to leave. Although this man still accepted psychopharmaceuticals that helped him manage his psychotic symptoms, the cultural acceptance and ritual management of his experiences seemed to help him live more peacefully with his experiences than Leroy.

A second contribution of an applied neuroanthropology, then, could be to study the effects of meaning-making for people with a psychotic disorder and their neural effects. Is there a detectable difference in neural activation patterns, for example, when a person whose psychotic experiences can be explained meaningfully (e.g., as a visit from spirits [McGruder 2004]) talk about their symptoms versus when a person who has no access to meaning-making (e.g., a person involuntarily medicated) describes their experiences? Are there differences in neural activation patterns between these two groups when they "hear" voices? Do family members respond more empathically to photographs of their loved one when the affliction is thought to be spiritual, rather than a biochemical imbalance?

This brings us to a third focus for an applied neuroanthropology of psychosis. Anthropologists have long suggested that ritual processes found in different contexts help people to use culturally available symbols and meanings to make sense of embodied experiences (Obeyesekere 1990; Turner 2006; Turner 1967). Neuroanthropological studies might identify how rituals help people manage symptoms of a psychotic disorder. The ritualized processes of yoga and loving-kindness meditation, for instance, appear to help people reduce negative symptoms of schizophrenia, as well as perceived stress, depression and anxiety (Duraiswamy et al. 2007; Johnson et al. 2009). An applied neuroanthropological study may reveal how these practices effect changes in the brain over time, as preliminary research suggests they do. Such practices may, for example reduce circulating biomarkers of oxidative stress or alter relevant neural circuitry to prevent initial or recurrent psychotic episodes in vulnerable people. The salience of the intervention for people, which anthropologists can capture ethnographically, may be an important factor in facilitating neural change. This kind of neuroanthropological study could observe how locally meaningful cultural practices generate well-being in bodies and brains. Ritual interventions during neurodevelopmentally sensitive periods prior to the "first break" may help reroute neurodevelopmental trajectories away from pathological functioning. Ritual practices may also achieve this without disrupting young people's everyday lives, but we need neuroanthropological studies to explore this concept further.

In the United States, where people are less likely to recover from a psychotic disorder, or return to the kind of life they may have been expected to live before they became ill, the culture of institutions charged with their care often fail to help people manage their stress, and rarely help them understand and integrate their psychotic experiences into their own life narratives and local moral worlds (Hopper 2007). Neuroanthropological studies may convince the public and policymakers that culture profoundly shapes people's everyday experiences—and also, consequently, their brains. The relevance of these findings for the everyday lives of people at-risk of developing psychotic disorders and people trying to avoid the recurrence of a psychotic episode may be particularly profound. For them, the stakes are high and resources are typically limited. Using transdisciplinary teams of neuroscientists and anthropologists to investigate the interplay of culture, brains, and experience, an applied neuroanthropology provides us with more comprehensive tools with which to understand, treat, and prevent psychotic disorders.

NOTE

Acknowledgments. The author would like to thank Daniel Lende, Greg Downey, Kim Hopper, and Tali Ziv for their comments on earlier drafts. This article was made possible by support from the Center to Study Recovery in Social Contexts P20 MH078188 from the National Institute for Mental Health and grant number 5-T32-AT000052 from the National Center for Complementary and Alternative Medicine (NCCAM) at the National Institutes of Health.

Its contents are solely the responsibility of the authors and do not necessarily represent the official views of NIMH or NCCAM.

REFERENCES CITED

Arseneault, LouiseAmerican Psychiatric Association
  2000 Diagnostic and Statistical Manual of Mental Disorders: DSM-IV-TR. Washington, DC: American Psychiatric Association.
Arseneault, Louise, Mary Cannon, Helen L. Fisher, Guillherme Polanczyk, Terrie E. Moffitt, and Avshalom Caspi
  2010 Childhood Trauma and Children's Emerging Psychotic Symptoms: A Genetically Sensitive Longitudinal Cohort Study. American Journal of Psychiatry 168(1):65–72.
Bauer, Susanne M., Hans Schanda, Hanna Karakula, Luiza Olajossy-Hilkesberger, Palmira Rudalevicience, Nino Okribelashvili, Harnoon R. Chaudhry, Sunday E. Idemudia, Sharon Gscheider, and Kristina Ritter
  2010 Culture and the Prevalence of Hallucinations in Schizophrenia. Comprehensive Psychiatry 52(3): 319–325.
Bleuler, Eugen
  1911 Dementia Praecox Oder die Gruppe der Schizophrenien. Leipzig, Germany: Deuticke.
Burns, Johnathan K., Khatija Jhazbhay, Tonya Esterhuizen, and Robin Emsley
  2011 Exposure to Trauma and the Clinical Presentation of First-Episode Psychosis in South Africa. Journal of Psychiatric Research 45(2):179–184.
Collins, Pamela Y., Vikram Patel, Sara Joestl, Dana March, Thomas R. Insel, Abdallah S. Daar, Isabel A. Bordin, E. Jane Costello, Maureen Durkin, Christopher Fairburn, Roger I. Glass, Wayne Hall, Yueqin Huang, Steven E. Hyman, Kay Jamison, Sylvia Kaaya, Shitij Kapur, Arthur Kleinman, Adesola Ogunniyi, Angel Otero-Ojeda, Mu-Ming Poo, Vijayalakshmi Ravindranath, Barbara J. Sahakian, Shekhar Saxena, Peter A. Singer, Dan J. Stein, Warwick Anderson, Muhammad A. Dhansay, Wendy Ewart, Anthony Phillips, Susan Shurin and Mark Walport
  2011 Grand Challenges in Global Mental Health. Nature 475(7354):27–30.
Compton, Michael T., and Beth Broussard
  2009 The First Episode of Psychosis: A Guide for Patients and Their Families. New York: Oxford University Press.
Corin, Ellen, Rangaswami Thara, and Ramachandran Padmavati
  2004 Living through a Staggering World: The Play of Signifiers in Early Psychosis in South India. In Cambridge Studies in Medical Anthropology, vol. 11: Schizophrenia, Culture, and Subjectivity: The Edge of Experience. Janis H. Jenkins and Robert J. Barrett, eds. Pp. 110–145. Cambridge: Cambridge University Press.
Dean, Brian
  2011 Understanding the Role of Inflammatory-Related Pathways in the Pathophysiology and Treatment of Psychiatric Disorders: Evidence from Human Peripheral Studies and CNS Studies. The International Journal of Neuropsychopharmacology 14(7):997–1012.
Dobbs, David
  2010 The Making of a Troubled Mind. Nature 468:154–156.
Duraiswamy, Ganesan, Jagadisha Thirthalli, H. R. Nagendra, and B. N. Gangadhar
  2007 Yoga Therapy as an Add-On Treatment in the Management of Patients with Schizophrenia—A Randomized Controlled Trial. Acta Psychiatrica Scandanivica 116(3):226–232.
Estroff, Sue E.
  2004 Subject/Subjectivities in Dispute: The Poetics, Politics, and Performance of First-Person Narratives of People with Schizophrenia. In Cambridge Studies in Medical Anthropology, vol. 11: Schizophrenia, Culture, and Subjectivity: The Edge of Experience. Janis H. Jenkins and Robert J. Barrett, eds. Pp. 282–302. Cambridge: Cambridge University Press.

Farmer, Paul

    2004 An Anthropology of Structural Violence. Current Anthropology 45(3):305–325.

Fisher, Helen, Craig Morgan, Paola Dazzan, Thomas K. Craig, Kevin Morgan, Gerard Hutchinson, Peter B. Jones, Gillian A. Doody, Carmine Pariante, and Peter McGuffin, Robin M. Murray, Julian Leff, and Paul Fearon

    2009 Gender Differences in the Association between Childhood Abuse and Psychosis. The British Journal of Psychiatry 194(4):319–325.

Gecici, Omer, Murat Kuloglu, Ozkan Guler, Omer Ozbulut, Erhan Kurt, E., Sinay Onen, Okan Ekinci, Delik Yesilbas, Ali Caykoylu, Murat Emul, Gazi Alatas, and Yakup Albayrak

    2010 Phenomenology of Delusions and Hallucinations in Patients with Schizophrenia. Bulletin of Clinical Psychopharmacology 20(3):204–212.

Geertz, Clifford

    1973 Thick Description: Toward an Interpretive Theory of Culture. *In* The Interpretation of Cultures: Selected Essays. Pp. 3–30. New York: Basic.

Hopper, Kim

    2007 Recovery from Schizophrenia: An International Perspective: A Report from the WHO Collaborative Project, the International Study of Schizophrenia. New York: Oxford University Press.

Howes, Oliver D., and Shitij Kapur

    2009 The Dopamine Hypothesis of Schizophrenia: Version III the Final Common Pathway. Schizophrenia Bulletin 35(3):549–562.

Ignatieff, Michael

    1978 A Just Measure of Pain: The Penitentiary in the Industrial Revolution 1750–1850. London: Macmillan.

Jenkins, Janis H.

    2010 Psychopharmaceutical Self and Imaginary in the Social Field of Psychiatric Treatment. *In* Pharmaceutical Self: The Global Shaping of Experience in an Age of Psychopharmacology. Janis H. Jenkins, ed. Santa Fe: School for Advanced Research Press.

Jenkins, Rachel, Joseph Mbatia, Nicola Singleton, and Bethany White

    2010 Prevalence of Psychotic Symptoms and Their Risk Factors in Urban Tanzania. International Journal of Environmental Research and Public Health 7(6):2514–2525.

Johnson, David P., David L. Penn, Barbara L. Fredrickson, Piper S. Meyer, Ann M. Kring, and Mary Brantley

    2009 Loving-Kindness Meditation to Enhance Recovery from Negative Symptoms of Schizophrenia. Journal of Clinical Psychology 65(5):499–509.

Kaur, Tejal, and Kristin S. Cadenhead

    2010 Treatment Implications of the Schizophrenia Prodrome. Current Topics in Behavioral Neurosciences 4:97–121.

Kelleher, Ian, and Mary Cannon

    2011 Psychotic-Like Experiences in the General Population: Characterizing a High-Risk Group for Psychosis. Psychological Medicine 41(1):1–6.

Kelly, B. D.

    2005 Structural Violence and Schizophrenia. Social Science and Medicine 61(3):721–730.

Kirkbride, James B., and Peter B. Jones

    2011 The Prevention of Schizophrenia: What Can We Learn From Eco-Epidemiology? Schizophrenia Bulletin 37(2):262–271.

Lucas, Rod

    2004 In and Out of Culture: Ethnographic Means to Interpreting Schizophrenia. *In* Cambridge Studies in Medical Anthropology, vol. 11: Schizophrenia, Culture, and Subjectivity: The Edge of Experience. Janis H. Jenkins and Robert J. Barrett, eds. Pp. 146–166. Cambridge: Cambridge University Press.

McEwen, Bruce S.

    1998 Stress, Adaptation, and Disease: Allostasis and Allostatic Load. Annals of the New York Academy of Science 840(1):33–44.

McGorry, Patrick
2011 Transition to Adulthood: The Critical Period for Pre-Emptive, Disease- Modifying Care for Schizophrenia and Related Disorders. Schizophrenia Bulletin 37(3):524–530.

McGruder, Juli
2004 Madness in Zanzibar: An Exploration of Lived Experience. *In* Schizophrenia, Culture, and Subjectivity: The Edge of Experience. Janis H. Jenkins and Robert J. Barrett, eds. Pp. 255–281. Cambridge: Cambridge University Press.

Metzner, Jeffrey L., and Jamie Fellner
2010 Solitary Confinement and Mental Illness in U.S. Prisons: A Challenge for Medical Ethics. Journal of the American Academy of Psychiatry and the Law Online 38(1):104–108.

Miller, Brian J., Peter Buckley, Wesley Seabolt, Andrew Mellor, and Brian Kirkpatrick
2011 Meta-Analysis of Cytokine Alterations in Schizophrenia: Clinical Status and Antipsychotic Effects. Biological Psychiatry 70(7):663–671.

Morgan, Craig, Helen Fisher, Gerard Hutchinson, James Kirkbride, Thomas K. Craig, Kevin Morgan, Paola Dazzan, Jane Boydell, Gillian A. Doody, Peter B. Jones, Robin M. Murray, Julian Leff, and Paul Fearon
2009 Ethnicity, Social Disadvantage and Psychotic-Like Experiences in a Healthy Population Based Sample. Acta Psychiatrica Scandinavica 119(3):226–235.

Myers, Neely
2011 Update: Schizophrenia across Cultures. Current Psychiatry Reports 13(4):305–311.

Neugeboren, Jay
1997 Imagining Robert: My Brother, Madness, and Survival. New York: Henry Holt.

Niwa, Minae, Atsushi Kamiya, Rina Murai, Ken-Ichiro Kubo, Aaron J. Gruber, Kenji Tomita, Lingling Lu, Shuta Tomisato, Hanna Jaaro-Peled, and Saurav Seshadri, Hideki Hiyama, Beverly Huang, Kazuhisa Kohda, Yukihiro Noda, Patricio O'Donnell, Kazunori Nakajima, and Akira Sawa
2010 Knockdown of DISC1 by in utero Gene Transfer Disturbs Postnatal Dopaminergic Maturation in the Frontal Cortex and Leads to Adult Behavioral Deficits. Neuron 65(4):480–489.

Nudel, Cassandra, ed.
2009 Firewalkers: Madness, Beauty and Mystery. Charlottesville, VA: VOCAL.

Obeyesekere, Gannath
1990 The Work of Culture: Symbolic Transformation in Psychoanalysis and Anthropology. Chicago: University of Chicago Press.

Oh, Gabriel, and Arturis Petronis
2008 Environmental Studies of Schizophrenia through the Prism of Epigenetics. Schizophrenia Bulletin 34(6):1122–1129.

Owen, Michael J., Michael C. O'Donovan, and Irving I. Gottesman
2002 Schizophrenia. *In* Psychiatric Genetics and Genomics. Peter McGuffin, Michael J. Owen, and Irving I. Gottesman, eds. Pp. 247–266. London: Oxford University Press.

Pedrini, Mariana, Raffael Massuda, Gabriel R. Fries, Matheus A. de Bittencourt Pasquali, Carlos E. Schnorr, Jose C. F. Moreira, Antonio L. Teixeira, Maria I. R. Lobato, Julio C. Walz, Paolo S. Belmonte-de-Abreu, Marcia Kauer-Sant'anna, Flavio Kapczinski, and Clarissa S. Gama
2012 Similarities in Serum Oxidative Stress Markers and Inflammatory Cytokines in Patients with Overt Schizophrenia at Early and Late Stages of Chronicity. Journal of Psychiatric Research 46(6): 819–824.

Rhodes, Lorna A.
2004 Total Confinement: Madness and Reason in the Maximum Security Prison. Los Angeles: University of California Press.

Ruhrmann, Stephan, Frauke Schultze-Lutter, Raimo K. R. Salokangas, Markus Heinimaa, Don Linszen, Peter Dingemans, Max Birchwood, Paul Patterson, Georg Juckel, and Andreas Heinz, Anthony Morrison, Shôn Lewis, Heinrich Graf von Reventlow, and Joachim Klosterkötter Heinz
2010 Prediction of Psychosis in Adolescents and Young Adults at High Risk: Results from the Prospective European Prediction of Psychosis Study. Archives of General Psychiatry 67(3):241–251.

Rylko-Bauer, Barbara, Merrill Singer, and John Van Willigen
   2006 Reclaiming Applied Anthropology: Its Past, Present and Future. American Anthropologist 108(1): 178–190.
Saks, Elyn R.
   2007 The Center Cannot Hold: My Journey through Madness. New York: Hyperion.
Sartorius, Norman, and Hugh Schultze
   2005 Reducing the Stigma of Mental Illness: A Report for a Global Programme of the World Psychiatric Association. Cambridge: Cambridge University Press.
Thara, Rangasawamy, and Tirupati N. Srinivasan
   1997 Outcome of Marriage in Schizophrenia. Social Psychiatry and Psychiatric Epidemiology 32(7):416–420.
Thompson, Barbara L., and Pat Levitt
   2010 Now You See It, Now You Don't—Closing in on Allostasis and Developmental Basis of Psychiatric Disorders. Neuron 65(4):437–439.
Tranulis, Constantin, Lawrence Park, Laura Delano, and Byron Good
   2009 Early Intervention in Psychosis: A Case Study on Normal and Pathological. Culture, Medicine and Psychiatry 33(4):608–622.
Turner, Edith L. B.
   2006 Among the Healers: Stories of Spiritual and Ritual Healing around the World. Westport, CT: Praeger.
Turner, Victor
   1967 Betwixt and Between: The Liminal Period in Rites de Passage. *In* The Forest of Symbols: Aspects of Ndembu Ritual. Pp. 93–111. Ithaca, NY: Cornell University.
Van Os, Jim, Richard J. Linscott, Inez Myin-Germeys, Philippe Delespaul, and Lydia Krabbendam
   2009 A Systematic Review and Meta-Analysis of the Psychosis Continuum: Evidence for a Psychosis Proneness-Persistence-Impairment Model of Psychotic Disorder. Psychological Medicine 39(2): 179–195.
Van Winkel, Ruud, Gabriel Esquivel, Gunter Kenis, Marieke Wichers, Dina Collip, Odette Peerbooms, Bart Rutten, Inez Myin-Germeys, and Jim Van Os
   2010 REVIEW: Genome Wide Findings in Schizophrenia and the Role of Gene-Environment Interplay. CNS Neuroscience and Therapeutics 16(5):e185–e192.
Walker, Elaine, Vijay Mittal, and Kevin Tessner
   2008 Stress and the Hypothalamic Pituitary Adrenal Axis in the Developmental Course of Schizophrenia. Annual Review of Clinical Psychology 4(1):189–216.

POST-TRAUMATIC STRESS DISORDER AND NEUROANTHROPOLOGY: STOPPING PTSD BEFORE IT BEGINS

GINO L. COLLURA

DANIEL H. LENDE
University of South Florida

Post-traumatic stress disorder (PTSD) is a problem that affects many combatants in war, including a high percentage of military personnel serving in Iraq and Afghanistan. The high rates of PTSD among veterans has pushed research and intervention to address the serious mental and behavioral health problems associated with wartime trauma. However, these efforts have largely proceeded using biomedical and psychological approaches, without recognizing the institutional and social contexts of trauma, adaptation, and recovery. Moreover, biomedical and psychological approaches have serious shortcomings in recognizing how individual–environment interactions, meaningful interpretations, and sense of identity play a key role in the impact of trauma and development (or not) of PTSD. A neuroanthropological approach can use ideas of neural plasticity and the encultured brain to link culture, interpretation and identity, and the impact of trauma. This synthetic approach then permits a critique of present efforts in the U.S. military to increase resilience and prevent PTSD, and propose alternative strategies and research approaches to more effectively understand and address PTSD. [trauma, adversity, PTSD, military, combative culture, neuroanthropology]

NEUROANTHROPOLOGY, TRAUMA, AND COMBAT

Neuroanthropology combines cultural formations, biocultural responses, and neuroscience, which together serve to formulate a "big picture" of stress and trauma. This unique formulation of perspectives offers the proactive ability to recognize certain cultural formations that can increase the impact of trauma, hasten the development of post-traumatic stress disorder (PTSD), and worsen outcomes. People in combat zones, as well as people who engage in hazardous and life-threatening service such as first-line responders in emergency zones, experience higher rates of PTSD (Perkinogg et al. 2001; Sundin et al. 2010), and there is a critical need to understand how the interpretation of stress and adversity play into the development and alleviation of trauma. We argue that providing the tools to recognize and manage cultural constructions of stress and to draw on sources of personal identity and resilience offers the key to helping soldiers deal with trauma during and after military service. Alleviating the destruction and suffering caused by PTSD is the humanitarian goal that inspires this research.

ANNALS OF ANTHROPOLOGICAL PRACTICE 36, pp. 131–148. ISSN: 2153-957X. © 2012 by the American Anthropological Association. DOI:10.1111/j.2153-9588.2012.01096.x

The wars in both Iraq and Afghanistan have been catalysts for staggering levels of PTSD among U.S. troops. Currently, it is estimated that over 31 percent of U.S. military personnel are returning from deployment with the disorder (Sundin et al. 2010). Typically, most soldiers that face trauma on the battlefield are resilient and only suffer minor setbacks of mental distress before being able to "bounce back" into a functional role within the military or while reassimilating into civilian life (Bonanno et al. 2011). Yet, some develop PTSD and are diagnosed through criteria that include increased hypervigilance, uncontrollable outbursts of anger, inability to concentrate, recurrent visions or dreams about events experienced, sporadic sleeping patterns, and disabilities in acculturating with other members of society (Turnbull 1998).

Since the onset of both "Operation Iraqi Freedom" (OIF) and "Operation Enduring Freedom" (OEF), psychiatrists, psychologists, and other medical personnel have been searching for ways to respond to the increased prevalence of PTSD. The remedies developed have been largely reactive, seeking to diminish the lasting effects of PTSD postdeployment. Much less attention has been paid to developing a proactive, predeployment approach that examines how different service members negotiate adversity, stress, and trauma. In maintaining this institutional approach that addresses trauma after the fact, the military has neglected how to prepare its members for the adversity they will almost inevitably face during deployment.

This neglect is not because of a lack of recognition. PTSD has been given many names throughout history, including soldier's heart, cardiac weakness, traumatic shock, traumatic neurosis, nervous shock, shell shock, neurocirculatory asthenia, war psychoneurosis, battle fatigue, combat exhaustion, and, most recently, PTSD (Turnbull 1998; Young 1995).

In the face of a "stressor," individuals who subsequently develop PTSD often feel intense fear, helplessness, or horror, as indicated in the Diagnostic and Statistical Manual (DSM-IV-TR; American Psychiatric Association 2000). But this "event plus emotion" model is not adequate. First, the reaction to stress is framed largely in individual terms— people who become afraid or shocked by what they experienced. This approach leaves out the institutional forces that place individuals in harm's way. Second, an event-focused approach leaves out much of what we know about stress from both neuroscience and anthropology. Stressors that are uncontrollable and unpredictable—that individuals can do little to change and that can happen at any time—are worse than stressors that come at regular intervals and that can be moderated by an organism's behavior. Moreover, horror and fear are not just reactions to immediate physical threats, but also meaningful reactions—losing a unit member or seeing a child killed in combat is not the same as seeing an enemy combatant killed. We use systems of meaning to try to make sense of these terrible events, to say sacrifices were worth it or death is part of war. But oftentimes these justifications are not adequate. This disjuncture, where the senselessness and helplessness of an event are magnified, has a direct impact on individuals' ability to cope with trauma.

However, clinicians have transformed PTSD into a psychiatric disorder that is largely medicalized (Young 1995). In other words, reactions to trauma are defined almost exclusively in psychobiological terms—arousal, avoidance, and repetition. However, individuals who face trauma, particularly combat, develop altered understandings of themselves and their lives (Finley 2011; Hinton and Lewis-Fernandez 2010; Kienzler 2008; Polusny et al. 2011). Issues of reacculturation, familial integration, social awareness, substance abuse, depression, violent tendencies with loved ones, and the inability to express their traumatic experiences have lasting consequences, which not only affect the health of the soldier but also the family and friends of the soldier.

In anthropological terms, PTSD has a cascade of effects that create behavioral and social dynamics, which can increase, or decrease, the impact of trauma, hypervigilance, and arousal over time (Finley 2012). How these effects play out for the individual soldier and his or her spouse are important to take into consideration, especially when children are within the household and bear witness to it. For example, Sayers and colleagues (2009) showed that soldiers returning from either Afghanistan or Iraq showed a 60 percent increase in domestic abuse since returning from deployment, and 53.7 percent of the study population experienced some sort of shouting, pushing, or shoving with their partner after returning from a combative theater. Exposure to such events has the possibility of fostering "Second Hand PTSD" in which children are exposed to traumatic environments (Arzi et al. 2000). Furthermore, an alarming number of soldiers are becoming addicted to alcohol, drugs, and prescription medications after developing PTSD (Bray et al. 2010). The use of antianxiety and antidepressant medications (i.e., Paxil or Zoloft), often given by the Veterans Administration, is common among soldiers who have been diagnosed with PTSD (Bray et al. 2010). Such medications serve largely as a temporary band aid and have fostered an "assembly line" approach in treating PTSD symptoms and perpetuate addiction behaviors.

UNDERSTANDING PTSD: DISORDERED MACHINE OR ENCULTURED BRAIN?

The "encultured brain" is a core concept in neuroanthropology, referencing how our brains develop within a cultural milieu, shaping neural structure and function over the lifespan. This approach provides a framing for understanding how cultural experience can get under the skin, and increase vulnerability to stress and trauma. This view contrasts with a common paradigm in both cognitive science and clinical practice that approaches human neural function as essentially having the same processes as modern technology such as computers. For example, clinicians often apply a universal approach to understanding mental health issues in combat and trauma (Kienzler 2008); this approach further emphasizes an "assembly line" style of medical treatment. This type of functional view emphasizes cause-effect models of trauma, hardware–software dichotomies about the brain and mind, and treatment approaches emphasizing pharmaceuticals and standardized clinical care. In the mind-as-technology view, human experience and function can be broken down into component parts that can be isolated and fixed, with little attention paid to ethnographic inquiry and the complexities of the human condition.

Neuroanthropology, in contrast, emphasizes the importance of actually understanding how trauma, stress, and adversity are experienced and interpreted before, during, and after combat, because this interpretation matters at the neural level. In this approach, cognition is not a content-free process, simply running on whatever neural processor is installed and with whatever environmental input is provided. The idea that human beings "process" information and have the ability to "download" ideas is not an accurate model that serves our unique ability to interpret our environment. The importance of culture, meaning making, and institutional identities reflect the ways in which interpretation is played out and ultimately the effect that it has on the perspective set forth by each individual when faced with adversity.

FACING ADVERSITY: THE COMPREHENSIVE SOLDIER FITNESS APPROACH

Recently, the U.S. military has created a thrust toward a more "resilient" army. This concept of resilience and the ability to maintain a positive outlook throughout adverse conditions has gained a lot of recognition within clinical psychology and is being adopted as official military practice within the U.S. Army. The army has implemented a program entitled "Comprehensive Soldier Fitness" (CSF), designed principally by Dr. Martin Seligman from the University of Pennsylvania's Positive Psychology Center. The program seeks to lower PTSD, increase resilience, and augment the number of military personnel "who grow" after experiencing some sort of adversity on the battlefield (Seligman and Fowler 2011). The program looks at emotional, social, family, spiritual, and physical domains of influence on a soldier's resiliency; resiliency is defined as the ability for a soldier to adapt swiftly to adversity, stress, and combative trauma (Ballenger-Browning and Johnson 2010). The program, instituted across the U.S. Army, is still in its infancy. The long-term results are not yet known, although preliminary results show a decrease in the severity of anxiety related disorders and a somewhat better assimilation process stateside in a small percentage of participants (Gottman et al. 2011).

CSF utilizes the Global Assessment Tool (GAT) to track and monitor the resilience of soldiers while both stateside and deployed. The GAT contains 105 computer-based questions that evaluate what the army considers to be the five pillars of fitness: family fitness, spiritual fitness, emotional fitness, social fitness, and physical fitness (U.S. Army Comprehensive Soldier Fitness 2011). It is taken once every 90 days and is thought to expose areas where improvement can be made to one's resilience through enhanced training techniques in areas of character that are thought to be "malleable" (U.S. Army Comprehensive Soldier Fitness 2011). Overall, the GAT presents generalized assessments derived from concepts used within psychology, often with an individual and internal focus and without a specific assessment of the demands and strengths related to military life and deployment. Furthermore, as Peterson and colleagues (2011:16) acknowledge, the GAT only assesses "at ease psychosocial fitness. The real challenge of fitness is during challenge and crisis and would require . . . measuring a soldier's assets in actual use."

Deployment, from combat trauma to the everyday grind of service in an active war, to dislocation from family at home and local communities, changes the ways in which soldiers view themselves as well as their relationship with the world (Brewin et al. 2010; Finley 2011). CSF only takes a "snapshot" of soldiers' mental health. Subjective self-assessment in front of a computer does not represent an accurate means to assess inevitable changes during soldiers' service, particularly when in an active war zone. Moreover, the CSF program does not examine who these men and women were before they entered the armed forces and what social, cultural, emotional, and religious (if any) influences persuaded them to want to serve in the military, and how that might affect their ability to adapt to present circumstances and potential trauma.

PTSD AND WORKING WITH SOLDIERS

Using neuroanthropology to address the current challenge of high PTSD rates in the military could bear a significant amount of fruit. Utilizing ethnographic methods from anthropology, recognizing the need for enhanced qualitative and quantitative assessments, and introducing the importance of biocultural consequences owing to varying personnel background offer new opportunities to address the prevention of PTSD. However, it is important to recognize that applied work takes on ethical considerations beyond those involved in the typical protection of human subjects. Doing research with the military has the potential for complicity and cooptation of research to unintended ends (Gusterson 2007). Critical perspectives can work to question how the military engages with anthropologists and other social scientists, and the ways in which they use research for political and institutional ends, which might not align with soldiers' interests and certainly not with the interests of the many different parties involved in a war zone (Gusterson 2007; Rylko-Bauer and Singer 2011). For example, the military might establish "acceptable risks" for personnel with regard to exposure to trauma and who is vulnerable to PTSD, in ways that contrast with research findings or the views of the soldiers actually facing those risks. Research within an institution like the U.S. military requires this sort of critical positioning of the researcher, and a clear sense of the ethical goals at the center of the research (Rylko-Bauer and Singer 2011). For us, our main motivation in doing this research is the social and personal suffering of veterans returning from war, and the belief that a preventive approach can reduce that suffering by helping lower the rates of PTSD among veterans and improve the quality of their lives as well as the lives of their family and friends.

THE NEUROANTHROPOLOGY OF PTSD

Culture and PTSD

Culture matters in PTSD, from resources that foster social and emotional support to interpretations of symptoms and how to make sense of trauma. Sources of emotional and social support have been linked to positive adjustment following disasters and other traumatic events (Bonanno et al. 2011). Similarly, organizational and economic resources make a difference in how stressful events are interpreted, as something controllable or as something threatening and disruptive (Hobfoll 2002; Miller and Rasmussen 2010).

These sources of support and subjective interpretations emerge from cultural and social dynamics (Finley 2012; Panter-Brick and Eggerman 2011). Institutional constructions of "right" and "wrong" as well as the ability to make sense of different cultures and "acceptable" interpretations of combat all play a role in soldiers' interpretations of what happens to them, their comrades, and enemy combatants (Burnell et al. 2011). As Brewin (2011) shows, the memory disturbances associated with PTSD are shaped by negative appraisals of self and negative interpretations of memory symptoms; in turn, emotions like shame and interpretive frameworks work through sociocultural dynamics (Budden 2009; Finley 2012; Hinton and Lewis-Fernandez 2010).

These types of internalized cultural structures, and their relationship to military policy, are important factors in soldiers' take on adversity. The military can both help and hinder acquiring the support and understanding that prove a necessary buffer to adversities faced while deployed. Panter-Brick and Eggerman (2011) highlight how deep rooted cultural understandings of stress are always "in play," and in the context of deployed soldiers, will generally be more important for understanding combat functionality than the military training that service members go through predeployment. The training experienced within boot camp and soldier's subsequent MOS training (their job or occupation within the Army or Marines) often do not have the same influence as the constructed cultural views of trauma, stress, and adversity that military personnel have acquired while growing up.

Cultural models and interpretations acquired in childhood and adolescence frame the ways that individual soldiers interpret combat and adversity and serve as a cipher of how and why some individuals can cope with trauma and combat and some cannot (Hinton and Lewis-Fernandez 2010; Panter-Brick and Eggerman 2011). This point establishes the importance of looking at multiple cultural spheres as influential forces in the development and functionality of soldiers on the battlefield, including recognizing them as people outside the military and embracing the idea that they are not just "GIs." Being thought of as only a soldier with a specific function in combat may serve the military mission at a critical moment, but the aftereffects of trauma can last a lifetime unless the soldier can make some sense of his or her combative actions and losses endured.

This cultural view needs to be augmented by a consideration of the socioeconomic diversity of people coming into the armed forces. A large majority of U.S. recruits come from a low socioeconomic status (Kleykamp 2006). These recruits do not have any other means of going to college and have typically dealt with ranging levels of adversity because of the economic disadvantages that have surrounded them (Kleykamp 2006). This type of economic adversity leaves the military as a last resort option in which young men and women seek to receive education funding via the Montgomery GI Bill. The decision to enlist as a last resort alternative because of economic hardship creates a sense of forced military service in which deep-rooted motives such as patriotism, honor, sense of duty, and an overall true excitement about volunteering for service in a time of war can be artificially present. Such words to describe military service are often seen advertised in low socioeconomic environments as a means of recruitment and enticement for young men and women. Yet, the motives for joining are often fueled by the desire for military benefits; a sense of personal pride and recognition; as well as the constructed and often romanticized view of being a war hero.

Finley (2011), in her ethnography of veterans struggling with PTSD on their return from Iraq and Afghanistan, highlights the adaptive qualities that humans possess that enable them to function in differing environments. These qualities include possessing a sense of service to others as well as increasing social capital postdeployment, and yet go awry in veterans who seek to isolate themselves from others and lack the ability to speak about the overall impact that combative trauma has had on their personal lives. The contrast between civilian life expectations and living a life of war is immense. Recognizing the need for GIs to be with individuals who care and are willing to listen to them reaffirms the positive outcomes that are associated with smooth transitioning between the two identities. The separation and differing expectations between civil society and military combative culture leaves room for confusion that is not navigated easily and almost always calls for strong support systems as a means of reaffirmation of servitude, duty, and justification for trauma suffered.

Dislocation is a central analytical construct in Finley's research (2011, 2012). PTSD is marked by the physical and psychological sense of dislocation; for combat veterans, both the camaraderie with other soldiers and the sense of the person they once were before war are gone. Together, these jarring changes feed into a sense of dislocation in which they feel they are different from others and cannot connect interpersonally. For Finley, forms of treatment, rituals of memory, webs of relationships and social support, and understandings of what trauma means shape veterans' attempts at making sense of trauma and coping with PTSD.

This ethnographic research highlights the social component of camaraderie and why it is that service members are known to suffer PTSD from enduring the loss of a fellow soldier, although they may have only known their comrade for a short amount of time. It is the strength of social interactions and what soldiers mean to one another, which buttress the ways that soldiers interpret what is going on within the battlefield. These intense relationships and forms of interpreting adversity carry over into civilian life once returning from deployment, and can create difficult situations when trying to adjust back to social norms. No longer are these service members faced with imminent danger; there are no improvised explosive devices (IEDs) lurking underneath a piece of pavement, Taliban snipers waiting to take a fatal shot, or the sound of incoming mortar fire. Rather, soldiers are surrounded with domestic issues (paying the bills, becoming employed, communicating emotions with loved ones), and are expected to deal with such issues with ease and confidence, as if they were never deployed to a combat zone for well over a year.

Identity

Identity matters in PTSD. As Berntsen and Rubin (2007) show, the degree to which traumatic memory forms a part of one's personal identity is directly correlated with the severity of PTSD symptoms, even when controlling for mental health problems like depression and anxiety. Furthermore, Jobson and O'Kearney (2008) shows cultural differences in identity that are linked to PTSD through interpretive frames, for example, how self is defined in relation to others and to culturally important goals. Anthropological research has established that for some combat personnel, fostering an identity as "indestructible" or as "Rambo" (as taught in boot camp) can create an identity crisis when faced with trauma and interpreting combat and loss (Finley 2011). This crisis can provoke or worsen mental health issues such as depression, substance abuse, PTSD, domestic violence, and suicide. What needs to be focused on within future resiliency training paradigms is the balance of cultural identities within the service member population. This issue of identity formation requires a closer look into the cultural constructs that are responsible for what stress and trauma mean to each individual soldier.

The cultural influences that young men and women have before going into the military help shape multiple facets to their identity. From the time a young man or young woman approaches a recruiter of the armed forces, they have a culturally constructed meaning of what serving in the military signifies. Through mass marketing campaigns and consistent exposure to governmental influences of how "glorious" military service is, many of these individuals develop a fantasy of military culture and the rewards that combat can bring. These influences are cultural constructs that are not only practiced on a daily basis but also are emphasized by recruiters, politicians, and segments of the U.S. population. They are wooed by the college incentive programs of enlisting, the benefits of a steady paycheck, and the opportunity of international travel. They are exposed to video games and movies that glorify the battlefield as a place of action and excitement, and imagine the characters of such entertainment as themselves operating as a hero as well as a person to be admired. Finally, they are encouraged to be an "Army of One," "Army Strong," "All That You Can Be," "A Global Force For Good," or "The Few. The Proud," all service mottos that have cultural interpretations of pride, honor, and servitude.

This cultural construction clashes with the realities of war once these young recruits enter into a theater of operation. Video games and mottos do not accurately depict the true nature of the combative military experience. Resources that might be drawn on to make sense of these experiences are often limited. From the military point of view, there is little room for the clashing of identities or the confusion of what one's place is on the battlefield. Nevertheless, this sort of clash and confusion inevitably happens.

When soldiers are initially trained to do things the "Army way" in boot camp, they are not allowed to build on their own identity as a person outside the military. This neglect can help foster disassociation (Seligman and Kirmayer 2008) and dislocation (Finley 2012), given that the identity and interpretations of an individual cannot be erased in a ten week period. There are tentacles of associations between their identity as a soldier and their identity as a son, daughter, mother, father, brother, sister, friend, and so forth. These associations attach meaning, and become essential when dealing with the vivid presence of death, violence, and dislocation. These expectations about combat and being a soldier, as well as how and even if to maintain a civilian identity, shape how service members interpret the loss, trauma, and adversity they meet once hitting the battlefield.

The contrast between what one thought the battlefield would be like and what it actually is can help produce disjunctures of identity and meaning making and foster soldier dysfunction. This dysfunction in turn can lead to increased levels of adversity for the individual, his or her comrades, and thus increase potential problems for entire units. Soldiers need to know that their loss and adversity mean something (Burnell et al. 2011). They need to feel and be defined by the fact that getting shot, blown up by an IED, or suffering the loss of their best friend in combat has meaning to it. Their ability to define meaning is correlated to their cultural understanding of honor, pride, and sacrifice. This sense of honor and sacrifice exist in contrast to horror and fear, two key components of initial reactions to trauma that can drive the development of PTSD (Finley 2012). We propose that as soldiers' ability to relate these positive meanings to traumatic experiences on the battlefield suffers a disjuncture, the possibility for PTSD can increase. This neuroanthropological view builds on research that shows that the feeling of loss and not having control of their environment causes a sense of distrust in their surroundings and is known to further increase symptoms of the disorder (Johnson et al. 2011).

The ability to "make sense" of adversity, trauma, sufferance, and loss in combat makes a large difference in how a soldier is going to deal with the inevitable flashbacks and memories after returning from deployment. This interpretive strength allows for a "big picture" to be formed and can help prevent the soldier from being defined by the trauma lived in combat. In making cultural connections with their unit members, Afghani and Iraqi citizens (combatants and noncombatants), family members, friends, as well as their surrounding environments, they will be able to maintain an image of why it is they are doing what they are doing and faced with such adversity on the battlefield.

Culturally specific understandings of trauma, idioms of distress, and the interpretation of trauma-caused symptoms all play a role in reactions to trauma (Hinton and Lewis-Fernandez 2010, 2011; Zur 1996). During deployment, interpretations of war will differ from one soldier to another. For example, if two soldiers are involved in a firefight and are side by side throughout the duration of the engagement, the story of significance that one soldier gives will not be the same exact story of significance that the other soldier gives. Because of differing cultural backgrounds and interpretations of death, killing, previous violence experienced (both within the military as well as a civilian), and motivational factors for voluntary military service, the events lived within that firefight will resonate with different meanings. The idea that an enemy force is actually trying to kill them and their need to respond with such violence of action will have an altering affect in how each soldier describes what took place post engagement. If one soldier had multiple deployments under his belt and had been involved with multiple past firefights over a nine year span, and the other soldier was a first year service member and had never been in a firefight but had been exposed to gang violence and shootings as a civilian, the ways in which they negotiate and describe the transpired events will differ.

These cultural understandings of one's self and one's relationship to his or her environment can depend on age, experience, and maturity. Such maturity is reflected in how individuals handle adversity and combative stress. Many times, this is reflected by life experience, which normally equates to age. According to the National Center for PTSD, veterans from ages 18 to 24 years faced the greatest risk for receiving mental health or PTSD diagnoses in a study of 103,788 veterans returning from deployment in Iraq and Afghanistan (Litz and Schlenger 2009). Neuroanthropology explains such differentiation via the cultural awareness and environmental understanding that the 18–24-year-old age group has versus those who are older. Establishing a soldiers' cognitive understanding of their surroundings and the institutional constructs that convinced them to go to war is of paramount importance in establishing greater resilience. Being grounded and culturally affluent with one's self outside adversity as well as predeployment is an important way for soldiers to not feel overwhelmed, and allows them to keep trauma and adversity on the battlefield "in check" with the big picture of their complete identity.

Neural Dynamics and PTSD

Previous research has established the close links between the meaning of specific acts and experiences and neural function, for example, in the salience of drug use or the impact of dissociative experience (Lende 2005; Seligman and Kirmayer 2008). Recent neuroanthropological work on memory and knowledge traditions highlights how different medical knowledge practices can drive differential use and organization of memory systems in the brain (Hay 2012). Neuroscience research also shows that established memories can become labile when they are retrieved or reactivated, with subsequent consolidation shaped by the present context and use of the memory (Inda et al. 2011; Schiller and Phelps 2011). Together, this research on memory highlights the strong possibility that memory-related aspects of identity rely both on cultural traditions and present uses, shaping the consolidation and activation of basic memory processes in the brain. This framework shows how soldiers' lives during deployment will shape how they interpret trauma, from forming invasive memories to fitting experiences into a "big picture" of what trauma means.

Identity is not only related to memory but also to self. The neural correlates of self are found in the midline structures of the brain, including the anterior cingulate, insula, and prefrontal cortex (Medford and Critchley 2010; Modinos et al. 2009; Qin and Northoff 2011). In relation to our discussion of dissociation and dislocation above, the point by Qin and Northoff (2011:1221) on how self emerges in the relation between default-mode functioning and present engagement is particularly pertinent: "our data suggest that our sense of self may result from a specific kind of interaction between resting state activity and stimulus-induced activity." Dislocations in self, in particular between more resting state and consolidated aspects of self and present challenges to self (such as caused by threats to life or to core aspects of personal meaning), can emerge through these interactions in ways that potentiate the impact of trauma on encultured individuals.

Finally, biocultural connections exist between the interpretation of trauma and how different individuals embody adversity (Kirmayer et al. 2007). Varying allostatic loads and epigenetic modifications can play a significant role in the dysregulation of the hypothalamus–pituitary–adrenal axis (HPA axis; see Yehuda and Bierer 2009), one of the primary systems mediating reactions to stress and trauma. This HPA dysregulation has been linked in part to the 5-HTT (serotonin transporter) gene, which promotes the development of the human stress response system (Gross and Hen 2004). Serotonin matters because the neurotransmitter works as a modulator of emotions and of stress-response hormones in the amygdala (Wang et al. 2011). Allele length variance of the 5-HTT gene is directly linked with an increase in amygdala activity when humans are put in moments of anxiety; this has been linked with greater susceptibility to the development of PTSD (Gross and Hen 2004). These differences can shape how people react to and interpret trauma; for example, experiencing greater or lesser amounts of anxiety will color what a particular event means to a person.

These aspects of neural function play a significant role in the impact of trauma and the overall development of PTSD. As Finley (2012) argues, there is a rewiring of responses to stress and fear in individuals who spend extended periods of time at war, with increases in vigilance and decreased reaction time and an emphasis on less cognitive processing in situations perceived as threatening. This response pattern demonstrates cultural priming, where previous learned experiences provide an instant interpretive frame for stress and trauma, both in the immediate aftermath and over the long term. Using this approach, Finley (2012) reinterprets the core diagnostic features of PTSD—hyperarousal, reexperiencing, and avoidance—through a model of neuroanthropological stress framed by the horror, dislocation, and grief that veterans experience through war.

In sum, the comprehensive lens that is offered through neuroanthropology allows us to connect the psychobiological components of reactions to trauma to individual experiences and interpretations that develop within specific cultural environments and are shaped by local institutional dynamics. This approach also paves the way for applied anthropological research to begin making recommendations for dealing with PTSD in a proactive manner.

HANDLING ADVERSITY AND APPLIED NEUROANTHROPOLOGY

Instead of adopting a uniform interpretation of stress and resiliency, the approach presented here argues that soldiers need to develop and utilize their own interpretations of the stresses of deployment, including combat. Soldiers need a balanced identity that can incorporate their previous cultural background, their present service, and the organizational values of the armed forces. Furthermore, these two elements—interpretation and identity—are not isolated themselves; individuals function within specific units, which can have varying assigned missions, access to resources, and cohesion. In creating an environment to handle adversity, greater resilience can be attained through shared world views and social reinforcement (Eggerman and Panter-Brick 2010). Fostering hope and the ability to push through adverse situations helps support the men and women in the unit, and are elements that can help the group deal with losses. In this way, having an ability to make sense of actions and events is not just an internalized resource; interpretation happens between people and depends on available social and cultural resources.

Utilizing neuroanthropology creates an applicable and flexible way to take on PTSD proactively. Identifying the role of earlier cultural domains on subsequent interpretations of deployment, the potential force of institutionally constructed meanings during military service, and the role of identity as a form of resilience in PTSD are all largely missing from the explicit methods and theories employed by the U.S. military and most clinicians. Complementing the snapshot that programs like CSF offers soldiers at a specific time within their service with a solid understanding of who they are prior to enlistment can buttress the way in which soldiers interpret the trauma and adversity they face. Showing soldiers how to identify their own reasons for experiencing stress based on their identity outside of their institutionalized role can create a more mature soldier that could have the tools to negotiate the traumas of war.

By establishing a greater synergy between different domains of identity, soldiers should be more resilient to the dislocations caused by trauma and have a greater ability to make sense of stress and adversity. The next question becomes, how? We believe that focusing on an applied strategy that addresses the conjunction of identity and vulnerability, and the need for interpretive reminders in the face of inevitable dislocations, offers a potential answer. One idea that arises from the conjunction of sense of identity and vulnerability to PTSD is to develop an identity card that reflects their overall cultural identity, rather than a more limited institutional identity.

This concept is a simple one—capture important social roles, formative experiences, and personally relevant symbols and represent them on an encultured identity map for the individual soldier. Service members would create a small poster (e.g., small enough to fit inside their body armor) that would have reminders of their civilian life back home and of important social experiences and cultural values for the soldier. This reminder of the many cultural influences that make them a person will allow the soldier to not lose sight of who they are and why it is they are facing the trauma and adversity that surrounds them in theater. Furthermore, these cards give moments of hope as to what is waiting for them once they leave combat and serve as reminders of their holistic identity and pillars of meaning that construct their interpretations of combat and embodied trauma.

Historically, the military has utilized the "battle buddy system" which pairs two soldiers together to watch out for one another (Lorge 2008). This system was modified in a response to rising suicide rates shortly after Operation Iraqi Freedom (OIF) as well as Operation Enduring Freedom (OEF) sparked off. Using a combination of anthropology, psychotherapy, and education, a program might be built to help instruct soldiers on ways to enhance their interpersonal communication, listening skills, and other forms of basic cultural analysis beyond their assigned "battle buddy." This idea represents a longer-term project, with the basic premise that creating stronger communicative bonds between military personnel will help augment resilience. A consistent level of exposure to interpersonal communication and listening skills might allow for soldiers to become more culturally aware of all their fellow comrades, and consequently themselves. In sharing consistent interpretations of stress and adversity, tighter cultural bonds would hopefully be formed, resulting in a more cohesive unit that can execute their assigned tasks while also dealing with stress and adversity.

By implementing interventions that are rooted in meaningful interpretations (such as the two recommended here, among others), soldiers can potentially have the ability to foster a sense of heightened awareness to themselves and one another. Such ability could possibly be the beginnings of providing more consistent peer evaluation of each other's capacity to negotiate stress and handle consistent combative engagements that perpetuate PTSD.

RESEARCH METHODS OF NEUROANTHROPOLOGY

Research on PTSD in the military has highlighted the need for better understanding of what happens when soldiers are deployed (Peterson et al. 2011). Anthropology, with its emphasis on field-based research and the documenting of lived experience, offers a robust approach to examine how military personnel deal with war, including the wounds of war that come with trauma, overwhelming adversity, and a sense of dislocation. There is an urgent need for this type of research, and here we provide an overview of how such research can be carried out. An ideal approach would begin with participant-observation within military organizational culture, and includes studying and observing individuals preenlistment, while on duty, post trauma, and during the reintegration into society.

A mixed methods approach during deployment is especially important for examining stress, adversity, and resilience. Researchers can identify initial understandings that soldiers have of combat and monitor levels of stress and resilience through peer interactions, soldier self-description, and biological measures like cortisol. Such neuroanthropological research could provide the means to identify those cultural experiences and interpretations that lend themselves to the development of PTSD. Whether it is the cultural construction of false expectations of combat, the repeated exposure of traumatic events prior to enlistment, the lack of "malleable" socioemotional skills that make navigating stress more challenging, or the identification of biological predispositions that can attribute to the development of PTSD, a neuroanthropology framework offers the means to link these factors to what is happening to soldiers on the ground.

Open-ended interviews would allow individual soldiers to present their ideas of who they are, where they stand in the "big picture" of combat, and understanding the methods they use to make sense of trauma and adversity will help show how they have been conditioned based on cultural influences. When conducted on a unit level, focus group interviews could identify specific cultural interpretations as well as underlying models that serve as pillars of representation in specific units. Biomarkers, such as cortisol and salivary alpha amylase, could provide physiological indicators of stress during deployment, and be linked to epidemiological and qualitative assessments of stress and resilience. Both cortisol measurements and salivary alpha amylase give independent indicators of stress, which provide insight into events that are interpreted as stressful or an altered state of homeostasis in which stress levels are consistently increased in "controlled" environments. Combining these methods can provide a necessary qualitative and quantitative intersection of understanding ways in which to negotiate trauma and foster resilience.

Identifying the sources of strengths and ways in which soldiers negotiate the trauma as well as adversity around them has yet to be addressed and calls for the perspective that neuroanthropology readily offers. Research on the concept of strengths, generally conceived in a psychological sense, has grown over the past decade. Bartone (1999) showed how "hardiness" can be understood as a set of personal characteristics that is linked to resilience in the face of combat exposure and trauma in troops in the first Gulf War. Bartone describes hardiness as commitment to life and work, a greater sense of control over life, an acceptance of stressful and painful experience as part of living, and more openness to change and challenges. Peterson and colleagues (Park et al. 2004; Peterson et al. 2008) examined a more comprehensive inventory of strengths that indicated that traits like hope, zest, curiosity, creativity, and bravery were linked to life satisfaction and coping with trauma. Three types of factors stood out: (1) learning and creativity, (2) persistence and hope, and (3) positive emotions like kindness and zest. Furthermore, trait resilience—"seeing the positive side of a bad situation"—recognizes that resilient individuals are often characterized by being committed to what they are doing, feeling in control of problems, and approaching difficult situations as an opportunity to master new challenges, rather than threats that must be endured (Ong et al. 2010).

This important research, however, has not examined specific strengths in military personnel, nor connected with the sort of on-the-ground qualitative insight anthropology can provide. Moreover, the implicit description of resilient versus nonresilient individuals ignores the natural heterogeneity in people, and does not ask the crucial question, how do these individuals actually accomplish being resilient? What strategies do they rely on? What resources do they draw on? How do they try to avoid negative outcomes? Qualitative research, as outlined above, can answer these questions in a broad sense. To specifically examine how these qualities might make a difference over deployment requires the development of quantitative assessments that can be track reactions to adversity and variations in interpretation and resilience. At present, there are both general measures of deployment risk and resilience (King et al. 2006) and psychological resilience (Connor and Davidson 2003; Johnson et al. 2011; Peterson et al. 2011). The development of novel scales offers the potential to complement these current resiliency measures by measuring the specific strengths of service members and other personnel serving in combat zones, as well as take into account sources of identity predeployment.

By combining qualitative and quantitative methods, neuroanthropological research can produce an overall picture of resiliency and strength. By working with military personnel before, during, and after deployment, such research could identify the strengths that soldiers have that heighten their ability to handle their duties and assignments while adapting effectively to life in a combat situation in a foreign theater. Alongside individual strengths, neuroanthropological research can examine the sources of strength that buttress service members' ability to cope. Unit morale, positive experiences with other soldiers, effective communication with loved ones at home, and other factors can make a major difference in dealing with adversity and trauma. By developing a clear understanding of strengths and sources of strength, such research could provide keen insight into specific training modalities to foster a proactive approach in dealing with adversity and trauma.

CONCLUSION

Utilizing neuroanthropology to guide the ways in which soldiers interpret adversity, trauma, and stress is going to be of vital importance as young recruits begin new careers in the military and soldiers continue to return from deployment suffering from the wounds of war. The goal of using neuroanthropology is to prevent and understand PTSD. The approach developed here seeks to enhance the manner in which health professionals address the disorder as well as the ways in which recruits are trained to interpret their surroundings, their sense of identity, and their reactions to trauma. No longer are the days when fresh military recruits are taught to keep their emotions bottled up and to "take it like a man." We have seen the product of such training and the long-term effects of creating a military trained in this manner. It is time that we tap into a new approach that takes seriously the connections between cultural interpretations, individual development and change, and neural function. The bridge that neuroanthropology provides between war and trauma and the social understanding of such events does not exist within any other academic discipline. Neuroanthropology aims to find which sociocultural factors shape the interpretations of stress and the biocultural consequences associated with military service. Yet, such an endeavor is going to require an interdisciplinary approach from all healthcare professionals and the ability to be open to one another's criticisms and critiques. This in itself requires researchers and professionals to have a sense of plasticity and cultural understanding of one another so that we can further our quest to improve the lives of our fellow human beings.

REFERENCES CITED

American Psychiatric Association
  2000 Diagnostic and Statistical Manual of Mental Disorders (4th edition, rev.) Washington, DC: American Psychiatric Association.
Arzi, Nir, Zahava Solomon, and Rachel Dekel
  2000 Secondary Traumatization among Wives of PTSD and Post-Concussion Casualties: Distress, Caregiver Burden and Psychological Separation. Brain Injury 14(8):725–736.
Ballenger-Browning, Kara, and Douglas Johnson
  2010 Key Facts on Resilience. Naval Center for Combat and Operational Stress Control. http://www.med.navy.mil/sites/nmcsd/nccosc/healthProfessionals/Documents/Resilience%20TWP%20formatted.pdf, accessed October 7, 2011.
Bartone, Paul
  1999 Hardiness Protects against War-Related Stress in Army Reserve Forces. Consulting Psychology Journal: Practice and Research 51(2):72–82.
Berntsen, Dorthe, and David Rubin
  2007 When a Trauma Becomes a Key to Identity: Enhanced Integration of Trauma Memories Predicts Posttraumatic Stress Disorder Symptoms. Applied Cognitive Psychology 21(4):417–431.
Bonanno, George, Maren Westphal, and Anthony Mancini
  2011 Resilience to Loss and Potential Trauma. Annual Review of Clinical Psychology 7(1):1–1.25.
Bray, Robert, Michael Pemberton, Marian Lane, Laurel Hourani, Mark Mattiko, and Lorraine Babeau
  2010 Substance Use and Mental Health Trends Among U.S. Military Active Duty Personnel: Key Findings From the 2008 DoD Health Behavior Survey. Military Medicine 175(6):390–399.

Brewin, Chris

    2011 The Nature and Significance of Memory Disturbance in Posttraumatic Stress Disorder. Annual Review of Clinical Psychology 7:203–227.

Brewin, Chris, Roman Garnett, and Bernice Andrews

    2010 Trauma, Identity, and Mental Health in UK Military Veterans. Psychological Medicine 41:1733–1740.

Budden, Ashwin

    2009 The Role of Shame in Posttraumatic Stress Disorder: A Proposal for a Socio-Emotional Model for DSM-V. Social Science and Medicine 69(7):1032–1039.

Burnell, Karen, Niall Boyce, and Nigel Hunt

    2011 A Good War? Exploring British Veterans' Moral Evaluation of Deployment. Journal of Anxiety Disorders 25(1):36–42.

Connor, Kathryn, and Jonathan Davidson

    2003 Development of a New Resilience Scale: The Connor-Davidson Resilience Scale (CD-RISC). Depression and Anxiety 18(2):76–82.

Eggerman, Mark, and Catherine Panter-Brick

    2010 Suffering, Hope, and Entrapment: Resilience and Cultural Values in Afghanistan. Social Science and Medicine 71(1):71–83.

Finley, Erin

    2011 Fields of Combat: Understanding PTSD among Veterans of Iraq and Afghanistan. Ithaca, NY: Cornell University Press.

    2012 War and Dislocation: A Neuroanthropological Model of Trauma among American Veterans with Combat PTSD. In The Encultured Brain: An Introduction to Neuroanthropology. Daniel H. Lende and Greg Downey, eds. Pp. 263–290. Cambridge, MA: MIT Press.

Gottman, John, Julie Gottman, and Christopher Atkins

    2011 The Comprehensive Soldier Fitness Program: Family Skills Component. American Psychologist 66(1):52–57.

Gross, Cornelius, and Rene Hen

    2004 The Developmental Origins of Anxiety. Nature Reviews Neuroscience 5:545–551.

Gusterson, Hugh

    2007 Anthropology and Militarism. Annual Review of Anthropology 36:155–175.

Hay, Cameron

    2012 Memory and Medicine. In The Encultured Brain: An Introduction to Neuroanthropology. Daniel H. Lende and Greg Downey, eds. Pp. 141–167. Cambridge, MA: MIT Press.

Hinton, Devon, and Roberto Lewis-Fernandez

    2010 Idioms of Distress among Trauma Survivors: Subtypes and Clinical Utility. Culture, Medicine and Psychiatry 34(2):209–218.

    2011 The Cross-cultural Validity of Posttraumatic Stress Disorder: Implications for DSM-5. Depression and Anxiety 28(9):783–801.

Hobfoll, Stevan E.

    2002 Social and Psychological Resources and Adaptation. Review of General Psychology 6(4):307–324.

Inda, Maria Carmen, Elizaveta V. Muravieva, and Cristina M. Alberini

    2011 Memory Retrieval and the Passage of Time: From Reconsolidation and Strengthening to Extinction. The Journal of Neuroscience 31(5):1635–1643.

Jobson, Laura, and Richard O'Kearney

    2008 Cultural Differences in Personal Identity in Post-Traumatic Stress Disorder. British Journal of Clinical Psychology 47(1):95–109.

Johnson, Douglas, Melissa A. Polusny, Christopher R. Erbes, Daniel King, Lynda King, Brett T. Litz, Paula P. Schnurr, Matthew Friedman, Robert H. Pietrzak, and Steven M. Southwick

    2011 Development and Initial Validation of the Response to Stressful Experiences Scale. Military Medicine 176(2):161–169.

Kienzler, Hanna

    2008 Debating War-Trauma and Post-Traumatic Stress Disorder (PTSD) in an Interdisciplinary Arena. Social Science and Medicine 67(2):218–227.

King, Linda, Daniel King, Dawn Vogt, Jeffrey Knight, and Rita Samper

    2006 Deployment Risk and Resilience Inventory: A Collection of Measures for Studying Deployment-Related Experiences of Military Personnel and Veterans. Military Psychology 18(2):89–120.

Kirmayer, Laurence J., Robert Lemelson, and Mark Barad

    2007 Understanding Trauma: Integrating Biological, Clinical and Cultural Perspectives. New York: Cambridge University Press.

Kleykamp, Meredith

    2006 College, Jobs, or the Military? Enlistment during a Time of War. Social Science Quarterly 87(2): 272–290.

Lende, Daniel H.

    2005 Wanting and Drug Use: A Biocultural Approach to the Analysis of Addiction. Ethos 33(1):100–124.

Litz, Brett T., and William Schlenger

    2009 PTSD in Service Members and New Veterans of the Iraq and Afghanistan Wars: A Bibliography and Critique. PTSD Research Quarterly 20(1):2–7.

Lorge, Elizabeth

    2008 Army Responds to Rising Suicide Rates. US Army Medical Department. http://www.behavioralhealth.army.mil/news/20080131armyrespondstosuicide.html, accessed October 10, 2011.

Medford, Nick, and Hugo D. Critchley

    2010 Conjoint Activity of Anterior Insular and Anterior Cingulate Cortex: Awareness and Response. Brain Structure and Function 214(5–6):535–549.

Miller, Kenneth, and Andrew Rasmussen

    2010 War Exposure, Daily Stressors, and Mental Health in Conflict and Post-Conflict Settings: Bridging the Divide between Trauma-focused and Psychosocial Frameworks. Social Science and Medicine 70(1):7–16.

Modinos, Gemma, Johan Ormel, and André Aleman

    2009 Activation of Anterior Insula during Self-Reflection. PLoS One 4(2):e4618. doi:10.1371/journal.pone.0004, accessed May 29, 2012.

Ong, Anthony, Thomas Fuller-Rowell, and George Bonanno

    2010 Prospective Predictors of Positive Emotions Following Spousal Loss. Psychology and Aging 25(3):653–660.

Panter-Brick, Catherine, and Mark Eggerman

    2011 Understanding Culture, Resilience, and Mental Health: The Production of Hope. The Social Ecology of Resilience 7:369–386.

Park, Nansook, Christopher Peterson, and Martin E. P. Seligman

    2004 Strengths of Character and Well-Being. Journal of Social and Clinical Psychology 23(5):603–619.

Perkinogg, Axel, Ronald Kessler, S. Storz, and Hans Ulrich Wittchen

    2001 Traumatic Events and Post-Traumatic Stress Disorder in the Community: Prevalence, Risk Factors and Comorbidity. Acta Psychiatrica Scandinavica 101:46–59.

Peterson, Christopher, Nansook Park, and Carl Castro

    2011 Assessment for the U.S. Army Comprehensive Soldier Fitness Program. American Psychologist 66(1):10–18.

Peterson, Christopher, Nansook Park, Nnamdi Pole, Wendy D'Andrea, and Martin Seligman

    2008 Strengths of Character and Post-Traumatic Growth. Journal of Traumatic Stress 21(2):214–217.

Polusny, Melissa, Christopher Erbes, Maureen Murdoch, Paul Arbisi, Paul Thuras, and Madhavi Reddy

    2011 Prospective Risk Factors for New-Onset Post-Traumatic Stress Disorder in National Guard Soldiers Deployed to Iraq. Psychological Medicine 41:687–698.

Qin, Pengmin, and Georg Northoff

    2011 How Is Our Self Related to Midline Regions and the Default-Mode Network? NeuroImage 57(3):1221–1233.

Rylko-Bauer, Barbara, and Merrill Singer
    2011 Political Violence, War, and Medical Anthropology. *In* A Companion to Medical Anthropology. Merrill Singer and Pamela Erickson, eds. Pp. 219–249. Malden, MA: Wiley-Blackwell.
Sayers, Steven, Victoria Farrow, Jennifer Ross, and David Oslin
    2009 Family Problems among Recently Returned Military Veterans Referred for a Mental Health Evaluation. Journal of Clinical Psychiatry 70(2):163–170.
Schiller, Daniela, and Elizabeth A. Phelps
    2011 Does Reconsolidation Occur in Humans? Frontiers in Behavioral Neuroscience 5:24.
Seligman, Martin E. P., and Raymond D. Fowler
    2011 Comprehensive Soldier Fitness and the Future of Psychology. American Psychologist 66(1):82–86.
Seligman, Rebecca, and Laurence J. Kirmayer
    2008 Dissociative Experience and Cultural Neuroscience: Narrative, Metaphor and Mechanism. Culture, Medicine and Psychiatry 32(1):31–64.
Sundin, Josefin, Nicola Fear, Amy Iversen, Roberto Rona, and Simon Wessley
    2010 PTSD after Deployment to Iraq: Conflicting Rates, Conflicting Claims. Psychological Medicine 40:367–382.
Turnbull, Gordon J.
    1998 A Review of Post-Traumatic Stress Disorder. Part I: Historical Development and Classification. Injury 29(2):87–91.
U.S. Army Comprehensive Soldier Fitness
    2011 Frequently Asked Questions. U.S. Army Comprehensive Soldier Fitness. http://csf.army.mil/faq.html, accessed November 2, 2011.
Yehuda, Rachel, and Linda M. Bierer
    2009 The Relevance of Epigenetics to PTSD: Implications for the DSM-V. Journal of Traumatic Stress 22(5):427–434.
Young, Allan
    1995 The Harmony of Illusions: Inventing Posttraumatic Stress Disorder. Princeton, NJ: Princeton University Press.
Wang, Zhewu, Dewleen Baker, Judith Harrer, Mark Hamner, Matthew Price, and Ananda Amstadter
    2011 The Relationship between Combat-Related Post-Traumatic Stress Disorder and the 5-HTTLPR/rs25531 Polymorphism. Depression and Anxiety 28(12):1067–1073.
Zur, Judith
    1996 From PTSD to Voices in Context: From an "Experience-Far" to an "Experience-Near" Understanding of Responses to War and Atrocity across Cultures. International Journal of Social Psychiatry 42(4): 305–317.

LIFE HISTORY AND REAL LIFE: AN EXAMPLE OF NEUROANTHROPOLOGY IN ABORIGINAL AUSTRALIA

VICTORIA K. BURBANK
University of Western Australia

A recent conceptual reworking of the developmental origins of health and disease model that places it within a life history framework is used to interpret some of the history of people living today in the remote Arnhem Land community of Numbulwar. This approach suggests some of the means by which their past circumstances may have had an impact on their current health. A combination of history, ethnography, and the neurobiology of stress and pregnancy provides a neuroanthropological approach for considering the manner in which environmental stressors, particularly those of social origin, may have intergenerational consequences for health. [stress, DOHaD, Aboriginal Australians, health, ethnography, neuroanthropology]

Neuroanthropology, an emerging subfield that seeks to integrate advances in neuroscience with anthropological theory and practice (Downey and Lende 2012) not only highlights the long asked question of just how the person is transformed by experience but also enables us to better address it. In this article, I do just that, turning to recent research on the neurophysiology of social stress and low birth weight to better understand the disturbing differences in mortality between Indigenous and non-Indigenous Australians. In doing so, I illustrate the utility of neuroanthropology for addressing real problems faced by real people in sociohistorical contexts that contribute to if not create those problems and join others whose work challenges determinist arguments about race and ill health (e.g., Dressler and Bindon 2000; Gravlee 2009; Kuzawa and Sweet 2008). Especially in times when so many media forms create and fan moral panics while perpetuating invidious social constructions and when political responses are often little more than self-interested knee jerk reactions, a considered etiology provides an important corrective for public discourse and policy decisions.

The social determinants of health framework originating in the work of Marmot and his colleagues has, in recent years, promised a particularly powerful way of understanding inequalities in health and wellbeing (Brunner and Marmot 1999). The attempts, prompted by this early research, to understand the mechanisms whereby environmental factors, especially those from the social environment, may not simply affect but transform human bodies and minds has created a new research orientation within the social sciences (e.g., Nguyen and Peschard 2003). Central to this emerging framework is the identification of the "flight-or-fight" circuitry as the principal means by which social factors result in ill health and disadvantage. Also central is a focus on the concept of "stress" (e.g., Sapolsky 1993, 2004). Currently, it is thought that maternal stress is translated into

ANNALS OF ANTHROPOLOGICAL PRACTICE 36, pp. 149–166. ISSN: 2153-957X. © 2012 by the American Anthropological Association. DOI:10.1111/j.2153-9588.2012.01097.x

a variety of physiological states that affect fetal and infant development with long-term consequences that may disadvantage the offspring, and even the grand-offspring of the stressed mother (e.g., Dunkel Shetter 2011; Gravlee 2009; Kuzawa and Quinn 2009). But just what people find stressful remains something of an open question. Although major events such as the Dutch Hunger Winter (Lumey 1992) or the 9/11 attacks on New York (Lauderdale 2006) appear to be associated with poor pregnancy outcomes in some populations, just why this is taking place has been far from clear. This neuroanthropological interpretation of some of the recent history of a group of Aboriginal people highlights the necessity of an ethnographic component for understanding the social determinants of health and wellbeing and, at the same time, the utility of considering neurophysiological factors in ethnography.

In great measure, Aboriginal people across the continent of Australia suffer from illnesses associated with an overactive stress system (e.g., Australian Bureau of Statistics 2005). At Numbulwar, the remote Aboriginal community at the heart of this discussion, health clinic personnel identified the "metabolic syndrome" as the main source of adult ill health; obesity, high blood pressure, Type 2 Diabetes and the related conditions of kidney failure and coronary heart disease were, and continue to be, widespread.[1] Community specific summaries of morbidity and mortality for remote communities in the Northern Territory of Australia are, unfortunately, nonexistent. However, in Ngukurr, a relatively nearby Aboriginal town to which the people of Numbulwar have long had social connections, Taylor and colleagues (2000:80) have estimated that "there are 4.5 times more deaths ... than would be expected if the mortality profile observed for the total Australian population applied." There is little to suggest that the situation at Numbulwar departs from this estimate in any significant way.[2]

In the field of Indigenous Australia, the injustices of colonization have been highlighted by anthropologists and others addressing issues of health inequality (e.g., Carson et al. 2007), but statistics such as these invite us to ask precisely how the destruction of a way of life creates a legacy of premature morbidity and mortality and how such consequences might be avoided in the future. To address these questions I have turned to a body of work that views health as a series of ongoing tradeoffs required of organisms by their circumstances (see Ellison 2005). This approach encourages us to ascribe the causes of poor health not so much to physiology as to environment, particularly the sociocultural environment. In taking this position, I am guided by recent conceptual reworkings of what is known most recently as "the developmental origins of health and disease" (DOHaD) model. This reconceptualization places the model within a life history framework, and invites us to consider the mechanisms of our species' life history strategies (Ellison 2005; Worthman and Kuzara 2005). This reconceptualization also allows us to circumvent a nature–nurture form of dichotomization found sometimes in the social determinants of health arena. For example, Gray and colleagues (2004) present the DOHaD model as an alternative to "the social exclusion" hypothesis. In contrast, the perspective I present grounds this discussion of Numbulwar's history in the neurological, physiological, and social. It becomes possible for us to see "social exclusion," for example, as a precursor of maternal constraint, that is, the capacity of a woman to nurture a fetus, that may contribute to later experiences of socially generated stress. This approach focuses our attention on aspects of the environment that stress mothers and, later, their offspring, whether such aspects are physical or social. It also allows us to consider the manner in which environmental stressors may have intergenerational consequence for health.

Human life history, that is, our species-specific pattern of birth, development, reproduction, and death, may be characterized as prolonged and plastic (e.g., Worthman 1999). An example of our plasticity may be seen in the fetal capacity to adapt to the uterine environment by modifying its rate and type of growth. Evidence suggests that when a fetus is undernourished, the placental blood supply is directed away from some developing organs to others. Thus, depending on gestational period, blood might be directed away from the developing kidneys to the brain, that supremely vital human structure. This individual's kidneys are likely to have fewer cells than those of a fetus better nourished during development; and kidneys with fewer cells are more likely to fail if later stressed (Barker 1994). As this example foreshadows, plasticity has its costs. It necessarily leads to what have been thought to be permanent changes in individual physiology, including brain physiology, although this view has been challenged (e.g., Gunnar and Quevedo 2007; Wyrwoll et al 2006). These changes may contribute to a greater disease burden in later life. Low birth weight (i.e., a less than expected newborn weight) has become the index of this future cost. Forms of adult ill health associated with low birth weight include coronary heart disease, stroke, hypertension, Type 2 diabetes (and obesity in association with this condition), depressive disorders and schizophrenia (Barker 2004; Eriksson et al. 2003; Thompson et al. 2001; Wahlbeck et al. 2001). All these conditions are found at Numbulwar.

Low birth weight, characteristic of a number of children at Numbulwar (Burbank and Chisholm 1989), is seen in the model I draw on as a consequence of uterine environments where resources are restricted or unpredictable. These kinds of uterine environment are seen, in turn, as the consequence of "poor or uncertain maternal nutrition, poor maternal health, and/or high allostatic load" (Worthman and Kuzara 2005:98). Allostatic load is what we call "stress," the cumulative biological cost of maintaining stability vis-à-vis changes in internal and external environments (McEwen and Wingfield 2003). Although nutrients in the placental blood supply may be what the fetal-placental unit responds to, more than maternal nutritional status may be responsible for this state (Gluckman et al. 2007). The experience of social stress, such as subjection to the power and control of others, may, in and of itself, diminish a woman's capacity to nourish her fetus although her diet is adequate.

In this model the neuroendocrine architecture, particularly that of the hypothalamic–pituitary–adrenal (HPA) axis, is the mechanism that allocates resources. Worthman and Kuzara (2005) review an extensive literature on birth weight, stress, and health outcomes. Given the pervasive role of the neuroendocrine architecture in body composition and function, they are not surprised to find associations between a birth weight continuum and variation in organ composition and function, body composition, metabolic regulation and functioning of components of the endocrine system. There is a greater likelihood that as low birth weight individuals develop, their bodies will contain, for example, more fat, less muscle, and fewer kidney cells than higher birth weight individuals. They are also likely to have greater resistance to insulin (Worthman and Kuzara 2005). This model suggests that a consideration of the physical, social, and cultural environments in which mothers may be well or ill nourished, in good or poor health, relatively secure and happy or anxious and depressed, is essential background for analyses of the current health environment.

NUMBULWAR AND ITS EARLY HISTORY

The materials for this history are scant in two respects. First, little is known about Aboriginal health prior to European colonization. Reconstructions must rely on the im-pressionistic reports of early contacts (largely from the southern part of the continent and Numbulwar is located in the north), knowledge of hunter-gatherer health more generally and skeletal remains. Scholars using these, very tentatively, conclude that Aboriginal peo-ple surviving the first five years of life were generally healthy and well nourished. They suffered little from infectious and chronic disease. They were more likely to suffer injury or death from accidents and, occasionally, violence (Beck 1985; Franklin and White 1991; Saggers and Gray 1991). Historical materials are also scarce. Most of the material I draw on has been provided by the work of Dr. Keith Cole a historian with close ties to the Anglican Church. Professor John Bern (personal communication, 2006) and Dr. Rose-mary O'Donnell (2007), both of whom work at Ngukurr, have also noted the dearth of historical materials for this area. I use this material to suggest the extent to which non-Aboriginal people controlled Aboriginal lives and the circumstances that made this control and subordination acceptable to Aboriginal people.

Numbulwar, then called the Rose River Mission, was established in August of 1952 by the Anglican Church Missionary Society (CMS). In accordance with the Common-wealth's Assimilation Policy, missionaries or other Westerners were in charge of its store, school, health clinic, church, and basic governance (Cole 1982; Young 1981). That the Mission was run in an authoritarian fashion is implied by Cole when he describes "mission discipline" as "strict," providing an example from the journal of John Mercer:

> Sunday 31.8.52 During the afternoon I had to request that a corroboree [a secular gathering for the purpose of dance] be discontinued. This will prove a helpful illustration to tomorrow's address on the fourth commandment. [Cole 1982:30]

This entry suggests the extent of mission control in the early decades of Rose River Mission:

> From June 1967 the catering for children was gradually phased out. Up till that time the children had been fed and given school clothes. The teacher at school had supervised showers, teeth cleaning, clothes changes and meals. The clothes had been washed by school laundresses and the older children had helped with serving and washing-up at meal times. As has been mentioned the system came under increased scrutiny by the missionaries. *They*

now decided that the parents should be given the responsibility of washing and mending school clothes, and a greater part in providing meals. [Cole 1982:54, emphasis added]

The subordination of Aboriginal people by these forms of control was likely accompanied and exacerbated by the "Europeans'" attitudes toward Indigenous people. Cole captures what this might have been when he discusses the CMS missions for "half-caste" children in the Northern Territory during his period:

Changes in community attitudes to part-Aborigines has been a feature of the past seventy years. In the early days men and women of compassion cared and acted while the white community despised and governments remained indifferent. Human bodies as well as human souls mattered to them. These people of compassion did what they thought was right. They took them away from meddling whites and unwholesome blacks, and taught them the "better" way of the white man. [Cole 1979:132]

Today Numbulwar is regarded as a "remote" Aboriginal community, inhabited by Indigenous people in an isolated part of the continent, maintained largely by government funding and a local desire, if not need, to reside there. Over the 30 years that I have conducted research in the community, Numbulwar's population has grown from roughly 400 to 1,000, fluctuating as people move between this "town" and other remote communities in the area, those of Bickerton Island, Groote Eylandt and Ngukurr, formerly the Roper River Mission. The language group most strongly identified with Numbulwar, as has always been the case, is that of the Nunggubuyu, speakers of Wubuy. Hunting and gathering still occupies some but does not support the population, there are few jobs to be had, and most of the Aboriginal people living there receive various forms of welfare. In the 1970s, governance of local affairs passed to an Aboriginal Council made up of representatives of the local clans. However, the community has always been assisted by a non-Indigenous town clerk recruited from outside Numbulwar and overseen by various Territory and Federal bodies. Similarly the community's teachers, doctors, nurses and directors of the various structures and programs that sustained it, are, with few exceptions, "whitefellas."

The Nunggubuyu seem to have been spared the harsher aspects of colonization buffered as they were, and continue to be, at least to a considerable extent, from settler culture by distance and a terrain not easily traversed, even on foot (Eastwell 1976; Thomson 1983). As far as I can tell, premission contact was largely restricted to visits from Macassans from the Celebes (now Sulawesi, Indonesia), who came to fish for trepang (Thomson 1983). These may have been stimulating and enriching encounters, if their traces in dance, loan words, and artifacts are any indication. However, to the west, south and north of Nunggubuyu countries, Aboriginal people were not so fortunate (Bauer 1964; Cole 1979; Merlan 1978; Morphy and Morphy 1984; Reid 1990; Thomson 1983). For example:

The tribes in the Roper River area had been decimated by the depredations of the pastoralists, and their tribal organisation had been smashed. The main tribes in the area, and those now severely depleted, were the Mara, Alawa, Wandarang, Ngandi, Ngalakan, the southernmost members of the Rembarrnga and Nunggubuyu tribes, and some of the Mangarayi tribe. [Cole 1985:57]

Residents at Numbulwar identify not only with Nunggubuyu but also with several other of these language groups, each with a different history of interaction with the colonial environmental. People who speak, or whose ancestors once spoke languages such as Anindiljuagwa, Mara, Ngandi, Ritharngu, and Wandarang are integrated into town life, often through intermarriage with Nunggubuyu people. Just as their language group identities vary, so we might imagine that their stress lineages vary in their potential for intergenerational harm (see Gunnar and Quevedo 2007). Regardless of language group, however, the Aboriginal people who first settled at Rose River Mission were required to adjust to circumstances that may have laid the ground for today's ill health.

STRONG CULTURE, STRONG BABIES

Neuroanthropology directs us to identify sociocultural factors that comprise much of the environment in which bodies become encultured. Because the human brain is so plastic, as are many other of our physiological systems, social arrangements and cultural practices that comprise our "developmental niche" (Super and Harkness 1986) can be expected to actually change our bodies and our minds (Downey and Lende 2012). Depression, chronic stress, and pregnancy anxiety have been identified as major precursors of low birth weight babies as well as those born prematurely (Dunkel Schetter 2011). The identification of sociocultural factors associated with these mental states is a critical step in attempts to reduce these conditions that may predispose the individual to a life of ill health and disability. It is also a critical step for an analysis of the pathways and mechanisms whereby a mother's mental or physical state transforms that of her unborn or newly born child (Kuzawa and Quinn 2009). Anthropology has a long tradition of documenting the unintended, and often deleterious, consequences of social arrangements imposed by those who are dominant in an intercultural setting, that is, one that contains divergent, and not always compatible or interacting, "experience, knowing and practice" (Merlan 2005:174). In this reconstruction of Numbulwar's early history, I trace several interventions into Aboriginal lives that together have created the developmental niches of current and past generations and may well be a major source of today's ill health.

Many of Numbulwar's residents are the children, grandchildren, or great-grand-children of polygynists (Chisholm and Burbank 1991). From the turn of the last century, missionaries in the area opposed this marriage form—along with the premenarcheal marriage age and practice of infant betrothal associated with it—and through a concerted and sustained campaign greatly reduced its practice (Burbank 1988). According to Cole (1977), CMS missionaries had long been concerned about the practice of polygyny, although it was not a concern they felt able to address until relatively late in mission history:

Mission pressures for (what they perceived to be) a more equitable distribution of women mainly to provide wives for unmarried men and so lessen fighting and quarrelling over women, were not felt to any great extent during the period 1908–1939. [Cole 1977:192]

Although the campaign against polygyny began at the first CMS mission at Roper River, according to a missionary present in the early days of Rose River Mission, it may be that activities at the Angurugu Mission on Groote Eylandt had the most immediate effect on marriage practices at Numbulwar (Burbank 1988:62). Describing mission initiatives at Groote Eylandt, Turner says:

In the period between 1944 and 1947 ... seven men belonging to Bickerton local groups who were married polygynously surrendered a total of eight wives to eight single Bickerton men. Another man gave up a wife, but after she had been married to the recipient, he reclaimed and kept her. [Turner 1974:51]

At Numbulwar, there was no formal redistribution of wives. However, the Aboriginal inhabitants of the mission were informed that polygyny was not consistent with a Christian way of life. Those that I have spoken with on the topic attribute its demise to the mission, although not always to the mission's policy of "one man, one wife." One woman told me, for example, that once they were living at the mission, some women simply left their husbands. Of course, if the missionaries felt as compelled to provide "sanctuary" to such women, as they did for girls under the age of 16 who were unwilling to go to their betrothed husbands, the missions may well have made separation possible (Burbank 1988:65–66).

By 2003, with only one or two exceptions, marriages were monogamous. Although the preponderance of monogamy in spite of men's continuing attempts to take additional wives suggests not only women's preference for this marriage form but also their ability to maintain it in their unions (Burbank 1994), their triumph may nevertheless be a source of the ill health characteristic of contemporary times. In a monogamous marriage, one woman may have to bear the reproductive load once borne by several. For at least a time in the recent past, some women have had more children at shorter intervals than did their mothers and grandmothers.

Mercer's stories about the early years of Rose River Mission include mention of the expected birth spacing at the time:

She should not have another baby whilst she was presently nursing a child, not yet walking or able to fend for itself. So you found that aboriginal children were about three years apart in age for mothers fed their babies for two years and they reached three years before they were able to fend for themselves. [Mercer 1978:45]

Genealogies, mission and health records allowing for comparison of birth averages of 31 polygynously and 41 monogamously married women, show a significantly greater number for the monogamous group, 6.05 children compared to 4.61. They also show a significant decrease, from 65.3 months to 39.76 months, in the mean interbirth interval for them (Chisholm and Burbank 1991:296).[3] A significant positive correlation between birth interval and birth weight in a sample of 75 children from birth to age five in 1988 has also been found; children born after longer intervals tended to be heavier (Burbank and Chisholm 1989:92).

Monogamy, however, need not be associated with a greater reproductive load for individual women as Western birth rates generally demonstrate. There are other factors to be considered here. A pronatalist ideology is one that may be crucial. At least during the late 1970s, this position appeared to be characteristic of men at Numbulwar:

> Some men have a wife and for three or four years she doesn't have a child. "Oh, this girl isn't having my kids. I'll get another wife." Then he marries another girl. Might be five or six months and his second wife has a baby. She is going to have a child so she can make a race and a big family. They see when they get old, see their wife having no children. "I'll have to get another." [Burbank 1980:104–105]

Several reasons that men might want to have children are suggested by this speaker. First among these might be the expectation that children will care for an elderly father, a reasonable expectation given the principle of reciprocity attached to parent–child relationships (Burbank 2006). I might also note the desire for a "big family" and for a "race" expressed in this text. In 1978, a woman explained to me that when Aboriginal women leave Numbulwar and marry non-Aboriginal men, people are not happy because "it makes not enough people." That is, a woman bearing children for a non-Aboriginal man is not bearing children for an Aboriginal man at Numbulwar. The possible motive of increasing the "race" is a poignant one, for it reminds us of the colonial violence at the margins of Nunggubuyu lands. The desire also suggests the extent to which the Nunggubuyu ancestors of people at Numbulwar were aware of this violence and passed this awareness on to younger generations. Although few speak of this, at least to me (Burbank 1994:23–24), a general awareness seems likely, especially given the connections of Numbulwar's people to Ngukurr. Should such violence have been interpreted along lines implied by use of the word "race" and the phrase "not enough people," that is, as genocidal, the pronatalist stance of local people would not be surprising (see also Spiro 1958).

There are also less speculative reasons for thinking that pronatalism has been a factor, at least until recently, in determining family size. Most sources suggest that pronatalism may originate more with men than women. In an analysis of fights occurring between 1977 and 1978 precipitated by the actions of seven men attempting to obtain additional wives, I found that four of these men's wives had no children, one wife had only one, and that two other wives were no longer fertile; in one of these cases, infertility was because of a woman's use of contraceptives (Burbank 1994). This is to say that in all of these cases, infertility might have been at least a contributing factor.[4] Conversations and interviews with 30 mothers and fathers in 1988 indicated that men were more likely to want larger numbers of children than their partners; all women interviewed wanted no more than they had at the time of the conversation (between two and four), whereas all the fathers wanted more than they had (between one and six; see Burbank and Chisholm 1992). In this material we can also see a source of gender difference in ideas about ideal family size: a male bias in pivotal social arrangements and a consequent desire for sons:

> I've got a part to play in ceremony too. I've got songs, ceremonial things. Land too. If I get old, I know that I've got a son, he might take responsibility of the ceremony and the country. Somebody who will take over and my family will go on and on. Instead of just having a family, we could have just lived on with no kids, that would have been the end of [my] family line. . . . With our first child we were really happy . . . and we decided to have another. Our real aim was to have a boy, but we didn't have that until we had three girls, then we had a boy, and I think we're finished. [Burbank and Chisholm 1992:183]

Circumstances of culture, history, and biology may have conspired with men against women in regard to family size. I have presented an example of fetal plasticity with reference to the number of cells in a kidney. A second example of human plasticity is seen in physiological systems that maintain a balance between a woman's own energy reserves and those dedicated to gestation or lactation. The label "maternal depletion syndrome" identifies a physiological state where this balance is upset. Insufficiently long birth spacing is one source of interference. Maternal depletion is thought to undermine the health of both mother and offspring; in the later case it may lead, among other things, to low birth weight (Ellison 2001; Shell-Duncan and Yung 2004).

Cole (1982) has emphasized the near coincidence of Numbulwar's establishment as the Rose River Mission with the Commonwealth's policy of assimilation, implemented in the Northern Territory's Welfare Ordinance of 1953: "Every endeavour was made to change them from being nomads into people living settled lives in communities. . . . They were taught health and hygiene and worthwhile trades and occupations" (Cole 1982:15).

In the mission's early years, most adult residents were required to work, although pregnant and lactating women were exempted. Together, the missionaries and their flock constructed an airstrip, sawmill, church, clinic, school, and houses (Young 1981). Indigenous residents were paid for their work according to the Montgomerie 1954 Annual Report: "No rations are issued to the people. They have to work for wages and may buy their flour and rice, etc. at the sales stores" (Cole 1982:34). Yet people were expected to obtain a substantial proportion of their food from the surrounding bush. Until 1958, supplies arrived by boat from Roper Mission only every six months. When they were low, Aboriginal residents were sent "walkabout" (Cole 1982; Young 1981).

Soon, however, food became plentiful. Reviewing early mission materials, Young (1981) paints a picture of this abundance:

> When mission construction was completed, attention turned towards increasing local food production, mainly for consumption within the community. This was so successful that it became apparent that Numbulwar could provide a considerable surplus, particularly in fruit, vegetables and eggs. In 1959/60 the market garden produced 4 tons of fruit and vegetables but in 1965/66 this had increased to over 40 tons, approximately a pound per day for every[one] on the settlement . . . [F]or a number of years Numbulwar exported eggs for workers for the Groote Eylandt Mining Company (GEMCO). In the absence of

a market, Numbulwar garden crops were distributed freely throughout the community or, on occasion, were left to rot. [Young 1981:174]

In 1956 over 150 dugong, yielding about 45,000 lbs of meat, were bought by the mission from the fishermen of Numbulwar. [Young 1981:194]

Once the mission became a sustainable community, people ceased moving from place to place in the manner of their hunting and gathering past. By the 1970s, when the outstation movement began and more people again travelled more extensively, they routinely used vehicles and motorized boats to do so.

The hunting and gathering lifestyle of groups like the Kung, or Ju/'hoansi, as reported by Howell (1979), is one associated with a particular pattern of fertility. This is characterized by a relatively late age of menarche, followed by a relatively prolonged period of subfecundity, and a completed reproductive history of four or five births spaced about four years apart by periods of lactational amenorrhea (Lancaster 1986).

Cowlishaw (1981) has argued on the basis of a compilation of biological, ethnographic, and historical material that this was probably the precontact reproductive pattern of Indigenous Australians. In support of Cowlishaw's (1981) argument, Saggers and Grey (1991) count Abbie's (1976) comparison of hemoglobin levels in remote dwelling Aboriginal people and "European" Australians. Only in the latter group was a sex difference found, that is, European women had lower hemoglobin levels than did European men. The absence of a sex difference in the Aboriginal group may be interpreted to mean that these women had "less frequent and shorter menstrual periods," indicating "less frequent ovulation" and hence lower fertility (Saggers and Grey 1991:24). Saggers and Gray also mention dietary restrictions to which Aboriginal women were subjected, patterns of breast feeding that may have reduced ovulation and the possibility that genital operations such as subincision reduced male fertility, although I am not aware of this operation ever having been a part of the series of male inductions into the religious life of the Nunggubuyu.

In the literature addressing hunter gatherer fertility in general, Bentley and colleagues point out that "forager, horticultural, and agricultural groups are all characterized by a high degree of heterogeneity in their fertility rates, and that it is not possible to predict fertility rates on the basis of subsistence technology alone" (1993:276–277). Nevertheless, following an analysis of "natural-fertility" populations, they concluded that "the intensification of subsistence technology is associated with increases in fertility. . . . Higher fertility is primarily associated with the intensification of agriculture." Although the people of Numbulwar have not become agriculturalists, their way of life on settlement at Rose River Mission increasingly became supported by the intensified technology associated with industrial societies.

Currently, women at Numbulwar appear to lead a physically less strenuous life than they or their ancestors did in hunting and gathering days. MacArthur's (1960) observations of subsistence practices in Arnhem Land in the 1940s included a hunting and gathering group on Bickerton, an island just a few kilometers off the coast from Numbulwar with an environment similar to that of the mainland. McArthur remarked of the women's food quest that it was "a job which went on day after day without re-lief," although "they rested quite frequently and did not spend all the hours of daylight searching for or preparing food" (MacArthur 1960:92). No comparable drain on women's energy expenditure appears to have arisen since settlement. With much of women's sub-sistence role rendered unnecessary by the availability of energy rich flour and sugar (see Altman 1984) and with the need to remain near at hand because children are at school, an institution that was established at Numbulwar in 1953, women's daily lives have taken a decidedly sedentary turn.

Bentley and colleagues have emphasized women's subsistence activities as "crucial [for fertility] given the relationship between women's energetic output and gonadal function" (Bentley et al. 2001:210). Factors to consider here would include the distance women travel, the loads they are required to carry (incl. dependent children), and the energy required by daily subsistence tasks, for example, digging for roots. An additional factor is "the level of temperatures to be endured" (Bentley 1985:86). This factor may well have affected the energetics of foraging in a climate that is hot and humid during most of the year. Although this literature makes it clear this is not always the case in a shift from a foraging to a horticultural subsistence strategy, the energetic demands of settled life for Numbulwar's women would seem to have been reduced considerably. Heat and humidity have much less of an effect on someone being driven less than a half-kilometer to the shop than on someone gathering food in areas that may be some kilometers from camp.

Cowlishaw (1981) also observed the increase in fertility, the lengthening of the fertile period and the decrease in birth spacing among women on missions and government settlements. In particular, she noted the association of this new fertility profile with changes in energy expenditure and diet. At Numbulwar, women have been consum-ing more calories than in the past. In April of 1979, Young surveyed the purchases made by Aboriginal people in Numbulwar's shop. Her survey indicated "excessive" con-sumption of "flour, bread and sugar" in particular and a daily caloric intake almost double that recommended. Although she admits that the use of shop expenditure to provide information on nutritional intake is very rough, the accuracy of her finding is suggested by increasing rates of obesity to be seen in men, women, and children (Young 1981).

What were the possibilities for women with bodies more receptive to pregnancies they may not have desired and that might have injured their health or that of the developing fetus? Contraceptive use would have been an option, but the mission run health service does not appear to have provided birth control methods, at least on a widespread basis, until the 1970s. An analysis of 232 live births to 73 mothers between 1925 and 1988 shows a decrease in the mean interbirth interval from over 50 months in the period 1925–49 to 26–29 months between 1965 and 1980. By 1988, a reversal of the interbirth interval appeared, increasing to 39 months (Burbank and Chisholm 1989). This increase was likely because of greater access to contraception.

On a recent trip to Numbulwar, I was able to ask a woman with a long experience of the health clinic about the availability of birth control devices:

VKB: When the missionaries were here could women get family planning from the clinic?

AW: In those days, I remember, for family planning, it never never been said. Only in traditional way that I been telling you. But in Western way family planning had not been brought out. The nurse knew and I was learning about it but we never talked to young woman or old woman because they couldn't understand. But now they know it. The nurse never said it. Later in the years, finally it came up. They can take loops [IUDs]. Later in the time when it started, I was interpreting, talking to the older ones. Young ones [use it] today. I had a group of women to discuss it with. Some didn't make sure they wanted it, but some did. Just the loops. They didn't have much to send out. Older ladies got loops because they had nother one coming, nother one coming. Just to have a rest.

VKB: Was that in the old clinic [building] or the new clinic?

AW: In the old clinic. You were in the caravan down with your *abuji* [kin term for FM, the year was 1978].[5]

The extent to which women employed traditional contraceptive practices, regarded as "women's business," is unknown. According to women like this speaker, the result of these is permanent infertility.

CONCLUSION

To say that until contraception was provided, the missionaries controlled Aboriginal women's fertility, is an exaggeration that nevertheless makes an important point. This kind of control may have had consequences beyond those of contributing to circumstances where women bore more children than was healthy or desired. In this depiction of the early years of Numbulwar, I find two intertwined sources of injury to subsequent generations, both related to HPA activity. First, assuming that Worthman and Kuzara (2005) are right when they suggest that the HPA axis' role in resource allocation is such that it responds to variations in the prenatal environment, we can posit a connection between the sociohistorical circumstances that may once have given rise to widespread maternal depletion and the poor health seen at Numbulwar today. The elevated production of glucocorticoids that accompanies undernutrition are thought to have lasting effects; included among these are the cluster of health conditions in the metabolic syndrome, so pervasive at Numbulwar today. Greater vulnerability to stress, such as "increased behavioral reactivity and sensitivity to novelty" (Worthman and Kuzara 2005:106), is another possible consequence.

A second source of today's ill health that I posit is the lack of control that women likely experienced because of repeated unplanned and possibly unwanted pregnancies. Elsewhere (Burbank 2011) I have discussed the incompatibility of having large numbers of closely spaced children with the highly responsive form of early childcare—often associated with hunting and gathering peoples—that women at Numbulwar both practice and expect of themselves. Given these expectations, yet another pregnancy, a significant and unwelcome intrusion felt to be completely out of a woman's control, may have been a major source of stress in and of itself (Dunkel Schetter 2011; Sapolsky 2004). The negative feelings experienced along with an unwanted pregnancy likely would have been even more intense when social subordination was experienced in association with an ascribed identity that had been the target of extreme violence, albeit much of this is now past. With this in mind, it is hard to imagine the Rose River Mission as anything other than an environment in which chronic stress was experienced by many of its Aboriginal residents. For pregnant women, fear for an unborn child, if not for themselves and their other children, may have made their experience all the more distressing.

It is becoming increasingly clear that while undernutrition may be the basis of the fetal origins of ill health and disease, this may not simply be because of what women eat. Recent work on the placenta's role in fetal development underlines its importance in many of these processes. Hypertension, for example, one of the components of the metabolic syndrome, may, by interfering with placental function, "severely limit fetal nutrient supply without a corresponding change in maternal nutrition" (Harding 2001:16). Similarly, stress may interfere with the placenta's capacity to buffer the effects of maternal HPA activity on the developing fetus, particularly in the case of "chronically stressed animals ... exposed to an acute stressor" (O'Donnell et al. 2009:289). The situation at Numbulwar may be just another example of what research increasingly shows: that psychosocial stress, in and of itself, has the potential to affect fetal development (Dunkel Shetter 2011; Worthman and Kuzara 2005). Thus, it is easy to imagine that the mothers of Numbulwar may be the fourth or fifth generation of women whose bodies and minds have been challenged in this way, if not by maternal depletion then by social disadvantage and other stressful experiences.

I think that the missionaries at Rose River, at least those I have known, were indeed "people of compassion," concerned with fairness and the wellbeing of Aboriginal people. Nevertheless, in hindsight it is easy to lay at least some of the blame for Aboriginal health at their door. But we would be better off looking not so much at what they did, as at what we are doing now, again with the best of intentions, to Aboriginal people, and others, today. In 2007, for example, the Australian federal government, in the last year of its 11 years of power, responded to a report on the sexual abuse of children in remote communities with the Northern Territory National Emergency Response. "Income management," the quarantining of welfare payments for essential items such as food and clothing, was one of the results, requiring suspension of Australia's *Racial Discrimination Act* as only some Aboriginal communities were subjected to it (Austin-Broos 2011). The "intervention," as the Response is often called, has been continued by the current federal government. A number of Aboriginal women have publically stated that "income management" is a beneficial arrangement. No longer are they subjected to forms of "demand sharing" (Peterson 1993) that may include violence by family members who want to spend their welfare checks on drugs and alcohol. There have also been media reports of improved nutrition for the children in these communities. Income management would seem to be a successful strategy for improving Aboriginal wellbeing. Yet, if we accept the argument I have been making, we must ask about the long-term consequences of imposed control of Aboriginal lives. The dissection of past well-meaning acts such as I have presented here should caution us against instituting other well-meaning but equally damaging forms of assistance. Enabling the people who must live with the consequences of decisions to make and implement those decision themselves is the alternative I would propose to many of Australia's current solutions to the "Aboriginal problem."

NOTES

Acknowledgments. This article is a revised segment of chapter 3 in Burbank 2011. I thank Palgrave Macmillan for permission to use this material here. I also thank Greg Downey and Daniel Lende for the invitation to contribute to this volume and the two anonymous reviewers for their suggestions and support.

1. I have been conducting anthropological research in this community since 1977.

2. Between 2003 and 2005, I conducted research on health and inequality at Numbulwar supported by an Australian Research Council Discovery Grant (#DP0210203) received with Professor Robert Tonkinson and Dr. Myrna Tonkinson, titled "Inequality, Identity and Future Discounting: A Comparative Ethnographic Approach to Social Trauma." This research included interviews with 20 Aboriginal people, men and women ranging in age from 18 to about 67. By 2007, three were dead, two had recovered from serious illness and two others had lost close kin, that is, over a third had been affected by severe medical conditions or death and none of the ill or dead had reached the age of 65.

3. The analysis excluded all spontaneous abortions, stillbirths, neonatal and infant deaths, and births in which the father was known to be different from the father of the preceding child.

4. In her cross-cultural study of "conjugal dissolution" Betzig (1989:662) found infertility second only to adultery in frequency as a reason for divorce.

5. Rather than IUDs, Implanon appears to be the contraceptive of choice today.

REFERENCES CITED

Abbie, Andrew A.
  1976 The Original Australians. Rev. edition. Sydney: Rigby.
Altman, Jon C.
  1984 Hunter-Gatherer Subsistence Production in Arnhem Land: The Original Affluence Hypothesis Re-Examined. Mankind 14(3):179–190.
Austin-Broos, Diane
  2011 A Different Inequality: The Politics of Debate about Remote Aboriginal Australia. Crows Nest, NSW: Allen and Unwin.
Australian Bureau of Statistics
  2005 The Health and Welfare of Australia's Aboriginal and Torres Strait Islander Peoples, 2005. http://www.aihw.gov.au/WorkArea/DownloadAsset.aspx?id=6442458575, accessed November 12, 2011.
Barker, David J. P.
  1994 Mothers, Babies, and Disease in Later Life. London: BMJ Publishing.
  2004 The Developmental Origins of Chronic Adult Disease. Acta Paediatric 93(s446):26–33.
Bauer, Francis H.
  1964 Historical Geography of White Settlement in Part of Northern Australia, Part 2, the Katherine-Darwin region. Canberra: CSIRO. Division of Land Research and Regional Survey.
Beck, Eduard J.
  1985 The Enigma of Aboriginal Health: Interaction between Biological, Social and Economic Factors in Alice Springs Town-Camps. Canberra: Australian Institute of Aboriginal Studies.
Bentley, Gillian R.
  1985 Hunter-Gatherer Energetics and Fertility: A Reassessment of the !Kung San. Human Ecology 13(1):79–109.

Bentley, Gillian R., Tony Goldberg, and Grażyna Jasieńska

    1993 The Fertility of Agricultural and Non-Agricultural Traditional Societies. Population Studies 47(2):269–281.

Bentley, Gillian R., Richard R. Paine, and Jesper L. Boldsen

    2001 Fertility Changes with the Prehistoric Transition to Agriculture: Perspectives from Reproductive Ecology and Paleodemography. *In* Reproductive Ecology and Human Evolution. Peter Ellison, ed. Pp. 203–231. New York: Aldine de Gruyter.

Betzig, Laura

    1989 Causes of Conjugal Dissolution: A Cross-Cultural Study. Current Anthropology 30(5):654–676.

Brunner, Eric, and Michael Marmot

    1999 Social Organization, Stress and Health. *In* Social Determinants of Health. Eric Brunner and Michael Marmot, eds. Pp. 17–23. Oxford: Oxford University Press.

Burbank, Victoria

    1980 Expressions of Anger and Aggression in an Australian Aboriginal Community. PhD Thesis, Department of Anthropology, Rutgers University.

    1988 Aboriginal Adolescence: Maidenhood in an Australian Community. New Brunswick: Rutgers University Press.

    1994 Fighting Women: Anger and Aggression in Aboriginal Australia. Berkeley: University of California Press.

    2006 From Bedtime to On Time: Why Many Aboriginal People Don't Especially Like Participating in Western Institutions. Anthropological Forum 16(1):3–20.

    2011 An Ethnography of Stress: The Social Determinants of Health in Aboriginal Australia. New York: Palgrave Macmillan.

Burbank, Victoria, and James Chisholm

    1989 Old and New Inequalities in a Southeast Arnhem Land Community: Polygyny, Marriage Age and Birth Spacing. *In* Emergent inequalities in Aboriginal Australia. Jon C. Altman, ed. Pp. 85–94. Oceania Monograph 38. Sydney: University of Sydney.

    1992 Gender Differences in the Perception of Ideal Family Size in an Australian Aboriginal Community. *In* Father-Child Relations: Cultural and Biosocial Contexts. Barry S. Hewlett, ed. Pp. 177–189. New York: Aldine de Gruyter.

Carson, Bronwyn, Terry Dunbar, Richard D. Chenhall, and Ross Bailie, eds.

    2007 Social Determinants of Indigenous Health. Crows Nest, NSW: Allen and Unwin.

Chisholm, James S., and Victoria K. Burbank

    1991 Monogamy and Polygyny in Southeast Arnhem Land: Male Coercion and Female Choice. Ethology and Socio-Biology 12(4):291–313.

Cole, Keith

    1977 A Critical Appraisal of Anglican Mission Policy and Practice in Arnhem Land, 1908–1939. *In* Aborigines and Change: Australia in the '70s. Ronald M. Berndt, ed. Pp. 177–198. Canberra: Australian Institute of Aboriginal Studies.

    1979 The Aborigines of Arnhem Land. Adelaide: Rigby.

    1982 A History of Numbulwar. Bendigo, VIC: Keith Cole Publication.

    1985 From Mission to Church: The CMS Mission to the Aborigines of Arnhem Land 1908–1985. Bendigo, VIC: Keith Cole.

Cowlishaw, Gillian

    1981 The determinants of fertility among Australian Aborigines. Mankind 13(1):37–55.

Downey, Greg, and Daniel Lende

    2012 Neuroanthropology and the Encultured Brain. *In* The Encultured Brain: An Introduction to Neuroanthropology. Daniel H. Lende and Greg Downey, eds. Pp. 55–141. Cambridge, MA: MIT Press.

Dressler, William W., and James R. Bindon

    2000 The Health Consequences of Cultural Consonance: Cultural Dimensions of Lifestyle, Social Support and Arterial Blood Pressure in an African American Community. American Anthropologist 102(2):244–260.

Dunkel Schetter, Christine

   2011 Psychological Science on Pregnancy: Stress Processes, Biopsychosocial Models, and Emerging Research Issues. Annual Review of Psychology 62:531–538.

Eastwell, H.

   1976 Associative illness among Aboriginals. Australian and New Zealand Journal of Psychiatry 10(1A): 89–94.

Ellison, Peter T.

   2001 On Fertile Ground. Cambridge, MA: Harvard University Press.

   2005 Evolutionary Perspectives on the Fetal Origins Hypothesis. American Journal of Human Biology 17(1):113–118.

Eriksson, Johan G., Tom Forsen, Jaakko Tuomilehto, Clive Osmond, and David J. P. Barker

   2003 Early Adiposity Rebound in Childhood and Risk of Type 2 Diabetes in Adult Life. Diabetologia 42(2):190–194.

Franklin, Margaret-Ann, and Isobel White

   1991 The History and Politics of Aboriginal Health. In The Health of Aboriginal Australia. Janice Reid and Peggy Trompf, eds. Pp. 1–36. Marrickville, NSW: Harcoutrt Brace Jovanovich.

Gravlee, Clarence C.

   2009 How Race Becomes Biology: Embodiment of Social Inequality. American Journal of Physical Anthropology 139(1):47–57.

Gray, Matthew C., Boyd H. Hunter, and John Taylor

   2004 Health Expenditure, Income and Health Status among Indigenous and Other Australians. Canberra: ANU Press. http://.anu.edu.au/caepr_sereis/no/moblie-devices/index.html, accessed October 12, 2011.

Gluckman, Peter D., Mark A. Hanson, and Alan S. Beedle

   2007 Early Life Events and Their Consequences for Later Disease: A Life History and Evolutionary Perspective. American Journal of Human Biology 19(1):1–19.

Gunnar, Megan, and Karina Quevedo

   2007 The Neurobiology of Stress and Development. Annual Review of Psychology 58:145–173.

Harding, Jane E.

   2001 The Nutritional Basis of the Fetal Origins of Adult Disease. International Journal of Epidemiology 30(1):15–23.

Howell, Nancy

   1979 Demography of the Dobe !Kung. New York: Academic.

Kuzawa, Christopher W., and Elizabeth A. Quinn

   2009 Developmental Origins of Adult Function and Health: Evolutionary Hypotheses. Annual Review of Anthropology 38:131–147.

Kuzawa, Christopher W., and Elizabeth Sweet

   2008 Epigenetics and the embodiment of race: Developmental origins of US Racial Disparities in Cardiovascular health. American Journal of Human Biology 21(1):2–15.

Lancaster, Jane B.

   1986 Human Adolescence and Reproduction: An Evolutionary Perspective. In School-Age Pregnancy and Parenthood: Biosocial Dimensions. Jane Lancaster and Beatrix Hamburg, eds. Pp. 17–38. New York: Aldine de Gruyter.

Lauderdale, Diane S.

   2006 Birth Outcomes for Arabic-Named Women in California before and after September 11. Demography 43(1):185–201.

Lumey, Lambert H.

   1992 Decreased Birthweights in Infants after Maternal in utero Exposure to the Dutch Famine of 1944–45. Paediatric and Perinatal Epidemiology 6(2):240–253.

MacArthur, Margaret

   1960 Food Consumption and Dietary Levels of Groups of Aborigines Living on Naturally Occurring

Foods. *In* Records of the Australian America Scientific Expedition, vol. 2. C. P. Mountford, ed. Pp. 90–135. Melbourne: Melbourne University Press.

McEwen, Bruce S., and John C. Wingfield
  2003 The Concept of Allostasis in Biology and Biomedicine. Hormones and Behaviour 43(1):2–15.

Mercer, John T.
  1978 Good Morning Lumbarra: Stories for Children Based upon the Experiences of a Missionary amongst Aborigines at Numbulwar in Arnhem Land, North Australia. Mt Tamborine, Qld: John T. Mercer.

Merlan, Francesca
  1978 "Making People Quiet" in the Pastoral North: Reminiscences of Elsey Station. Aboriginal History 2(1):70–106.
  2005 Explorations towards Intercultural Accounts of Socio-cultural Reproduction and Change. Oceania 75(3):167–182.

Morphy, Howard, and Frances Morphy
  1984 The "Myths" of Ngalakan History: Ideology and Images of the Past in Northern Australia. Man 19(3):459–478.

Nguyen, Vinh-Kim, and Karine Peschard
  2003 Anthropology, Inequality, and Sisease: A Review. Annual Review of Anthropology 32(1):447–474.

O'Donnell, Rosemary S.
  2007 The Value of Autonomy: Christianity, Organisation and Performance in an Aboriginal Community. Ph.D. dissertation, Department of Anthropology, University of Sydney.

O'Donnell, K. T., G. O'Connor, and V. Glover
  2009 Prenatal Stress and Neurodevelopment of the Child: Focus on the HPA Axis and Role of the Placenta. Developmental Neuroscience 31(4):285–292.

Peterson, Nicholas
  1993 Demand Sharing: Reciprocity and the Pressure for Generosity among Foragers. American Anthropologist 95(4):860–874.

Reid, Gordon
  1990 A Picnic with the Natives: Aboriginal-European Relations in the Northern Territory to 1910. Melbourne: Melbourne University Press.

Saggers, Sherry, and Dennis Gray
  1991 Aboriginal Health and Society: The Traditional and Contemporary Aboriginal Struggle for Better Health. St. Leonards, NSW: Allen and Unwin.

Sapolsky, Robert M.
  1993 Endocrinology Alfresco: Psychoendocrine Studies of Wild Baboons. Recent Progress in Hormone Research 48:437–468.
  2004 Social Status and Health in Humans and Other Animals. Annual Review of Anthropology 33:393–418.

Shell-Duncan, Bettina, and Stacie A. Yung
  2004 The Maternal Depletion Transition in Northern Kenya: The Effects of Settlement, Development and Disparity. Social Science and Medicine 58(12):2485–2498.

Spiro, Melford E.
  1958 Children of the Kibbutz: A Study in Child Training and Personality. New York: Schocken.

Super, Charles M., and Sara Harkness
  1986 The Developmental Niche: A Conceptualization at the Interface of Child and Culture. International Journal of Behavioural Development 9(4):545–569.

Taylor, John, John Bern, and Kate A. Senior
  2000 Ngurkurr at the Millennium: A Baseline Profile for Social Impact Planning in South-East Arnhem Land. Centre for Aboriginal Economic Policy Research. Research Monograph No. 18, Australian National University, Canberra.

Thompson, Christopher, Holly Syddall, Ian Rodin, Clive Osmond, and David J. Barker
  2001 Birth Weight and the Risk of Depressive Disorder in Later Life. British Journal of Psychiatry 179: 450–455.

Thomson, Donald

1983 Donald Thomson in Arnhem Land. South Yarra, VIC: Currey O'Neil.

Turner, David H.

1974 Tradition and Transformation: A Study of Aborigines in the Groote Eylandt Area, Northern Australia. Canberra: Australian Institute of Aboriginal Studies.

Wahlbeck, Kristian, Tom Forsen, Clive Osmond, David J. Barker, and Johan G. Eriksson

2001 Association of Schizophrenia with Low Maternal Body Mass Index, Small Size at Birth, and Thinness during Childhood. Archives of General Psychiatry 58(1):48–52.

Worthman, Carol M.

1999 Evolutionary Perspectives on the Onset of Puberty. *In* Evolutionary Medicine. Wenda Trevathan, E. O. Smith, and James J. McKenna, eds. Pp. 135–163. Oxford: Oxford University Press.

Worthman, Carol M., and Jennifer Kuzara

2005 Life History and the Early Origins of Health Differentials. American Journal of Human Biology 17(1):95–112.

Wyrwoll, Caitlin S., Peter J. Mark, Trevor A. Mori, Ian B. Puddey, and Brendan J. Waddell

2006 Prevention of Programmed Hyperleptinemia and Hypertension by Postnatal Dietary ω-3 Fatty Acids. Endocrinology 147(1):599–606.

Young, Elspeth A.

1981 Tribal Communities in Rural Areas: The Aboriginal Component in the Australian Economy. Canberra: Development Studies Centre, Australian National University.

FROM WHITE BULLETS TO BLACK MARKETS AND GREENED MEDICINE: THE NEUROECONOMICS AND NEURORACIAL POLITICS OF OPIOID PHARMACEUTICALS

HELENA HANSEN

MARY E. SKINNER
New York University

Synthetic opiates (opioids) have created among the most profitable markets worldwide. Two decades ago, FDA approval of Oxycontin® as a "minimally addictive" opioid pain reliever fueled an unprecedented rise in prescription opioid abuse. This was followed by a little known act of U.S. Congress enabling general physicians to use an opioid maintenance medication, buprenorphine, for addiction treatment in their private practices, leading to enormous growth in the U.S. addiction treatment market. Based on participant-observation and interviews among pharmaceutical executives, policy makers, patients and prescribers, this article describes the neuroeconomics and neuropolitics of new opioid maintenance treatments. This article contrasts the historical emergence of methadone clinics from the 1960s to the 1980s as a treatment for the Black and Latino urban poor, with the current emergence of buprenorphine, a maintenance opioid approved for prescription on doctor's offices, as a treatment for white, middle-class prescription opioid abusers. The article then traces the counterintuitive result of bringing addiction pharmaceuticals into the medical mainstream in an effort to reduce the stigma of addiction: a two tiered system of addiction treatment that reinforces stigma among the urban poor, and enhances the biological, political, and economic dependence of all classes on opioid markets, both legal and illegal. [addiction treatment, opiate maintenance, methadone, buprenorphine, race, class, political economy, pharmaceuticals]

The only addiction treatment pharmaceuticals that actually make money are the opioid agonists, like buprenorphine. Can you imagine a better commodity than one that is physiologically addictive, and that the physician tells the patient he or she must take indefinitely?

—Marc Galanter, President of the American Society of Addiction Medicine, 1999–2001

One of the concerns that we all have had is that buprenorphine was somehow going to help create a two-tiered treatment system, that is, a treatment system that the poor people and underserved and unemployed will get put into methadone treatment, and everybody else, the employed and people with money would be able to go onto buprenorphine. Has it happened? To some extent I think it has.

—Charles O'Keeffe, CEO of Reckitt Benckiser Pharmaceuticals, 1980–2002

ANNALS OF ANTHROPOLOGICAL PRACTICE 36, pp. 167–182. ISSN: 2153-957X. © 2012 by the American Anthropological Association. DOI:10.1111/j.2153-9588.2012.01098.x

A neuroanthropology of pharmaceuticals must not only account for the individual level biocultural interaction between physiologies and perception but also must attend to the structural level biocultural interaction between the marketing of bioactive commodities, on the one hand, and systems of social stratification, governmental control, and self-discipline, on the other hand. For example, a political economic component to biocultural analysis is key to explaining how concepts of racial difference and vulnerability to addiction come about through social forces. Such political economic perspectives have been key contributions of anthropology to the emerging field of neuroeconomics (Goodman and Leatherman 1999; Gravlee 2009; Leatherman and Goodman 2011; Schull and Zaloom 2011).

In this article, we trace the market logic of the development of a race and class stratified system of treatment for opiate dependence with opioid maintenance. We argue that the current state of opioid maintenance treatment in the United States can be understood using a biocultural lens, in which the physiological dependence causing properties of opiates and opioids (synthetic opiates) make them ideal commodities from a pharmaceutical corporation's perspective, but that the cultural associations of opioids and opiates with racial and class marginalization necessitated novel marketing and regulatory strategies to supply white, upper-income consumers with opioid maintenance. Ultimately, two neuroactive agents with similar pharmacological properties, methadone and buprenorphine, have vastly different systems of dissemination and regulation structured around them, in which one opioid (methadone) is a part of a clinical system that is subject to tight government regulation and surveillance of criminalized patients, and the other opioid (buprenorphine) is part of a deregulated private clinical system based on a view of opiate dependents as neurochemically deficient. These two clinical systems are the economic by-product of a racialized bipolarity in U.S. cultural frames for addiction, as a moral deficiency on one pole, and as a chronic neuroreceptor deficiency on the other pole. Science studies scholars of addiction neuroscience demonstrate that neuroscientific projects reformulate the social contexts of addiction as points of biological, rather than moral, lapse (Campbell 2010, 2011). Yet the example of buprenorphine and methadone highlights that these biologizing projects map onto race and class stratified institutional structures in which neurobiological amorality is inherently racialized and politicized (see Kirmayer and Gold 2011; Vrecko 2010a, 2010b).

Opioids are one of the largest selling classes of drugs in the world, with the United States consuming 80 percent of the world's opioids despite claiming only 4.6 percent of the world's population. In the United States, the opioid hydrocodone (sold as Vicodin®) has been the number one most prescribed drug for several years in the past decade (Manchikanti and Singh 2008). The physiologically addicting properties of opioids, along with their criminalization and past symbolic association with marginalized groups, make them a fruitful topic of inquiry for understanding the interaction between neuroeconomies and social systems of control. By neuroeconomics, we indicate the broad spectrum of systems of regulation and exchange that interact as psychoactive substances circulate in social life, ranging from the physiological (e.g., downregulation of neuroreceptors and endogenous neurotransmitters with exposure to pharmaceuticals) to the corporate (e.g., strategies to enhance supply and demand, governmental deregulation).

The recent history of industries of opioid dependence and treatment provides an illustrative example. Here we provide this history, based on in-depth 30–90 minute, topically directed, open-ended interviews with 56 policy makers, pharmaceutical executives, physicians and patients, as well as four years of participant-observation by the first author working as a psychiatry resident and fellow, and the second author working as a volunteer in a substance abuse treatment program. Participant-observation involved observing doctor–patient encounters, addiction medicine conferences, and working groups, as well as the daily work of agencies and community based organizations devoted to addiction treatment. The interview and observational data from this study indicate that categories of race and class not only shape pharmaceutical markets but also that pharmaceutical marketing, in turn, shapes the very categories of race and class as experienced in biomedical clinics. The race- and class-marking of different opioid formulations has allowed opioid manufacturers to extract profits from opposite ends of the social strata in the United States, while creating (in theory) biologically equivalent opioid dependence across strata. At the same time, this bioequivalence itself has been challenged by theorists of local biologies who argue that social context shapes both biological process and perception of biological process (Lock and Nyugen 2010). Whether or not the neurobiology of opiate dependence differs by strata in the United States, however, this dependence is experienced in contrasting ways at either end of the race and class-based stratified system, which reflects that people in the top and bottom strata have unequal abilities to resist surveillance, and unequal opportunities to enact consumer choice and privatization of their health care.

THE RISE OF PRESCRIPTION OPIOIDS

In 1996, Purdue Pharmaceuticals got FDA approval for a long-acting form of opioid painkiller, oxycodone, which it named Oxycontin®. Based on the logic that its time release capsule prevented the rapid rise in drug levels in the blood that gives opiate abusers intense pleasure through saturation of the opioid receptors in their brains, and based on time limited clinical trials of Oxycontin® with acute pain patients, Purdue marketed the drug as a "minimally addictive" opioid pain reliever, with a less than 1 percent risk of addiction, appropriate for long-term use in chronic pain (Van Zee 2009). It was to be the first of the opioid class to skirt the problem of addictive potential, but still retain its potent analgesic properties.

In addition to heavy investments in educational symposia, promotional gifts embossed with the Oxycontin® logo, and free Oxycontin® samples and coupons for patients, Purdue Pharmaceuticals hired a cadre of 671 drug representatives to bring the good news of this minimally addictive opioid to a call list of almost 100,000 physicians across the country. By 2003, half of Oxycontin® prescribers were primary care physicians, who used this designated magic bullet for everything from cancer to lower back pain. Several states including Maine and West Virginia reported increases in numbers prescription opioid abuse patients of 500 percent or more in the first five years after Oxycontin® was released, with similar increases in opioid overdose deaths (Van Zee 2009). Opiate naïve patients soon discovered that their need to use escalating doses for the same pain relief, and their discomfort when missing doses, meant that they had developed an opioid tolerance and dependence; patients with preexisting drug habits soon found they could crush the time-release capsule and inject or snort the contents for a dependable, "pharmaceutical grade" heroin-like rush (Butler et al. 2011; Cicero et al. 2005). Doctor and dentist shopping for additional Oxycontin® prescriptions, and vibrant black markets in Oxycontin® and sister prescription opioids Percocet® and Vicodin® became commonplace. In keeping with the demographics of the U.S. insured middle class who have easiest access to expensive new nongeneric, on-patent, nonformulary drugs, prescription opioid abuse was associated with a white, often privileged clientele; the Oxycontin® habits of celebrities such as Rush Limbaugh were featured in the popular press (CNN 2003). By 2004, prescription opioids had outstripped heroin as the major opiate of abuse in the United States, and by 2010 prescription medications became the most abused class of substances among U.S. high school seniors (National Institute of Drug Abuse [NIDA] 2011). Purdue Pharmaceutical executives, likely aware of the financial potential of the black market they had stoked with their wide-ranging drug promotion campaign (Singer 2008), paid $634 million in fines for criminal charges based on misrepresentation of Oxycontin's addictive potential (Van Zee 2009), a sum that was dwarfed by the $3 billion that Purdue gained in Oxycontin profits in 2009 alone.

The prescription opioid abuse epidemic of the late 1990s–2000s came on the heels of a rise in the number of middle class, white heroin users as well. Beginning in the late 1980s, newly planted heroin harvests in Colombia led Latin American cartels to compete with Middle Eastern and Asian heroin suppliers in a purity and price war that left street heroin dramatically purer, cheaper, and easier to snort, encouraging middle-class drug users in the United States to turn to heroin (Hamid et al. 1997). These middle-class heroin users, and the even larger cadre of prescription opioid abusers emerging in the 1990s, posed a problem for the U.S. addiction treatment system. Treatment adherence rates for opioid dependence in biomedical clinics were low, except those of methadone clinics, whose patients had higher retention rates and lower illicit drug use rates than those using medication-free treatment modalities (Mattick et al. 2003; Sees et al. 2000).

Opioid maintenance was not readily available either: since the 1914 Harrison Narcotic Act, individual physicians had been barred from treating opiate addiction with opioid maintenance. This historical segregation of opioid maintenance from the mainstream of clinical medicine was partially challenged by methadone researchers at Rockefeller University, Vincent Dole, Marie Nyswander, and Mary Jeanne Kreek, who in 1966 began publishing their clinical trials of methadone maintenance in mostly African American heroin dependent patients from Harlem (Dole et al. 1966). Their research team made a strong biological argument for methadone maintenance: that opiate dependence was a disease of opiate receptor deficiency, analogous to diabetes, requiring opioid replacement therapy, just as diabetes requires insulin. Ultimately the measured outcomes of interest were not biological, however; they were social. It was the dramatically lower rates of crime committed by patients after methadone treatment, and their high rates of employment six months into methadone maintenance, that got national attention. Based on these findings, by 1971 President Nixon launched a network of methadone clinics as part of his War on Drugs to combat a raging heroin problem among returning Vietnam veterans, and among African Americans and Latinos in inner cities (Kuehn 2005).

Thus, methadone was associated with Blacks and Latinos living in poverty, with crime and with the rundown neighborhoods in which methadone clinics were permitted to operate. Methadone treatment was often given in settings more resembling correctional facilities than medical clinics. Tightly regulated by the DEA and often segregated from biomedical campuses, the clinics required daily onsite dosing under the observation of a nurse and guards, regular urine testing, and sanctions for violation of clinic rules. As one addictions specialist working as a high ranking official in the Bush I administration of the 1990s told us of middle-class opioid dependent patients: "People with good jobs didn't want to wait in line for methadone with people just off the street." Furthermore, he explained, he did not want those with stable jobs and lives to be exposed to the illicit drug trade that is often found outside methadone clinics, where some patients barter their weekend take-home doses for the benzodiazepine sedatives (like Xanax[®] and Valium[®]) that they combine with methadone to achieve a boosted euphoria. Buprenorphine, prescribed monthly in private doctors' offices, offered a clean clinical atmosphere removed from poverty, ethnic minorities, and street crime.

The prescription opioid abuse epidemic of the late 1990s–2000s also came on the heels of President George H. W. Bush's Decade of the Brain, a decade during which NIDA devoted its research agenda to biotechnological treatments for addiction and basic science locating the cause for addiction in the brain and biology of individuals (Vocci et al. 2005). At the end of the Decade of the Brain, in 2000, a widely cited article was published by leading addictions researchers in the Journal of the American Medical Association (JAMA) entitled "Drug Dependence, A Chronic Medical Illness" (McLellan 2000). It demonstrated that chemical addictions were comparable to diabetes, asthma, and hypertension in terms of heritability, contribution of environment, and treatment adherence. The article argued that these similarities called for addiction to be treated as a chronic physiological disease, in general medicine (as opposed to psychiatric) settings, with pharmaceuticals. This flew in the face of the received wisdom both inside and outside of medicine, that addiction was a problem of morale if not morality, requiring psychotherapy or support groups to address the emotional and characterological roots of self-destructive behavior. Addiction treatment had long been excluded from "real" medicine, with widespread neglect of addictions in U.S. medical training (Soyka and Gorelick 2009), despite the fact that addiction is one of the leading causes of death in the United States (CASA National Center on Addiction and Substance Abuse at Columbia University 2009). In fact, addicted people are barely considered patients, as most physicians in opinion surveys say they would prefer not to treat people with addiction (Soyka and Gorelick 2009). In reaction to these attitudes, addiction specialists across the country used the JAMA article to campaign for placing addictions treatment in the mainstream of biomedicine, with the idea that fully biomedicalizing addiction, treating it in the same clinics, and in the same way as other chronic diseases—that is, with long-term medication, would destigmatize addiction, end decades of punitive addiction treatment, and desegregate addiction treatment from mainstream medicine.

OFFICE-BASED OPIOID MAINTENANCE AS NEUROECONOMIC STRATEGY

In pursuit of this vision of fully biomedicalized addiction treatment, in 2002 the FDA approved the synthetic opiate buprenorphine for maintenance treatment of opiate dependence in private, buprenorphine-certified doctor's offices. Two years prior to this, the U.S. Congress passed a law that legalized office-based treatment of opiate dependence with Schedule III narcotics (Jaffe and O'Keeffe 2003). This law—the Drug Abuse and Treatment Act, or DATA 2000, did not name buprenorphine specifically, but a former Office of Narcotic and Drug Control Policy official who had a central role in crafting the legislation explained to us in an interview that the law was designed with buprenorphine in mind. Accordingly, buprenorphine's manufacturer, along with prodrug maintenance legislators and researchers, pressured the FDA and DEA to make buprenorphine a Schedule III drug, which would categorize it as at low to moderate risk of creating dependence, and subject to less surveillance than high risk schedule II narcotics (such as Oxycontin®). Pharmacologically similar to methadone, in that it blocks opiate receptors in the brains of addicted patients, buprenorphine can be prescribed monthly for use at home, while methadone is restricted to DEA regulated clinics that require direct observation of patients taking their doses. Officially, the manufacturer, Reckitt Benckiser Pharmaceuticals gained approval for office-based use of buprenorphine based on buprenorphine's pharmacological advantages over methadone. It is a weaker opioid than methadone, and is therefore less likely to cause overdose. Also, it is manufactured with another drug, naloxone, which causes withdrawal if it is injected, rather than dissolved under the tongue as prescribed. Based on these differences, Reckitt Benckiser Pharmaceuticals persuaded the FDA that buprenorphine is a safer and less abusable drug than methadone, and can therefore be taken at home.

A less official version of the story involves the selling of office-based buprenorphine to the DEA and the FDA based on its race- and class-specific market. The DEA had long been opposed to the unregulated use of opioids, and the popular imagery of methadone as a treatment associated it with criminality, and with Black and Latino poverty. The emerging prescription opioid epidemic presented an optimal market for office-based buprenorphine maintenance. Not only was the patient population middle class and insured, with access to private physicians who could prescribe buprenorphine, but also the whiteness and class background of its targeted clientele reduced federal anxieties about buprenorphine's potential street sales. The potential for buprenorphine to be diverted to the streets and create yet another opioid black market had long been a preoccupation of the DEA. As explained to us by a pharmaceutical researcher who contracted to collect pharmaceutical diversion data, Reckitt Benckiser Pharmaceuticals voluntarily established an extensive monitoring system involving a national network of local law enforcement offices and regional researchers to collect diversion data. This data was for private use by the Reckitt Benckiser, but the company agreed to share it with the DEA. In a form of public–private partnership, the manufacturer collected data not only on illicit sales of buprenorphine but also collected analogous data on a host of other commonly abused prescription drugs, providing valuable pharmaceutical diversion information for the Federal government. This diversion monitoring apparatus, and resource sharing agreement, predisposed the DEA to schedule buprenorphine at level III (Campbell and Lovell 2012). Congressional hearings identifying the growing ranks of opiate dependent "suburban youth"—coded language for middle class and white—as the clientele for buprenorphine (Netherland 2010) also likely contributed to the DEA's less restrictive scheduling of buprenorphine. This qualified buprenorphine for office-based treatment under the DATA 2000 act, in contrast with other opioids including Methadone, Oxycontin®, Percocet® and Vicodin®, all of which are Schedule II, considered higher risk, with restrictive dispensing rules.

The sociocultural specificity of buprenorphine as a white middle-class drug in the United States, and the importance of this identity for overcoming a century of U.S. governmental and public resistance to the use of opioids to treat opiate addiction, is clear when looking to other countries. France was one of the first countries to adopt buprenorphine maintenance as a treatment for opiate dependence, and now has one of the highest buprenorphine prescription rates in the world (Fatseas and Auriacombe 2007). Since 1996, the French government promoted buprenorphine use among primary care doctors for opiate dependence, and its prescription was less regulated than in the United States; physicians were not required to complete buprenorphine certification to prescribe it. The social identity of buprenorphine and the political reasons for its promotion are different than those of the United States: from its introduction in France, advocates for buprenorphine were activist primary care doctors caring for impoverished immigrant heroin injectors in suburban low income housing developments. They saw buprenorphine treatment as an HIV prevention tool consistent with the public health philosophy of harm reduction: a philosophy that has met with considerable resistance in the United States since the beginning of the HIV epidemic. As a result, the majority of buprenorphine maintenance patients in France are low income immigrant heroin injectors (Lovell 2006). And despite the seamless argument made by the buprenorphine manufacturer to the U.S. FDA, that buprenorphine is less abusable than methadone, because as a weaker opioid receptor agonist it causes less euphoria, buprenorphine has become the most abused opioid in France and in other countries including Finland (Aalto et al. 2007) and Malaysia. In fact, in Malaysia it is the buprenorphine formulation that is manufactured in combination with the opioid antagonist naloxone—the very formulation that was claimed to cause withdrawal when injected—that is the most abused formulation: Malay injectors claim they feel negligible discomfort from naloxone (Bruce et al. 2009). In the United States, the fact that buprenorphine is used by middle class, less socioeconomically dislocated opiate dependent people than methadone users may itself contribute to the lower rates of buprenorphine misuse than of methadone. But in addition, the association of buprenorphine with the white middle class may have shielded it from scrutiny of the international literature on buprenorphine's abuse and diversion; scrutiny that might have challenged the manufacturer's claims to the U.S. FDA.

ETHNIC MARKETING AND THE NEUROECONOMICS OF STIGMA

From the beginning of buprenorphine's release, under the trade name Suboxone®, for treatment of opiate dependence, signs of the manufacturer's targeting of white, middle-class prescription opioid dependent consumers were evident. Because of negotiations with the manufacturer, the DEA required physicians to complete an eight hour certification course in the use of buprenorphine for opiate dependence, and certified prescribers had to have a special prescribing number to write buprenorphine prescriptions. This was the first time such a training and certification requirement had been placed on physicians to use a particular drug. Because this requirement severely limited the number of eligible prescribers, most of whom turned out to be specialists in private practice, rather than primary care doctors in public clinics, the U.S. Federal Substance Abuse and Mental Health Services Administration worked with the manufacturer to develop an online referral system that patients seeking buprenorphine treatment could use to identify a certified prescriber. This system presumed a clientele with regular access to information about new biomedical treatments for addiction, and with the computer literacy to seek treatment by searching for online resources.

Suboxone® was advertised primarily over the internet, with public service announcements launched on the website of the National Alliance for Advocates of Buprenorphine Treatment (naabt.org), a nonprofit that is financially sponsored by Reckitt Benckiser Pharmaceuticals. These public service announcements featured people like Mike, a white diner owner living in Ohio with his wife and two children. Mike, an all-American who tells his story seated in between two U.S. flags that adorn the wall of his diner, is a singer in his church choir and is coach of his son's baseball team. Tearful, he relates becoming inadvertently addicted to his opioid painkillers after a back injury sustained while repairing his diner. As Mike tells it, "I didn't think it could happen to me," but he was relieved when he found a buprenorphine-prescribing private physician who "got me my life back" using new treatment technology.

Yet, for all of the excitement about buprenorphine as a new treatment for opiate dependence, buprenorphine was an old drug. It was first introduced in the early 1970s as an analgesic, developed in the laboratory of a British chemical firm, then Reckitt-Coleman. Reckitt-Coleman, now Reckitt-Benckiser, was and is a major manufacturer of household products including Easy Off®, Woolite®, and Lysol®. Burprenorphine was the only prescription pharmaceutical to which Reckitt-Coleman held patent rights, and in time, the company would create a single drug subsidiary, Reckitt-Benckiser Pharmaceuticals, to manage buprenorphine's marketing. Initially Reckitt-Coleman promoted buprenorphine as a minimally addictive opioid pain reliever, based on early clinical trials indicating that it created less dependence than morphine. However these early findings did not hold up postmarketing against clinical experience, and buprenorphine was not the blockbuster that the manufacturer had hoped. Researchers from the National Institute on Drug Abuse saw buprenorphine as a potential treatment for opiate dependence, but as a former NIDA researcher who worked on the early (1970s) clinical trials of buprenorphine for opiate dependence explained to us in an interview, the company was not interested at that point in being associated with a stigmatized condition like addiction.

By the early 1990s, however, the drug had still not found market niche as a pain reliever, and NIDA officials reapproached the manufacturer to discuss marketing buprenorphine for opiate dependence. As part of the Decade of the Brain's focus on the neurochemistry of addiction, NIDA had made development of pharmacological treatments for addiction a national priority, and buprenorphine was one of the only promising drugs on the horizon. To entice the company into the addiction treatment market, NIDA ultimately awarded $23 million in grants for clinical trials of buprenorphine for opiate dependence, collaborated with the manufacturer and key legislators to pass the DATA 2000 act, and later persuaded the FDA to approve buprenorphine for office-based opioid maintenance treatment. In addition, NIDA officials facilitated a patent extension for buprenorphine through 2009 to protect the manufacturer's profits under an orphan drug designation that was originally intended to stimulate drug development for tropical diseases in low-income countries (Jaffe and O'Keeffe 2003). The strategy paid off handsomely for Reckitt Benckiser. With multiple governmental subsidies in place, Reckitt Benckiser went on to increase its sales of Suboxone steadily at 50 percent per year, and to earn $3.4 billion between 2005 and 2010 in the United States and Australia (Reckitt Benckiser Pharmaceuticals 2009, 2010).

Buprenorphine is actually the latest entry in a long line of opioid medications marketed by pharmaceutical companies as nonaddictive pain relievers and treatments for opiate addiction; nonaddictive opioids have long been the Holy Grail of pharmaceutical discovery. For instance, heroin was marketed by Bayer corporation in 1898 as a nonaddictive pain medicine and treatment for morphine addiction (Courtwright 2001). By the 1940s, heroin addiction was first treated with methadone, an opioid synthesized in Germany during WWII as a pain medication; with time, however, illicit markets for methadone developed and methadone's own addictive potential was acknowledged (Kuehn 2005). By 1996, after FDA approval, Oxycontin was heavily promoted as a nonaddictive treatment for pain. Then in 2002, buprenorphine, having failed to sell as a nonaddictive pain reliever because it was shown to be addictive, was marketed among primary care doctors by Reckitt Benckiser pharmaceuticals as a treatment for Oxycontin addiction.

At the same time, buprenorphine's approval was novel. It represented the first time since the 1914 Harrison Act that generalist doctors were permitted to use opioids to treat opiate addiction. Addiction specialists hail it as a sea change in the culture of medicine: treating addiction in the same settings as other chronic medical conditions, and desegregating addiction treatment from the rest of clinical medicine. This breakthrough in federal law was the result, on the one hand, of a campaign on the part of addiction advocates in federal agencies, who saw in buprenorphine a route to less stigmatizing forms of pharmaceutical intervention than methadone. On the other hand, it was the result of Reckitt-Benckiser Pharmaceuticals search for a new market niche for buprenorphine. The targeting of white middle-class consumers helped buprenorphine's manufacturer to reduce the stigma associated with addiction treatment, minimizing risk to their profits and their public image.

For addiction treatment advocates, buprenorphine marked the coming of a golden age of smart drugs that could crack even the stubborn problem of addiction, the problem that pulls even the most technically skilled doctors into a moral and social morass, as their interventions are continually met with relapse and resistance. But as smart as buprenorphine might be, as one noted buprenorphine researcher admitted to me, the most important difference between buprenorphine and methadone is that buprenorphine is not called methadone. It does not call up the image of homeless black and brown people waiting outside makeshift clinics on the other side of the tracks, and therefore does not have the same DEA restrictions.

And in fact buprenorphine users are different than methadone users. A national survey of buprenorphine users published four years after buprenorphine's FDA approval identified users as 92 percent white, over half employed at baseline, over half with at least some college education, and 75 percent prescription opiate addicted. The survey compared these percentages to those of methadone patients, who nationally were only 53 percent white, 29 percent employed at baseline, and 19 percent with some college education, most of whom injected heroin (Stanton et al. 2006). My own quantitative research with collaborators at the Nathan Kline Institute for Psychiatric Research, studying New York City as the U.S. city with the largest number of opiate dependent people, found that even after a major New York City initiative to promote the use of buprenorphine in public clinics, the vast majority of buprenorphine prescriptions are written in high income, mostly white neighborhoods, while the majority of methadone clinic patients live in low income, largely Black and Latino neighborhoods (Hansen n.d.).

NEUROPOLITICS ON THE GROUND

Ironically, the attempt to fully biomedicalize opiate addiction, and thereby eliminate the stigma of addiction, by treating it with long-term pharmaceuticals in physicians' offices, has led to forms of ethnic marketing that heighten stratification and stigma by race. It has produced what sociologist of racial genetics Troy Duster would call the molecular reinscription of race (Duster 2006), in this case via pharmaceuticals. Rather than mainstreaming marginalized addicts, biomedicalization of addiction has in many cases led to a physiologically reinforced hierarchy of power, a hierarchy bitterly resented by both our methadone and buprenorphine maintained informants in the clinics we observed for this study.

One of our main research sites was the only public clinic in its large metropolitan region to offer buprenorphine maintenance. This created the novel situation of a group of low income black and Latino patients on buprenorphine treatment, counter to the pervasive trend of white, middle-class buprenorphine usage. But escape from restrictive methadone clinics did not necessarily mean freedom and equality for this group of Medicaid insured and uninsured patients. Raul, a 54-year-old Puerto Rican man had received years of methadone treatment, managed to switch to buprenorphine, but found himself dependent on local pharmacists that he found racist. When they delayed ordering his buprenorphine, he ran out of his home supply and experienced withdrawal, a reminder that despite his take-home prescriptions he still did not control his fate: as he said, "I'm hooked—I'm still hooked!"

Despite buprenorphine's promise of enhanced autonomy for patients, buprenorphine patients in our study were still preoccupied with the locus of control around their prescriptions and how they took their medication. Patients obsessed over how often they scheduled doctors' visits, who decided how many times a day they took buprenorphine and at what dose, whether and how they took other medications or drugs along with buprenorphine. They struggled to reconcile feeling "normal" on buprenorphine, with being physiologically dependent on a powerful opioid. They aspired to be drug free, and many attempted to taper themselves off of buprenorphine against the advice of their doctors. Some patients had their own political-economic critique of buprenorphine maintenance, pointing out that they were enriching drug companies by staying on long-term treatment for a condition defined as a chronic physiological disease.

We also found ethnic, racial, and socioeconomic differences in how patients related to providers. White, educated patients often took comfort in the rituals of professional consultation offered in a doctor's office. Many talked about the technical competence and credentials of their doctors, they described themselves in terms of their diagnoses and their responsibility to get treated. African American and Latino patients, most of them Puerto Rican or Dominican, did not always accept physicians' authority based on their credentials but often focus on their doctors' interpersonal qualities and whether they can be trusted. Most working-class patients, including white patients, were attuned to how welcoming and socially accessible their doctors are. They also told stories of institutional violence by hospital staff. Several patients reported that they never mention their addiction when they go to the hospital for physical problems, because if they do the staff will not treat their pain, and may not even examine or treat their presenting condition. One man described his hospitalization for severe phlebitis when he was actively injecting heroin: "I learned about rounds. Rounds is when the head doctor comes in with about 10 other people first thing in the morning, yanks off my gown, points to a huge boil on my butt and tells them I'm an addict."

Prescribers, for their part, worked hard keep buprenorphine in the cultural frame of a prescription medication, rather than a pleasure giving opioid. They reminded patients to take it at the same time, every day, as prescribed, preventatively "like a vitamin," and not to manage the dosing themselves. Doctors spent time assessing whether patients felt pleasure from their doses, which would be an indication to lower their dose, and assessing whether patients were sharing, or diverting their buprenorphine for sale, which would be illegal. The neuroeconomic structures of opioid sales and regulation put these physicians in a double bind of treatment: they could not approach their patients solely from the point of view of their patients' symptoms and suffering, but had to balance these concerns with their awkward role as gatekeeper to a highly profitable commodity, potentially implicating them as physicians in illegalities, and calling on them to judge the boundary between legitimate relief of suffering and undue pleasure.

This type of discussion went along with disciplining of drug users into clinical routines: staff meetings were consumed with talk about behavioral contracts regarding consequences for missed appointments, late arrival for appointments, and lost prescriptions. A clinic administrator joked that her patients never came for scheduled visits but called her on their cell from a car downstairs when they needed a prescription, as if she was a dealer. One astute addictions specialist identified the issue as trust. As she put it, it's understandable that people who are routinely denied medical treatment because they use substances would hesitate to give control over to a doctor. And we interpreted this to mean that it is difficult to destigmatize addiction by biomedicalizing it, if biomedical institutions have been such potent sources of discrimination against addicted people.

CONCLUSION: THE CONTINUED (NEURO) ECONOMIC CENTRALITY OF RACE

As science studies scholar Dorothy Roberts wrote of race in the United States, race may be the reason that the United States does not have a national health plan (Roberts 2011). In other words, the industrial fabric of the United States, and particularly its consumer base, rests on a foundation of racial, as well as class, stratification that sustains the capitalist individualism of our time. Prescription opioids and their treatments are a recent chapter in this continued story of marking one treatment sector by nonwhite race to unmark (mainstream into biomedicine) another sector using white race. The biomedical sector of the U.S. economy, just like other sectors of the economy, relies on race to indicate the status of biomedical goods and services, and to channel consumers accordingly. Racialized patterns of biomedical treatment are a product not only of income related disparities in insurance coverage and ability to pay but also are the product of segmented marketing strategies in which high end goods and services are marketed based on the exclusivity of their clientele. Those biomedical goods and services marketed to a largely white, upper-income clientele are presented as race-free, technological advances based on pure science stripped of social baggage (such as the partial opiate receptor agonist theory of buprenorphine's lower abusability), whereas those marketed to marginalized ethnicities carry the mark of social contexts and less biological, and therefore less universal, indications (such as criminality and employment as outcome measures for buprenorphine treatment).

Particular to opioid pharmaceuticals, however, are their neuroactive properties. A new cohort of people, having become dependent on opioid analgesics that are directly marketed to them and to their physicians, is now faced with treatment consisting of physiological dependence on another opioid (buprenorphine) that is directly marketed to them. Unlike methadone patients, this more affluent group of prescription opioid abusers are too politically and financially empowered to tolerate the obvious governmental surveillance and control epitomized by methadone; they are led into a profit-driven system of consumption and dependence through the use of free market techniques that give the upper hand to addictive commodities that yield neurophysiologically guaranteed returns. Buprenorphine thus conforms to a prevailing trend of privatization and commodification of health care through development and marketing of targeted molecular technologies;

to what sociologist Adele Clarke calls biomedicalization (Clarke et al. 2003). Methadone clinics fall into an older tradition of reframing problems formerly thought of as social or moral deficits into medical terms, involving treatment in settings that are often publicly funded and that discipline newly recognized "patients" into a paternalistic clinical subjectivity, a process that Peter Conrad has called medicalization (Conrad 2005). Yet even the process of medicalization of methadone is incomplete: the physical segregation of methadone clinics from the rest of medical practice, the direct regulation of methadone clinics by the DEA, the requirement of directly observed dosing and regular urine narcotic testing for methadone patients, and the continued political challenges to the legitimacy and legality of methadone maintenance as a treatment modality indicate that methadone treatment lies somewhere between the clinic and the penal colony, blurring the distinction between clinical and correctional forms of social control for lower income, heroin injecting addicts.

The biopolitics of opioid analgesics, now among the most consumed, profitable and therefore socially influential commodities in the United States, if not the world, are characterized by ethnic, racial, and socioeconomic market segmentation. Both the abused opioid—injected heroin versus oral prescription Oxycontin®—and the treatment for its abuse—buprenorphine versus methadone—involve the sharp social distinction and segmentation of pharmacologically similar agents. This ethnicity- and class-marked segmentation, a pervasive element of U.S.-based capitalism, both perpetuates and creates social stratification: buprenorphine patients are more mainstreamed and biomedicalized than methadone patients; in particular, white and higher income buprenorphine patients are defined as consumers or patients by the privatized health care industry, while methadone patients are symbolically criminalized in high surveillance publicly funded clinics segregated from the medical mainstream. The segmented market for addiction medicine thus acts to reconcile standing tension between alternate framings of addiction, as a biomedical versus moral disorder, by distinguishing between two populations, and distinguishing between two socially distinct (albeit pharmacologically almost identical) addictions: heroin and prescription opioids.

Ultimately these findings point to the need for intervention on the structures underpinning disparate neurological experience, those that fuel inequalities in the consumption and prescription of neuroactive substances. Neuroeconomic analyses that synthesize political economic with cultural explanations for variation in addiction experiences and treatment point to the hand of corporate industries in shaping local biologies; the "biosocial differentiation" takes place through interactions of social and biological processes over time that sediment into variation by population (Lock and Nguyen 2010). Missing in many medical anthropological studies of the biologically formative power of social process, however, has been a focus on corporations and industrial cultures (Benson and Kirsch 2010). The power of industrial cultures has been demonstrated in a wide range of biological sites, from the "bioethnic conscription" of research subjects in the burgeoning industry of genetic medicine (Montoya 2007) to the interwoven cartels of licit and illicit drug trade (Singer 2008). In the case of addiction treatment, the disparate tracks of methadone and buprenorphine call attention to segmented marketing practices, pharmaceutical industry deregulation, and the hidden power of racial segregation as part of an economy of distinction in contemporary U.S. markets as points of intervention in neuroeconomic inequality.

REFERENCES CITED

Aalto, Mauri, Jukka Halme, Jukka-Pekka Visapaa, and Mikko Salaspuro
  2007 Buprenorphine misuse in Finland. Substance Use and Misuse 42(6):1027–1028.
Benson, Peter, and Stuart Kirsch
  2010 Capitalism and the Politics of Resignation. Current Anthropology 51(4):459–486.
Bruce, Douglas R., Sumathi Govindasamy, Laurie Sylla, Adeeba Kamarulzaman, and Frederick L. Altice
  2009 Lack of Reduction in Buprenorphine Injection After Introduction of Co-Formulated Buprenorphine/Naloxone to the Malaysian Market. American Journal of Drug and Alcohol Abuse 35(2): 68–72.
Butler, Stephen F., Ryan A. Black, Theresa A. Cassidy, Taryn M. Daily, and Simon H. Budman
  2011 Abuse risks and routes of administration of different prescription opioid compounds and formulations. Harm Reduction Journal 8(1):29. http://www.harmreductionjournal.com/content/8/1/29, accessed January 30, 2012.
Campbell, Nancy D.
  2010 Toward a Critical Neuroscience of "Addiction." BioSocieties 5(1):89–104.
  2011 The Metapharmacology of the "Addicted Brain." History of the Present 1(2):194–218.
Campbell, Nancy D., and Anne M. Lovell
  2012 The History of the Development of Buprenorphine as an Addiction Therapeutic. Annals of the New York Academy of Sciences 1248:124–139.
CASA National Center on Addiction and Substance Abuse at Columbia University
  2009 Shoveling Up II: The Impact of Substance Abuse on Federal, State, and Local Budgets. http://www.casacolumbia.org/articlefiles/380-ShovelingUpII.pdf, accessed May 11, 2012.
Cicero, Theodore J., James A. Inciardi, and Alvaro Munoz
  2005 Trends in Abuse of Oxycontin® and Other Opioid Analgesics in the United States: 2002–2004. Journal of Pain 6(10):662–672.
Clarke, Adele E., Janet Shim, Laura Mamo, Jennifer R. Fosket, and Jennifer R. Fishman
  2003 Biomedicalization: Technoscientific Transformations of Health, Illness, and U.S. Biomedicine. American Sociological Review 68(2):161–194.
CNN
  2003 Rush Limbaugh Admits Addiction to Pain Medication. CNN Entertainment, October 10. http://articles.cnn.com/2003–10–10/entertainment/rush.limbaugh_1_wilma-cline-rush-limbaugh-inaccuracies-and-distortions?_s=PM:SHOWBIZ, accessed electronically November 23, 2011
Conrad, Peter
  2005 The Shifting Engines of Medicalization. Journal of Health and Social Behavior 46(1):3–14.
Courtwright, David T.
  2001 Dark Paradise: Opiate Addiction in America Before 1940. Cambridge, MA: Harvard University Press.
Dole, Vincent P., Marie E. Nyswander, and Mary Jeanne Kreek
  1966 Narcotic Blockade. Archives of Internal Medicine 118(4):304–309.
Duster, Troy
  2006 The Molecular Reinscription of Race: Unanticipated Issues in Biotechnology and Forensic Science. Patterns of Prejudice 40(4–5):427–441.
Fatseas, Melina, and Marc Auriacombe
  2007 Why Buprenorphine Is So Successful in Treating Opiate Addiction in France. Current Psychiatry Reports 9(5):358–364.
Goodman, Alan, and Tom Leatherman
  1999 Building a New Biocultural Synthesis. Ann Arbor, MI: University of Michigan Press.

Gravlee, Clarence C.

    2009 How Race Becomes Biology: Embodiment of Social Inequality. American Journal of Physical Anthropology 139(1):47–57.

Hamid, Ansley, Richard Curtis, Kate McCoy, Judy McGuire, Alix Conde, William Bushell, Rose Lindenmayer, Karen Brimberg, Suzana Maia, Sabura Abdur-Rashid, and Joy Settembrino

    1997 The Heroin Epidemic in New York City: Current Status and Prognoses. Journal of Psychoactive Drugs 29(4):375–391.

Hansen, Helena, Carole Siegel, David Bertollo, Danae DiRocco, and Marc Galanter

    N.d. Buprenorphine and Methadone in New York City: Two Tiers of Treatment? Unpublished MS, New York University.

Jaffe, Jerome, and Charles O'Keeffe

    2003 From Morphine Clinics to Buprenorphine: Regulating Opioid Agonist Treatment of Addiction in the United States. Drug and Alcohol Dependence 70(supp. 2):3–11.

Kirmayer, Laurence J., and Ian Gold

    2011 Re-Socializing Psychiatry: Critical Neuroscience and the Limits of Reductionism. *In* Critical Neuroscience: Handbook of the Social and Cultural Contexts of Neuroscience. Suparna Choudhury and Jan Slaby, eds. Pp. 305–330. Oxford: Wiley-Blackwell.

Kuehn, Bridget M.

    2005 Methadone Treatment Marks 40 Years. JAMA 294(8):887–889.

Leatherman, Tom, and Alan H. Goodman

    2011 Critical Biocultural Approaches in Medical Anthropology. *In* A Companion to Medical Anthropology. Merrill Singer and Pamela I. Erickson, eds. Pp. 29–47. Malden, MA: Wiley-Blackwell.

Lock, Margaret, and Vinh-Kim Nguyen

    2010 An Anthropology of Biomedicine. Malden, MA: Wiley-Blackwell.

Lovell, Anne M.

    2006 Addiction Markets: The Case of High Dose Buprenorphine in France. *In* Global Pharmaceuticals: Ethics, Markets and Practices. Adriana Petryna, Andrew Lakoff, and Arthur Kleinman, eds., Durham, NC: Duke University Press

Manchikanti, Laxmaiah, and Angelie Singh

    2008 Therapeutic Opioids: A Ten-Year Perspective on the Complexities and Complications of Escalating Use, Abuse, and Nonmedical Use of Opioids. Pain Physician 11(supp. 2):63–88.

Mattick, Richard, Courtney Breen, Jo Kimber, and Marina Davoli

    2003 Methadone Maintenance Therapy versus No Opioid Replacement Therapy for Opioid Dependence. Cochrane Database Systems Review 2003(2):CD002209.

McLellan, A. Thomas, David C. Lewis, Charles P. O'Brien, and Herbert D. Kleber

    2000 Drug Dependence: A Chronic Mental Illness. JAMA 284(13):1689–1695.

Montoya, Michael J.

    2007 Bioethnic Conscription: Genes, Race and Mexicana/o Ethnicity in Diabetes Research. Cultural Anthropology 22(1):94–128.

National Institute of Drug Abuse (NIDA)

    2011 Prescription Drug Abuse: A Research Update from the National Institute on Drug Abuse. May 2011. http://drugabuse.gov/tib/prescription.html, accessed November 23, 2012.

Netherland, Julie C.

    2010 Becoming Normal: The Social Construction of Buprenorphine and New Attempts to Medicalize Addiction. Ph.D. dissertation, Department of Sociology, City University of New York Graduate Center.

Reckitt Benckiser Pharmaceuticals

    2009 Powering Ahead: Annual Report and Financial Statements 2009. http://annualreport2009.rb.com/Home, accessed April 28, 2012.

    2010 Driving Innovative Growth: Annual Report and Financial Statements 2010. http://www.rb.com/Investors-media/Investor-information/Online-Annual-Report-2010, accessed April 28, 2012.

Roberts, Dorothy

2011 Fatal Invention: How Science, Politics, and Big Business Re-Create Race in the Twenty-First Century. New York: New Press.

Schull, Natasha D., and Caitlin Zaloom

2011 The Shortsighted Brain: Neuroeconomics and the Governance of Choice in Time. Social Studies of Science 41(4):515–538.

Sees, Karen L., Kevin L. Delucchi, Carmen Masson, Amy Rosen, H. Westley Clark, Helen Robillard, Peter Banys, and Sharon M. Hall

2000 Methadone Maintenance vs. 180-Day Psychosocially Enriched Detoxification for Treatment of Opioid Dependence: A Randomized Controlled Trial. JAMA 283(10):1303–1310.

Singer, Merrill

2008 Drugging the Poor: Legal and Illegal Drug Industries and the Structuring of Social Inequality. Long Grove, IL: Waveland Press

Soyka, Michael, and David A. Gorelick

2009 Why Should Addiction Medicine Be an Attractive Field for Young Physicians? Addiction 104(2):169–172.

Stanton, Arlene, Caroline McLeod, Bill Luckey, Wendy Kissin, and L. J. Sonnefeld

2006 Expanding Treatment of Opioid Dependence: Initial Physician and Patient Experiences with the Adoption of Buprenorphine. American Society of Addiction Medicine, March 2006. Presentation. http://www.buprenorphine.samhsa.gov/ASAM_06_Final_Results.pdf, accessed March 10, 2010.

Van Zee, Art

2009 The Promotion and Marketing of OxyContin: Commercial Triumph, Public Health Tragedy. American Journal of Public Health 99(2):221–227.

Vocci, Frank, Jane Acri, and Ahmed Elkashef

2005 Medication Development for Addictive Disorders: The State of the Science. American Journal of Psychiatry 162(8):1432–1440.

Vrecko, Scott

2010a Birth of a Brain Disease: Science, the State and Addiction Neuropolitics. History of the Human Sciences 23(4):52–67.

2010b Neuroscience, Power and Culture: An Introduction. History of the Human Sciences 23(10):1–10.

POVERTY POISONS THE BRAIN

DANIEL H. LENDE
University of South Florida

The concept of "poverty poisons the brain" has become a major area of research in neuroscience and the health sciences, and an increasingly utilized metaphor to argue for the importance of addressing inequality and poverty in the United States. This article systematically presents the research behind poverty poisons the brain, which includes the impact of socioeconomic status on human development, the developmental models used to understand how poverty impacts children, and the proximate social factors and brain mechanisms that represent the core causal model behind this research. This overview examines the uses of this research for neuroanthropology, highlighting the impact of inequality and how experience becomes embodied. Nevertheless, a simplistic cause–effect approach and the reduction of the social to the biological often hamper this type of research. A critical approach to how poverty poisons the brain provides the basis for making the shift to a more robust neuroanthropological approach to poverty. Neuroanthropology can utilize social embodiment, the dynamics of stress, and the production of inequality to transform research on poverty and children, and to make policy recommendations, do applied research, and craft and test interventions to deal with the pernicious impact of poverty. [poverty, human development, stress, inequality, critical theory]

In February 2008, Paul Krugman, Nobel laureate economist and *New York Times* columnist, wrote an op-ed entitled, "Poverty Is Poison." He summarized research presented at the American Association for the Advancement of Science annual conference by Martha Farah, a University of Pennsylvania neuroscientist, and her colleagues. These data showed that "unhealthy" levels of stress hormones in poor children can harm neural development. Krugman then argued:

> The effect is to impair language development and memory—and hence the ability to escape poverty—for the rest of the child's life. So now we have another, even more compelling reason to be ashamed about America's record of failing to fight poverty [Krugman 2008].

This theme of connecting neuroscience research with the discussion of poverty is one that has repeated itself several times in the intervening years. In 2009, Gary Evans and Michelle Schamberg, scientists at Cornell, published "Childhood Poverty, Chronic Stress, and Adult Working Memory" in the *Proceedings of the National Academy of Sciences*. At the popular *Wired* magazine site, journalist Brandom Keim followed suit with "Poverty Goes Straight to the Brain." The opening to Keim's article reads,

ANNALS OF ANTHROPOLOGICAL PRACTICE 36, pp. 183–201. ISSN: 2153-957X. © 2012 by the American Anthropological Association. DOI:10.1111/j.2153-9588.2012.01099.x

Growing up poor isn't merely hard on kids. It might also be bad for their brains. A long-term study of cognitive development in lower- and middle-class students found strong links between childhood poverty, physiological stress and adult memory [Keim 2009].

In Keim's reporting, being "bad for kids' brains" deserves separate emphasis, beyond poverty itself.

At the start of 2012, journalist Nicholas Kristof penned his own *New York Times* op-ed, "A Poverty Solution that Starts with a Hug." Once again the equation of poverty, stress, and damaged brain development in childhood comes into play. His piece opens, "Perhaps the most widespread peril children face isn't guns, swimming pools or speeding cars. Rather, scientists are suggesting that it may be 'toxic stress' early in life, or even before birth." This time the public conclusion draws not just on research, but on what Kristof calls a "landmark warning" from the American Academy of Pediatrics. This well-respected group of pediatricians had just published a policy statement in their own journal, *Pediatrics*: "Early Childhood Adversity, Toxic Stress, and the Role of the Pediatrician: Translating Developmental Science into Lifelong Health."

Pediatricians are now armed with new information about the adverse effects of toxic stress on brain development, as well as a deeper understanding of the early life origins of many adult diseases. As trusted authorities in child health and development, pediatric providers must now complement the early identification of developmental concerns with a greater focus on those interventions and community investments that reduce external threats to healthy brain growth [Committee on Psychosocial Aspects of Child and Family Health et al. 2012:e224].

I call this consistent linkage of children living in poverty and negative brain development the "poverty poisons the brain" model (Lende 2008). This model provides a powerful framing for thinking about how "experience gets under the skin" and how social factors like class and race negatively impact individuals. The poverty poisons the brain model is also "compelling" to people who argue in public about poverty—toxic stress is presented as a terrible peril early in life because it is bad for brain development.

This article will present the research behind "poverty poisons the brain," critically analyze the model and its social uses, and finally examine how to make it into a more robust neuroanthropological approach. The first half moves through the basic research paradigm behind poverty poisons the brain, which uses multifactorial etiology and a nested model of causation to understand how poverty does affect the brain. This research offers potential strengths for neuroanthropologists interested in how culture and society shape development. Similarly, research in biological and medical anthropology that examines individual outcomes with respect to social conditions can gain theoretical and applied insights for work that examines poverty, health disparities, and other similar domains. The second half of the article examines the poverty poisons the brain paradigm in a critical light. By placing important social dynamics in the background, this research often hides both actual poverty and the political economy of inequality from view. The approach can reinforce essentialist understandings of social class, and assume that

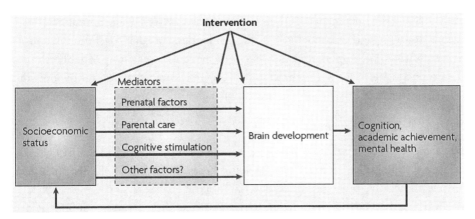

FIGURE 1. The Basic "Poverty Poisons the Brain" Model. Notice the unidirectional arrows leading from left to right, such that SES becomes the proximate mediators, which then turns into brain development, and finally individual outcomes. The accompanying text reads: "Socioeconomic status (SES) has effects on cognition, academic achievement and mental health. Research on brain development enables us to identify the differences in the cognitive and affective neural systems that underlie the effects of SES on cognition, academic achievement and mental health. In addition, neuroscience research in animals and humans can provide biologically plausible candidate mediators for explaining the cause–effect relationships between SES and neural development. These mediators include prenatal factors, parental care and cognitive stimulation, as well as other possible mechanisms. It is also likely that the effects of SES during early childhood on cognition, academic achievement and mental health will influence adult socioeconomic advancement." *Source*: Hackman and colleagues (2010).

by fixing poisoned brains, social problems can largely be solved. I finish by outlining research questions and additional model elements that could transform this approach in ways that match the holistic and comparative fundamentals at the core of anthropology.

FROM POVERTY TO THE BRAIN

Overview

Research linking poverty and the brain starts by establishing that there is a problem first—that lower socioeconomic status (SES) during childhood does indeed lead to negative outcomes in adults. That established, the research presents a developmental framework to understand that linkage. Next comes the heart of the poverty poisons the brain story—the combination of proximate environmental factors that shape childhood development and internal neurological mechanisms that translate proximate factors into structural and functional brain changes and associated capabilities and deficits. As shown in Figure 1, the core of the model is centered on local mediators and brain development.

In the move to considering the proximate factors shaping development, SES is generally placed to one side. SES is not seen as a proximate mechanism that can interact directly with people's brains and bodies; rather, SES is embodied through social relationships, personal experiences, and local material and social conditions that can impact the individual. This reduction generally strikes researchers as normal and appropriate—SES is a macro factor, and can only interact through local factors that constitute the broader SES indicator. More importantly, the brain is seen as only intersecting with SES through these individual-level factors, such that psychology, environmental health, and individual development become the primary lenses to explain how the poisoning actually happens.

SES and Negative Outcomes

Researchers generally establish that there is a significant problem in the first place that is in need of an explanation. Indeed, there is robust evidence that links SES in Western settings to negative outcomes (Duncan et al. 1994; Noble et al. 2007). Researchers are then careful to define SES. It is presented as an indicator of status and position in society, and often gets measured in two basic ways in western countries, level of income and level of education (not coincidentally, these are among the easiest aspects of SES to measure). Still, researchers hedge their bets by acknowledging that SES is a "complex construct" which derives from "household income, material resources, education and occupation, as well as related neighborhood and family characteristics" (Hackman et al. 2010:651). As another example, Evans et al. (2012) describe SES as having "associated physical/material, financial, educational, and social environmental features" but label its "primary constituents" as "income, education, [and] occupation."

Researchers also highlight the specific types of negative outcomes that are linked to lower SES. These generally fall into three areas: physical health, mental and behavioral health, and intelligence and academic success. Lower childhood SES is linked to lower ratings of health, greater cardiovascular disease, and increased mortality in adulthood (Adler and Stewart 2010). For mental and behavioral health, Hackman and colleagues document that, "children and adolescents from low-SES backgrounds show higher rates of depression, anxiety, attention problems and conduct disorders, and a higher prevalence of internalizing (that is, depression- or –anxiety-like) and externalizing (that is, aggressive and impulsive) behaviours, all of which increase with the duration of impoverishment" (Hackman et al.:652). On the intelligence side, lower SES is associated with lower IQ scores, less academic success, and less language ability. Recent research is pointing to links from childhood adversity to lower intelligence and cognitive success over the lifespan, which in turn is linked to greater mortality (Jokela et al. 2009).

The Causal Models Linking SES to Negative Outcomes

The link between SES and different types of negative outcomes is supported by multiple studies. The next step in this research has been to account for why there is this association between SES and negative outcomes: What mechanisms account for it? How does SES specifically lead to negative outcomes? This research first assumes that the linkage is a causal relationship, that SES does have direct and indirect effects on success and health. Then a model involving human development and multifactorial etiology is used to examine the causal factors. One of the most recent versions of this combination is the American Academy of Pediatrics' explicit embrace of an "ecobiodevelopmental" framework, which combines together an ecological model of development with a biodevelopmental focus on the child (Committee on Psychosocial Aspects of Child and Family Health et al. 2012).

The overall model is one that combines a distal to proximate conceptualization of the developing child, where multiple causes can come into play to influence development. In practice, the poverty poisons the brain research establishes that distal factors—SES —matters, and then moves to focus on the proximal factors that mediate the impact of SES in local environments like the home. Then it also examines the internal mechanisms, particularly the neurobiological systems, that are seen to account for the negative outcomes. In other words, the causal flow goes from SES to local mediators, and from local mediators to the altered development of the brain, and finally that altered development accounts for the negative outcomes experienced by the person later in life (see Figure 1). In this causal flow, the reason that neuroscience matters is that "in contrast to sociological and epidemiological approaches, neuroscience can identify the underlying cognitive and affective systems that are influenced by SES . . . [and provide] candidate mechanisms for the cause-effect relationships between SES and neural development" (Hackman et al. 2010:651).

Development

Theories of human development play a central role in advanced versions of the "poverty poisons the brain." These models go beyond asserting that "toxic stress" or some other cause is to blame for damaged brains. Rather, these developmental models aim to account for how experiences during development actually lead to positive and negative changes in neural development, function, and capability. There are four basic causal models used. Although they are often used in conjunction to explain specific outcomes, they are nonetheless distinct in how they understand the role of development in shaping biology (Hackman et al. 2010). These four models emphasize different dimensions of development: early experience, cumulative experience, selective achievement, and interactive experience. Each draws on research in human development that establishes how sensitive periods, an increasing number of risk factors, and behavior can shape the functioning of the person.

The first model—emphasizing the role of early experience—is often described as an embedding or developmental origins model. The key point is that early experience embeds itself in biological function during critical formative periods, leading to altered development over the lifespan. For poverty, it is clear that early experiences of deprivation are influential over the lifespan, often leading to health problems and reductions in lifetime income (Adler and Stewart 2010; Hackman et al. 2010). The second model is typically described as an accumulation of risk factors or adverse experiences. For example, the longer children spend in poverty, the worse in general are the adult outcomes across a range of indicators, from cardiovascular health to academic achievement to adult income (Adler and Stewart 2010; Hackman et al. 2010). In contrast to an emphasis on formative early experiences, the second model focuses on the developmental pathways children take, where pathways marked by adversity can lead to negative outcomes. The cumulative negative effects pave the way to bad health and adult capacity.

The selectionist model is one of the most determinist. It posits that individuals are born with certain traits and capacities and that these neural limits lead to a selective effect (Hackman et al. 2010). High-skill individuals end up with greater SES, whereas individuals born with lower abilities end up in lower classes. The selective effective is often seen as twofold: low-SES parents had lesser ability, however measured, and their cognitive abilities got passed onto their child; the child, in turn, was only able to progress so far along the SES scale because he or she did not have the same level of brain power as other children.

Although this model, put so baldly, might seem more a part of social discourse—we live in a meritocracy, people get their just desserts, and so forth—it actually appears more often in psychology and neuroscience research than might be expected. For example, recent work on neuroimaging and addiction among siblings compared to controls highlights a lack of executive control, or the ability to inhibit behavior, as a central feature in the risk of developing substance abuse (Ersche et al. 2012). "Abnormalities in fronto-striatal brain systems implicated in self-control" among confirmed addicts and their nonaddicted siblings point to an "underlying neurocognitive endophenotype" for addiction (Ersche et al. 2012:601). The implication is that this shared trait comes from family, and thus from genetics; in the media, this turns into the explanation for why individuals with low executive function, marked by abnormal brains, end up as substance abusers (Hamilton 2012; Szalavitz 2012). As Hamilton (2012) puts it, "Addicts' brains may be wired at birth for less self-control."

The final model is an interactive model, where behavior and feedback from the environment place individuals in different developmental niches. By changing the proximal environments that shape development, individuals thereby change their own growth and development (Worthman 2010). This feedback effect from the local environment can have both positive and negative effects. For example, a child that seeks out supportive relationships that he or she does not have at home can buffer the negative effects of the home environment. In contrast, an individual that seeks out drug-using friends to escape from home can create a cascade of negative effects on his development. The interactive model is the one needing the most development, and closest to a neuroanthropological approach that aims to link social and cultural research with brain function, child development, and the enculturation and socialization of brains (Odden 2009; Worthman 2009). Ideas about neural plasticity and neural reuse, links between experiences in the environment and epigenetic regulation of development, the concept of a zone of proximal development and of important sociocultural niches with human development can come together in this type of interactive developmental approach.

Proximate Mechanisms

Hackman and colleagues (2010) provide comprehensive coverage of the proximate mechanisms that research has shown relate to brain development and negative outcomes. These include parenting quality, in utero environment, home environment, toxin exposure (e.g., lead), nutrition, and stress (both chronic and acute). Research on how these proximal factors directly interact with the developing child generally focuses on direct insults or problems, for example, exposure to lead having a negative impact on brain development and leading to lowered cognitive ability, or how a lack of resources, whether malnutrition or books, can place limits on development.

Nevertheless, some researchers recognize that neighborhood quality can make a difference, and provide a link to understanding how inequality and deprivation affect childhood outcomes. Hertzman and Boyce (2010) outline one major study they have undertaken in British Columbia on early child development and neighborhood socioeconomic characteristics. In this research, evidence shows that more than 40 percent of the variance for health vulnerabilities, as measured by early development indicators, can be attributed to neighborhood socioeconomic characteristics. Furthermore, inequality can get under the skin through the experience of social status. Hertzman and Boyce write that, "Findings on the health correlates of subjective social status and peer group subordination suggest that the health disparities associated with SES may be at least partially attributable to differences in individuals' sense of identity, respect, and position within societies, small or large, marked by nonegalitarian structures and values" (Hertzman and Boyce 2010:332).

However, in most neuroscience research, the main proximal factors considered are social relationships and educational opportunities. For example, descriptions of the home environment often focus on "familial conflict and problematic parental behaviour," including "harsh and inconsistent discipline, less sensitivity to the needs of the child, [and] reduced verbal communication" (Hackman et al. 2010:654). In other words, they are bad parents, while SES remains a distal cause: "The important point is that broader social and economic context can influence the quality of parental care, which then influences the activity of the neural systems that regulate stress reactivity and cognition in offspring" (Hackman et al. 2010:655).

The other area that often receives attention is "the level of cognitive stimulation in the home" (Hackman et al. 2010). Stimulation includes "the availability of books (and other literacy resources), computers, trips, and parental communication. Together, these factors can explain the effects of SES on cognitive ability in children (for example, on reading and mathematics skill), even when maternal IQ has been controlled for" (Hackman et al. 2010:655). Thus, SES gets reduced to parenting and home quality, which are then associated with the negative outcomes. However, this causal move effectively washes SES from sight; the availability of books is the relevant indicator, not how greater or lesser SES might affect access to books, computers, and museum trips.

Finally, researchers focus on local stressors in the environment and local experiences with status as two ways that SES can impact the developing individual. As McEwen and Gianaros describe it, "the chronic experience of low SES at the individual level could involve enduring financial hardships, a sense of insecurity regarding future prosperity, and the possible demoralizing feelings of marginalization or social exclusion attributable to comparative social, occupational, or material disadvantage" (McEwen and Gianaros 2010:192). They also highlight subjective social status, the person's "perception of her or his relative standing or ranking in a social hierarchy" (McEwen and Gianaros 2010:192), as something that can affect emotional and physiological processes, thus implicitly making the negative experience of subjective social status into a problem of stress.

Internal Mechanisms

To understand how "experience gets under the skin" researchers focus on biological mechanisms that mediate experience and can change over time because of this experience. Hertzman and Boyce (2010) provide a useful two-piece framework for understanding this process—social causation and biological embedding. Social causation, unlike the typical cause–effect relation taught in basic science, is nonlinear and often nonspecific. A child might have a general vulnerability to adversity, and subsequently, dynamic interactions with the environment affect the cumulative impact of experience on development. Social causation often involves mundane experiences and relies on repeated exposures over time. This linkage of dynamic interactions and mundane experiences can lead to contingent lines of causation, for example, divorce leading to a drop in earning power leading to more economic stress leading to more drinking by a parent. Finally, social causation involves interpretive processes—meaning and emotion matter in experience. The impact of an adverse experience often depends as much on how the person interprets it as it does on some intrinsic aspect of the event itself.

Hertzman and Boyce (2010) present biological embedding as the complement to social causation. Biological embedding occurs when experience alters biological function, which can lead to long-term stable changes over development. Biological embedding does not work indiscriminately; rather, Hertzman and Boyce (2010) propose that biological systems have to meet several basic characteristics for embedding to occur: (1) the system in question can be influenced by daily experience and (2) responds to experience over the lifecourse; (3) its functioning (or dysfunction) has significant impacts on health, learning, and/or behavior, and (4) the differences in outcome can derive in part from early experience. Although Hertzman and Boyce highlight several systems that meet these criteria—the autonomic nervous system and the prefrontal cortices, for example—they present stress and the hypothalamic–pituitary–adrenal (HPA) axis as the best model for how biological embedding happens.

The American Academy of Pediatrics (Committee on Psychosocial Aspects of Child and Family Health et al. 2012) also places "toxic stress" at the center of how early childhood adversity affects childhood development and adult health and capability. Toxic stress is defined largely in biological terms: "excessive or prolonged activation of the physiologic stress response systems" and "disruptive physiologic responses (ie, toxic stress) that produce 'biological memories' that increase the risk of health-threatening behaviors and frank disease later in life" (Committee on Psychosocial Aspects of Child and Family Health et al. 2012:e225). Although "stable, responsive relationships" with caregivers can buffer early adversity, the American Academy of Pediatrics highlights stress as the principal mediating cause of inequality, writing that growing evidence "links childhood toxic stress to the subsequent development of unhealthy lifestyles (eg, substance abuse, poor eating and exercise habits), persistent socioeconomic inequalities (eg, school failure and financial hardship), and poor health (eg, diabetes and cardiovascular disease)"

(Committee on Psychosocial Aspects of Child and Family Health et al. 2012:e225). Toxic stress becomes the focal point of rhetoric, research, and policy.

Stress is not an idle choice—it does represent an excellent system to demonstrate that poverty can indeed poison the brain. At a mechanistic level inside the person, the physiology of stress involves both brain and body and is often driven by reactions to environmental stressors, both real (e.g., a fistfight) and perceived (e.g., thinking a fistfight could happen). Thus, the physiology lends itself to metaphorical understanding, as a way to think and talk about how poverty is damaging. But the technical details back that talk up. To use the language of McEwen and Gianaros, "stress processes arise from bidirectional patterns of communication between the brain and the autonomic, cardiovascular, and immune systems via neural and endocrine mechanisms underpinning cognition, experience, and behavior" (McEwen and Gianaros 2010:190). McEwen and Gianaros (2010) then present the concept of allostasis, in which short-term activation of the stress system to deal with adversity can lead to long-term costs because of wear-and-tear with chronic stress, as a way to understand how a relatively constant condition like SES can produce negative effects over time.

Stress also becomes a way to both examine and evoke other biological mechanisms that play a role in how development adapts to experience, both positively and negatively. The loss of neuroplasticity through glucocorticoid exposure as a fetus or infant is one main way researchers like McEwen and Gianaros (2010) and Hackman et al. (2010) explain how the poisoning happens—high levels of glucocorticoids can lead to greater neuronal loss and less proliferation of connections among neurons, leading to a less-effective brain. Epigenetics is another major way to talk about how stress, and experience more broadly, can alter brain development. Lupien and colleagues (2009) argue that through epigenetics, genes get expressed differently because of timing and exposure to stress coupled with previous exposure to adversity. Recently, Essex and colleagues (2011) demonstrated differential DNA methylation, a crucial epigenetic mechanism, in adolescents exposed to childhood adversities earlier in life.

Beyond stress, researchers also focus on the mechanistic links between childhood poverty and adverse outcomes with respect to academic achievement. Generally, the link is made between compromised language acquisition and cognitive development and later IQ–cognitive ability and educational success. For example, a recent prospective study by Najman and colleagues concluded, "Children experiencing family poverty at any developmental stage in their early life course have reduced levels of cognitive development, with the frequency that poverty is experienced predicting the extent of reduced cognitive scores" (Najman et al. 2009:284). Similarly, Hackman and Farah write, "Language ability differs sharply as a function of SES . . . SES gradients have been observed in vocabulary, phonological awareness and syntax at many different stages of development" (Hackman and Farah 2009:65).

A final area where internal mechanisms can play a role is in behavior, particularly the impact of poverty on mental and behavioral health, where greater rates of problems are found among low SES children and adolescents (Hackman et al. 2010). Often these problems are linked to the effect of early maltreatment and conflict-filled relations in the home, which can impact the development of emotional regulation and cognitive control in the limbic and prefrontal areas of the brain. There is also evidence that directly links the experience of lower SES to threat appraisal and fear within the individual, pointing to a more direct way that inequality might shape children's brains (McEwen and Gianaros 2010). In this research, lower perceived parental social standing was linked to greater amygdala reactivity to angry faces and lower subjective social status was associated with reduced volume in the anterior cingulate cortex. As McEwen and Gianaros argue, these areas affect the regulation of behavior, and compromised function here can "increase vulnerability to psychiatric and medical syndromes characterized by dysregulated emotion-related behaviors and physiology" (McEwen and Gianaros 2010:207).

In summary, the mechanistic approaches use stress, epigenetics and neuroplasticity, language acquisition, and emotion regulation as ways that social causes can alter biological function through biological embedding. A key system here is the HPA axis, and the concept of "toxic stress" that can drive continued overactivation of the axis with an associated impact on the brain. Toxic stress becomes how poverty poisons the brain.

APPROACH TO INTERVENTIONS

Hackman and Farah write, "societal investment in reducing the impact of childhood poverty on cognitive ability is far more efficient [early in life] than programs designed to reverse its effects later in life" (Hackman and Farah 2009:71). This basic point—that the greatest payoff comes from early investment, and that this early investment can help mitigate lifelong effects of poverty—is the strongest policy point that emerges from the "poverty poisons the brain" model.

Beyond this important conclusion, different researchers propose different interventions for early childhood. Hackman and Farah (2009) highlight providing additional income to families of poor children, which has been linked to improved language function. They also argue that interventions can directly target specific neurocognitive systems, describing the example of the "Tools of the Mind" program, a computerized game aimed at enhancing executive function in children. Hackman et al. (2010) paint in broader brushstrokes, mentioning direct changes to SES, improving access to medical care and nutritional supplements, and also direct interventions through cognitive training and enhancement. They also present "poverty poisons the brain" as a public health problem that requires shaping the environments of these children. "Precedence should be given to improving care for children and to providing enriching environments during pre- and postnatal development. Therefore, policies and programmes that reduce parental stress, enhance parental emotional well-being and provide adequate resources for parents and communities should be prioritized" (Hackman et al 2010:656).

McEwen and Gianaros (2010) present an approach aimed specifically at reducing chronic stress and allostatic load. They highlight basic things like increasing physical activity and social integration, both of which can buffer the person against chronic stress. They argue that pharmaceutical interventions should be considered, even with potential side effects. Finally, they point to "top-down effects of policies," where "education, housing, taxation, setting of a minimum wage, and addressing occupational health and safety and environmental pollution regulations are all likely to affect the brain and health via a myriad of mechanisms" (McEwen and Gianaros 2010:212).

The American Academy of Pediatrics is most explicit on the policy side, advocating a "broad-based, multisector commitment" that aims to reduce toxic stress in children (Committee on Psychosocial Aspects of Child and Family Health et al. 2012). Part of this commitment can come through pediatricians themselves, who should shift to this new approach emphasizing toxic stress while continuing to draw on their strengths in developmental approaches to health, understanding the importance of prevention, and having a powerful role as advocates for change. Besides more extensive training about toxic stress, the Academy recommends recognizing the limits of an office-based approach to "full address the new morbidities effectively" (Committee on Psychosocial Aspects of Child and Family Health et al. 2012:e226) and the urgent need for the development of more evidence-based strategies.

Although these broad-based approaches are often advocated, it is clear that medications and brain-based training are already at the forefront of what will count as "effective interventions." These types of intervention studies are easy to construct as "evidence based," requiring a double-blind approach that washes away the complexity of engaging specific communities or aiming for large-scale programs to achieve change.

"POVERTY POISONS THE BRAIN"–USES FOR NEUROANTHROPOLOGY

Before turning to a critical analysis of the "poverty poisons the brain" approach, I want to highlight four potential uses for neuroanthropologists concerned with the links between inequality, development, children, and health. First, the interactive elements of the overall approach offer useful conceptual tools for neuroanthropologists. Social causation, the interactive model of development, biological embedding, and neuroplasticity and epigenetics provide a cascading approach to understanding just how poverty poisons the brain, and thus how unequal social outcomes and health disparities come to be. Second, the "poverty poisons the brain" model gets at central anthropological questions, such as how do culture and social structure shape the individual. This research highlights the need for us to think seriously about how experience gets under the skin, from processes of enculturation to the impact of inequality. Anthropologists like Gravlee (2009) and Worthman (2009) are actively examining the embodiment of social inequality and the development of emotion regulation through childhood experience. The "poverty poisons the brain" approach offers ways to further link embodiment to development, and thus produce even more robust anthropological models for how social inequality and cultural experience shape us into the people we are.

Third, "poverty poisons the brain" offers a powerful rhetorical model that anthropologists might use to argue publicly about the need to address systemic inequality, structural violence, and health disparities. As a metaphor, it can help policy makers and the public understand the high costs that these systemic social inequalities can create, and also to tease out and explain away some of the obvious objections—that behaviors like drug use or violence are to blame, or that these people simply reached some preordained limits, and resources would be better spent elsewhere. Inequality is toxic is a compelling line, and locating that toxicity inside people—inside their brains—can help researchers convince often-skeptical audiences that social forces do indeed matter and should be addressed. Negative outcomes like drug use and low educational achievement are just that, outcomes linked to toxic stress and other neurobiological reactions to what children face. Although this approach does offer a double-edged sword, which will become apparent below, "poverty poisons the brain" can cut through to issues that anthropologists consider central to applied efforts.

Fourth, the "evidence-based" approach offers potential uses for anthropologists. The American Academy of Pediatrics emphasizes prevention, collaborating with the community, and thinking outside the office setting. Anthropologists, armed with a neuroanthropological approach, can help design interventions that can make a difference in families' and children's lives. These types of interventions can be just as easily subjected to an evidence-based approach as brain-based training. Thus, "poverty poisons the brain" can help frame an overall approach to developing effective applied anthropology that can show demonstrable effects and thus become incorporated into the work of broader societal institutions like the American Academy of Pediatrics.

THE NEUROANTHROPOLOGY OF "POVERTY POISONS THE BRAIN"

A Critical Failing

The first and most obvious problem with "poverty poisons the brain" is how it effectively works to conceal the social forces—both the actual poverty suffered by people and the systemic effects and politics of inequality—from view. This flaw is almost enough to undercut the entire approach. Although these researchers do aim to highlight the pernicious effects of poverty during childhood on the rest of the lifecourse, they don't actually focus on poverty much. As Figure 1 shows explicitly, SES becomes prenatal factors, parental care, and cognitive stimulation, which in turn becomes brain development, and that leads to cognition, academic achievement, and mental health. The effect is to wash away social considerations and theory from the model, and thus essentialize social difference in the family and the individual. As researchers move from social inequality to the proximate factors, neighborhood quality and SES get reduced to low-quality parenting, household conflict, and other local manifestations of "toxic stress." The social level of analysis gets left behind, even though in reality, the social is part-and-parcel of the household and the child's experience.

Researchers like Hackman and Farah do warn that the neuroscience is open to "blaming the victim," writing "Characteristic differences between individuals of higher and lower SES have been used by some to argue that low SES individuals are intrinsically less deserving or less valuable members of society. The biological nature of the differences documented by cognitive neuroscience can make these differences seem all the more 'essential' and immutable" (Hackman and Farah 2009:71). Nevertheless, they seem blithely unaware of how their own models facilitate such blaming. How else are we supposed to read the transition from SES to brain development and academic achievement? Simply contradicting ideas about "fixed, innate programs" and stating "there is little evidence to suggest differences are essential or immutable" is not good enough. As ethnographic research on the "disease model" of addiction has shown, social actors like law enforcement can easily incorporate supposedly liberating biology-based models to justify increased criminalization and prosecution of drug users (Garriott 2011). After all, they have a disease—a biological problem, whether that pathology came through an innate genetic program or "specific causal pathways by which socioeconomic deprivation can affect brain function" (Hackman and Farah 2010:71).

The same model—where socioeconomic deprivation comes down to brain function—also supports existing approaches to dealing with brain problems, from pharmaceuticals to education that "treat" or "enhance" brain function. A massive capitalist enterprise already exists for developing pharmaceuticals for children. A new market is rapidly taking shape for "brain training" initiatives to shape the newly conceived "plastic" brain, building on existing therapeutic and educational enterprises. All these endeavors will take the "poverty poisons the brain" model and seek to both profit and assert societal control through this new causal metaphor to understand children's development.

Thus, neuroanthropologists who plan to use a "poverty poisons" approach need to be aware of the double-edged sword of the metaphor. We are not the only actors who will use it, and although it might cut toward confronting inequality, it also cuts toward essentializing difference and favoring already existing forms of social control and biology-driven management of "poisoned brains." To counteract these considerable drawbacks, neuroanthropologists must be explicit on making the "poverty poisons" model into one that moves far beyond a focus on how SES gets lodged in the brain, thereby losing social theory through an intrinsic focus on the individual. Three ways exist to reform this approach, and make it into something that can do considerable anthropological work.

The Social Embodiment of Inequality

One way to bring the social into view is to recognize, as I wrote above, that inequality itself (and not just "the impact" of inequality) will be manifest in the environment and in development. The embodiment of inequality offers an approach to better understand how proximate factors and dynamics include social and cultural forces (Gravlee 2009; Krieger 2005). Such an approach can draw on (1) radical contextualization, where the use of ethnography, studying up, and biosocial analysis can help highlight how social processes underpin health disparities (Chapman and Berggren 2005); (2) the anthropology of adverse environments, which incorporate "a range of physical, social, and temporal factors that are highly localized and sensitive to community-level influences on growth and health" (Moffat and Galloway 2007:676); (3) the social embodiment of biology, to understand how context and environment can get under the skin (Gravlee 2009; Kuzawa and Sweet 2009); (4) risk focusing, where culture plays a fundamental role in the cumulative experience of disadvantage over development (Schell 1992); and (5) the everyday practices of privilege, discrimination, and status that play a role in perpetuating inequality (Schultz et al. 2006; Stephens and Gillies 2012; Sweet 2010). Together, these approaches offer the way to understand, first, how the social is present in the everyday life of inequality, and second, to connect that to a much wider range of proximate factors and local environments that shape development and embodied biology.

FROM "TOXIC STRESS" TO THE DYNAMICS OF STRESS AND INEQUALITY

Stress is the lynchpin around which much of the "poverty poisons the brain" discourse revolves. "Toxic stress" does the poisoning, while the HPA axis is exhibit number one to show how connected the brain is to the body and the environment, and thus vulnerable to poverty. The main problem is that "toxic stress affects vulnerable biology" does not change either reductive cause–effect thinking or move beyond a mechanical conceptualization of what stress is. Still, decades of research on stress provide the grounding for a better model of stress that can link easily to social theory and to the everyday reality of inequality.

First, anthropological research has consistently linked the experience of social status to stress, such that incongruity with social norms (McDade 2008), a lack of consonance with societal ideals (Dressler 2011), the sense of social alienation and social worth (Blakey 1998), negotiating social conflicts in relationships (Flinn 2007), and the inability to achieve major social goals for a "good life" (Brown et al. 2009) all impact stress. Second, anthropologists have also reformulated environmental stressors as cultural, particularly through the interpretive frameworks brought to bear to understand and cope with adversity (Eggerman and Panter-Brick 2010; Snipes et al. 2007). Together, this research shows that the ability to realize collective goals in one's life, not being able to "find a way out" of difficult social situations or conflicting demands, and feelings of despair and hope matter deeply in what stress is and does.

The next step is to link this anthropological work on stress with psychological and neurobiological research. This research, often done with animal models or in controlled situations in university laboratories, resonates deeply with the anthropological research. This research highlights how uncertainty and unpredictability are stressful; that a lack of control, or the ability to do something about one's situation, exacerbates stress; and that lower social status, particularly in social interactions where that status is judged and reinforced, is intrinsically stressful (Matthews and Gallo 2011; Miller et al. 2009; Sapolsky 2005). These findings are remarkably close to the anthropological work. Uncertain and unpredictable interactions with people of higher status (e.g., waiting for the other shoe to drop); a lack of control and feeling despair; few if any means to do anything about one's social situation—the joint social and neural dynamics make stress poisonous. "Toxic stress" is toxic not simply through the accumulation of stressors, but because there is a match between sociocultural forces and neuropsychological forces.

Thus, a neuroanthropology of poverty shows that poverty is not bad simply because of lower social status, increased environmental stressors, and a lack of resources. Poverty is bad because it unites individual and societal lack of control, creates unpredictable adversity, sets conditions that leave people unable to respond, and creates a sense of helplessness and despair. Yet there is a flip side to this neuroanthropological approach. The dynamic view also provides recommendations for what to do. Given people options, reducing uncertainty, and generating more equal relations are all ways to change the neuroanthropology of stress. Doing that requires tackling inequality in both its proximate and societal dimensions.

THE PRODUCTION OF SOCIAL FACTS

The flow of causality in the basic "poverty poisons the brain" model is from SES to the individual brain, where changes in neural structure and function are then assumed to largely account for individual outcomes like educational achievement. This reductionist approach assumes that assembling a group of underachieving, brain-compromised individuals is the central key to understanding how social class and inequality come about. These researchers overlook how the brain can and does play a role in the social production and reproduction of class and patterns of social inequality and health disparity. Indeed, if we think about Bourdieu's habitus, that internal collection of habits and tastes and practices, the brain becomes a particularly important way to understand how we actually come to have a habitus, rather than simply assume that it is given, sui generis, by social forces (Downey 2010; Hay 2009). The brain contributes to the production and reproduction of our social lives, and that perspective offers a truly important way to understand how poverty, social experience, and brain development come together in helping to create social class and the reproduction of social structure. The social organization of inequality happens through how social forces shape our neuroplastic and embodied brains. Opening up questions for how this process happens is a crucial next step for really understanding what we mean by "poverty poisons the brain."

As neuroscience shows, poverty literally can be anatomy, something that cannot be fixed simply by money or by declarations of human rights. This view challenges typical liberal policy. Inequality runs through families, through development and through behavior and biology. Standard liberal solutions often assume that changing the environment—affecting policy or providing better information—is enough. It is not. People themselves take part in reproducing inequality. It is in their bones, in their hearts, in the brains. This reality makes both "blame the victim" and social justice approaches equally viable. To move beyond this easy dichotomy, a good first step is to draw on the multifactorial etiology approach to understanding the conjunction of social environments, behavioral biology, and human development. A crucial next step is to incorporate measures of higher level social causes into this model, and to also develop measures that better examine the sociocultural dimensions and neuroanthropological processes present at the proximate level of explanation. This second step opens up an evidence-based approach to showing how the social matters at all levels represented in Figure 1, and for showing better how poverty truly does poison the brain. Alongside this empirical approach, it is important to develop multilevel and multisited interventions that are tied together by a holistic applied anthropology focused on the neuroanthropology of poverty.

However, better measurements and interventions using a multifactorial model will not solve the culture versus biology or mind–body dichotomies present in both anthropology and neuroscience. Understanding the role that the brain plays in generating social structure is not as simple as recognizing that neuroscience can contribute to our under-standing of concepts like habitus or aid in understanding how inequality gets reproduced generation to generation. It also requires a wholesale shift in how many anthropologists and many neuroscientists conceive of the brain. The mechanistic research done by neuroscience is often done from the perspective of the brain, for example, that stress is largely psychobiological, an internal and individual state shaped by the "fight-or-flight" evolution of the stress system. This view might be useful in the laboratory, the scientific gaze to fix on a certain neurological function. But it is not how the brain works in the real world. The social and the meaningful become part of how the brain functions. That requires a fundamental shift in how we understand what the brain does.

One of the most problematic issues with "poverty poisons the brain," and much of brain research in general, is that the brain becomes a fetish. We point to the neuroanatom-ical changes in the brain, and then say, this stuff about poverty being bad for children must be true. Recall the opening of the *Wired* piece, "Growing up poor isn't merely hard on kids. It might also be bad for their brains." Here children are placed to one side in favor of our new marker of individuality, the brain. Social relationships between people, from the structural to the everyday, become reduced to how they are expressed, mediated, and transformed by mechanical processes—objects—within the brain. Referencing the brain as the central mediator of poverty hides the larger truths of inequality and distorts our understanding of what poverty really is. To take a more extreme example to illustrate the same point, it is like saying slavery is both harmful to people and morally wrong because it impacts brains.

The brain has become like property, something a person possesses and that poverty—somehow separate from the person, a naturalized thing that causes stress—negatively impacts. This view is in need of a radical change. The social system does flow through the brain, among other material and symbolic substrates; the brain works in such a way that its function is, at least in part, social. Put differently, taking the perspective of human meaning and social relations as the way to understand brain function is an area in need of urgent development.

The brain is not anatomy alone. Taking the combination of neuroscience and an-thropology seriously means that social environments, in all their complexity, become as important as any brain part. Still, anthropology does need to go through an un-settling shift in our understanding of inequality, given the central role that devel-opment and neural function do play in what poverty is and means for people. In anthropology, often social forces become the privileged way we understand social suffer-ing. Neuroanthropology challenges that view. The embodiment that runs through the brain—this sociobiological embedding of our experiences and our social relations—is indeed a core cause, a central hub, around which inequality is created. The embodied brain is not just a fundamental place of suffering, it is a fundamental cause of social suffering. The way our brains work, their openness to social causation and biological embedding; the way the dynamics of the stress system can meet the dynamics of the social system—these mean that suffering from poverty is not reducible to social theory alone. People suffer through their embodied brains, through despair and toxic stress and destructive behavior. The brain suffers poverty. We can build research that examines how and why neuroanthropological dynamics play a role in social suffering, the reproduction and impact of inequality, and the disparities in health and well-being that children experience by growing in unequal conditions.

REFERENCES CITED

Adler, Nancy E., and Judith Stewart
  2010 Health Disparities across the Lifespan: Meaning, Methods, and Mechanisms. Annals of the New York Academy of Sciences 1186(1):5–23.
Blakey, Michael L.
  1998 Beyond European Enlightenment: Toward a Critical and Humanistic Human Biology. *In* Building a New Biocultural Synthesis: Political-Economic Perspectives on Human Biology. Alan H. Goodman and Thomas L. Leatherman, eds. Pp. 379–406. Ann Arbor: University of Michigan Press.
Brown, Ryan A., David H. Rehkopf, William E. Copeland, E. Jane Costello, and Carol M. Worthman
  2009 Lifecourse Priorities among Appalachian Emerging Adults: Revisiting Wallace's Organization of Diversity. Ethos 37(2):225–242.
Chapman, Rachel R., and Jean R. Berggren
  2005 Radical Contextualization: Contributions to an Anthropology of Racial/Ethnic Health Disparities. Health 9(1):145–167.
Committee on Psychosocial Aspects of Child and Family Health, Committee on Early Childhood, Adoption, and Dependent Care, and Section on Developmental and Behavioral Pediatrics, Andrew S. Garner, Jack P. Shonkoff, Benjamin S. Siegel, Mary I. Dobbins, Marian F. Earls, Andrew S. Garner, Laura McGuinn, John Pascoe, and David L. Wood
  2012 Early Childhood Adversity, Toxic Stress, and the Role of the Pediatrician: Translating Developmental Science Into Lifelong Health. Pediatrics 129(1): e224–e231.
Downey, Greg
  2010 "Practice without Theory": A Neuroanthropological Perspective on Embodied Learning. Journal of the Royal Anthropological Institute 16(supp. 1):22–40.
Duncan, Greg J., Jeanne Brooks-Gunn, and Pamela K. Klebanov
  1994 Economic Deprivation and Early Childhood Development. Child Development 65(2):296–318.
Dressler, William W.
  2011 Culture and the Stress Process. *In* A Companion to Medical Anthropology. Merrill Singer and Pamela Erickson, eds. Pp. 119–134. New York: Wiley-Blackwell.
Eggerman, Mark, and Catherine Panter-Brick
  2010 Suffering, Hope, and Entrapment: Resilience and Cultural Values in Afghanistan. Social Science and Medicine 71(1):71–83.
Ersche, Karen D., P. Simon Jones, Guy B. Williams, Abigail J. Turton, Trevor W. Robbins, and Edward T. Bullmore
  2012 Abnormal Brain Structure Implicated in Stimulant Drug Addiction. Science 335(6068):601–604.
Essex, Marilyn J., W. Thomas Boyce, Clyde Hertzman, Lucia L. Lam, Jeffrey M. Armstrong, Sarah M. A. Neumann, and Michael S. Kobor
  2011 Epigenetic Vestiges of Early Developmental Adversity: Childhood Stress Exposure and DNA Methylation in Adolescence. Child Development. doi:10.1111/j.1467–8624.2011.01641.x, accessed February 24, 2012.
Evans, Gary W., Edith Chen, Gregory Miller, and Teresa Seeman
  2012 How Poverty Gets Under the Skin: A Life Course Perspective. *In* The Oxford Handbook of Poverty and Child Development. Valerie Maholmes and Rosalind B. King, eds. Pp. 13–36. New York: Oxford University Press.
Evans, Gary W., and Michelle A. Shamberg
  2009 Childhood Poverty, Chronic Stress, and Adult Working Memory. Proceedings of the National Academy of Sciences 106(16):6545–6549.

Flinn, Mark V.

    2007 Why Words Can Hurt Us: Social Relationships, Stress, and Health. *In* Evolutionary Medicine and Health. Wena Trevathan, E. O. Smith, and James J. McKenna, eds. Pp. 247–258. Oxford: Oxford University Press.

Garriott, William

    2011 Policing Methamphetamine: Narcopolitics in Rural America. New York: New York University Press.

Gravlee, Clarence C.

    2009 How Race Becomes Biology: Embodiment of Social Inequality. American Journal of Physical Anthropology 139(1):47–57.

Hackman, Daniel A., and Martha J. Farah

    2009 Socioeconomic Status and the Developing Brain. Trends in Cognitive Science 13(2):65–73.

Hackman, Daniel A., Martha J. Farah, and Michael J. Meaney

    2010 Socioeconomic Status and the Brain: Mechanistic Insights from Human and Animal Research. Nature Reviews Neuroscience 11(9):651–659.

Hamilton, Jon

    2012 Addicts' Brains May be Wired at Birth for Less Self-Control. Morning Edition, National Public Radio. http://www.npr.org/blogs/health/2012/02/03/146307907/addicts-brains-may-be-wired-at-birth-for-less-self-control, accessed February 3, 2012.

Hay, M. Cameron

    2009 Anxiety, Remembering, and Agency: Biocultural Insights for Understanding Sasaks' Responses to Illness. Ethos 37(1):1–31.

Hertzman, Clyde, and Tom Boyce

    2010 How Experience Gets Under the Skin to Create Gradients in Developmental Health. Annual Review of Public Health, 31(1):329–347.

Jokela, Markus, G. David Batty, Ian J Deary, Catharine R. Gale, and Mika Kivimäk

    2009 Low Childhood IQ and Early Adult Mortality: The Role of Explanatory Factors in the 1958 British Birth Cohort. Pediatrics 124(3):e380–e388.

Keim, Brandon

    2009 Poverty Goes Straight to the Brain. Wired Science. March 30. http://www.wired.com/wiredscience/2009/03/poordevelopment/, accessed February 3, 2012.

Krieger, Nancy

    2005 Embodiment: A Conceptual Glossary for Epidemiology. Journal of Epidemiology of Community Health 59(5):350–355.

Kristof, Nicholas D.

    2012 A Poverty Solution that Starts with a Hug. New York Times. January 7. http://www.nytimes.com/2012/01/08/opinion/sunday/kristof-a-poverty-solution-that-starts-with-a-hug.html, accessed February 9, 2012.

Krugman, Paul

    2008 Poverty is Poison. New York Times. February 18. http://www.nytimes.com/2008/02/18/opinion/18krugman.html, accessed February 3, 2012.

Kuzawa, Christopher W., and Elizabeth Sweet

    2009 Epigenetics and the Embodiment of Race: Developmental Origins of US Racial Disparities in Cardiovascular Health. American Journal of Human Biology, 21(1):2–15.

Lende, Daniel

    2008 Poverty Poisons the Brain. Neuroanthropology: For a Greater Understanding of an Encultured Brain and Body. http://neuroanthropology.net/2008/02/18/poverty-poisons-the-brain/, accessed February 3, 2012.

Lupien, Sonia J., Bruce S. McEwen, Megan R. Gunnar, and Christine Heim

    2009 Effects of Stress throughout the Lifespan on the Brain, Behaviour and Cognition. Nature Reviews Neuroscience 10(6):434–445.

Matthews, Karen A., and Linda C. Gallo

    2011 Psychological Perspectives on Pathways Linking Socioeconomic Status and Physical Health. Annual Review of Psychology 62(1):501–530.

McDade, Thomas

  2008 Beyond the Gradient: An Integrative Anthropological Perspective on Social Stratification, Stress, and Health. *In* Health, Risk and Adversity. Catherine Panter-Brick and Agustín Fuentes, eds. Pp. 209–235. New York: Berghahn.

McEwen, Bruce S., and Peter J. Gianaros

  2010 Central Role of the Brain in Stress and Adaptation: Links to Socioeconomic Status, Health, and Disease. Annals of the New York Academy of Sciences 1186(1):190–222.

Miller, Gregory, Edith Chen, and Steve W. Cole

  2009 Health Psychology: Developing Biologically Plausible Models Linking the Social World and Physical Health. Annual Review of Psychology 60(1):501–524.

Moffat, Tina, and Tracey Galloway

  2007 Adverse Environments: Investigating Local Variation in Child Growth. American Journal of Human Biology 19(5):676–683.

Najman, Jake M., Mohammad R. Hayatbakhsh, Michelle A. Heron, William Bor, Michael J. O'Callaghan, and Gail M. Williams

  2009 The Impact of Episodic and Chronic Poverty on Child Cognitive Development. The Journal of Pediatrics 154(2):284–289.e1.

Noble, Kimberly G., Bruce D. McCandliss, and Martha J. Farah

  2007 Socioeconomic Gradients Predict Individual Differences in Neurocognitive Abilities. Developmental Science 10(4):464–480.

Odden, Harold L.

  2009 Interactions of Temperature and Culture: The Organization of Diversity in Samoan Infancy. Ethos 37(2):161–180.

Sapolsky, Robert M.

  2005 The Influence of Social Hierarchy on Primate Health. Science 29(308):648–652.

Schell, Lawrence M.

  1992 Risk Focusing: An Example of Biocultural Interaction. *In* Health and Lifestyle Change, vol. 9. Rebecca Huss-Ashmore, Joan Schall, and Mary Hediger, eds. Pp. 137–147. Philadelphia: University of Pennsylvania Museum of Archaeology and Anthropology.

Schulz, Amy J., Clarence C. Gravlee, David R. Williams, Barbara A. Israel, Graciela Mentz, and Zachary Rowe

  2006 Discrimination, Symptoms of Depression, and Self-Rated Health among African American Women in Detroit: Results from a Longitudinal Analysis. American Journal of Public Health 96(7):1265–1270.

Snipes, Shedra A., Beti Thompson, Kathleen O'Connor, Ruby Godina, and Genoveva Ibarra

  2007 Anthropological and Psychological Merge: Design of a Stress Measure for Mexican Farmworkers. Culture, Medicine and Psychiatry 31(3):359–88.

Stephens, Christine, and Annemarie Gillies

  2012 Understanding the Role of Everyday Practices of Privilege in the Perpetuation of Inequalities. Journal of Community and Applied Social Psychology 22(2):145–158.

Sweet, Elizabeth

  2010 "If Your Shoes Are Raggedy You Get Talked About": Symbolic and Material Dimensions of Adolescent Social Status and Health. Social Science and Medicine 70(12):2029–2035.

Szalavitz, Maia

  2012 Siblings Brain Study Sheds Light on the Roots of Addiction. Time Healthland, February 3. http://healthland.time.com/2012/02/03/siblings-brain-study-sheds-light-on-the-roots-of-addiction/, accessed February 12, 2012.

Worthman, Carol M.

  2009 Habits of the Heart: Life History and the Developmental Neuroendocrinology of Emotion. American Journal of Human Biology 21(6):772–781.

  2010 The Ecology of Human Development: Evolving Models for Cultural Psychology. Journal of Cross-Cultural Psychology 41(4):546–562.

BIOSKETCHES OF CONTRIBUTORS–Neuroanthropology and Its Applications

Victoria K. Burbank is Professor of Anthropology at the University of Western Australia. She is a psychological anthropologist who has worked in the Arnhem Land community of Numbulwar since 1977. Her publications on Numbulwar include *Aboriginal Adolescence: Maidenhood in an Australian Community* (1988), *Fighting Women: Anger and Aggression in Aboriginal Australia* (1994), and *An Ethnography of Stress: The Social Determinants of Health in Aboriginal Australia* (2011).

Gino L. Collura, M.A., Latin American and Caribbean studies (concentration in international relations), is currently a Ph.D. student at the University of South Florida. He is specializing in medical anthropology and neuroanthropology under the auspices of Dr. Daniel Lende. His concentrations are trauma, resilience, combative stress, post-traumatic stress disorder, and identity. He is a former business owner and consultant and has worked as an executive protection specialist.

Greg Downey (greg.downey@mq.edu.au) is Senior Lecturer in Anthropology at Macquarie University in Sydney, Australia. He has been conducting ethnographic and psychological research on sports, dance, and skill acquisition since 1992 in Brazil, Australia, New Zealand, and the United States. His first book, *Learning Capoeira: Lessons in Cunning from an Afro-Brazilian Art* (Oxford, 2005), was a study of the Afro-Brazilian dance and martial art, and he has published extensively on capoeira, no-holds-barred fighting, coaching, dance, music and other skills. Downey is especially interested in the ways physical education and training regimes in different cultures generate distinctive physiological capacities, behavior patterns, sensory abilities, and skill sets. His current research is on rugby training in Australia, New Zealand, and among Pacific Islanders. He is cofounder of the Neuroanthropology.net weblog, now part of the Public Library of Science (PLoS) Blogs, and coeditor of the 2012 MIT Press volume, *The Encultured Brain: An Introduction to Neuroanthropology*.

Katie Glaskin is Associate Professor of Anthropology at the University of Western Australia. She has coedited two books, *Customary Land Tenure and Registration in Australia and Papua New Guinea* (2007) and *Mortality, Mourning and Mortuary Practices in Indigenous Australia* (2008). Her geographic research areas include Northwest Australia, where she has worked with Indigenous Australians since 1994, and Japan, where she lived during 2007. Her research interests include property, personhood, dreams, sleep, and creativity; humanoid robots, emotion and empathy; and culture in litigated settings. Her current projects include a coedited book on the anthropology of sleep and a legal ethnography of an Australian native title claim.

ANNALS OF ANTHROPOLOGICAL PRACTICE 36, pp. 202–204. ISSN: 2153-957X. © 2012 by the American Anthropological Association. DOI:10.1111/j.2153-9588.2012.01100.x

James Griffith, M.D., is Interim Chair of the Department of Psychiatry and Behavioral Sciences at George Washington University. He directs the general psychiatry residency program. His books include *The Body Speaks: Therapeutic Dialogues for Mind–Body Problems* (1994, with Melissa Elliot Griffith); *Encountering the Sacred in Psychotherapy: How to Talk with People about Their Spiritual Lives* (2002, with Griffith); and *Religion That Heals, Religion That Harms: A Guide for Clinical Practice* (2010).

Helena Hansen, M.D., Ph.D., in cultural anthropology from Yale, is a board certified psychiatrist. Her research interests focus on mainstreaming addiction treatment into general medicine settings, the corporate marketing of psychopharmaceuticals to ethnic and social groups and how this shapes utilization, and the effects of changes in social welfare and disability benefit eligibility criteria on patients' health outcomes and self-perception.

Nathaniel Kendall-Taylor is Director of Research at the FrameWorks Institute. In this role, he employs social science theory and research methods from anthropology to improve the ability of public policy to positively influence health and social issues. This involves studying how cognitive theory can be applied in understanding how people interpret information and make meaning of their social worlds. His past research has focused on child and family health and in understanding the social and cultural factors that create health disparities and affect decision making. As a medical anthropologist, Kendall-Taylor has conducted fieldwork on the coast of Kenya studying pediatric epilepsy and the impacts of chronic illness on family well-being. He has also applied social science methods in research in Azerbaijan and Kazakhstan and has conducted ethnographic research on motivation in "extreme" athletes. Kendall-Taylor has a B.A. from Emory University and master's and doctoral degrees from the University of California, Los Angeles.

Brandon A. Kohrt, M.D., Ph.D., is Medical Anthropologist and Resident in general psychiatry at George Washington University, Department of Psychiatry and Behavioral Sciences, in Washington, D.C. He has conducted research in Nepal for 16 years. He studies the intersection of mental health and human rights, including the mental health of child soldiers and torture survivors. In the United States, he provides clinical services to torture survivors and refugees. He started a mental health clinic for Bhutanese refugees in 2009. He received the Physicians for Human Rights' Navin Narayan Health and Human Rights Leadership Award for his work with torture survivors. He wrote the documentary film, *Returned: Child Soldiers of Nepal's Maoist Army* (2008).

Daniel Lende (dlende@usf.edu) is Associate Professor of Anthropology at the University of South Florida. His work focuses on the integration of neuroscience and anthropology, behavioral health, addiction, stress and trauma, and applied anthropology. He has done mixed-method research in Colombia and the United States. He is cofounder of the Neuroanthropology.net blog, now part of the Public Library of Science blogs, and coeditor of the 2012 volume *The Encultured Brain: An Introduction to Neuroanthropology* from MIT Press. His work has also appeared in *Ethos*, *Addiction*, *Qualitative Health Research*, and *Addiction Research and Theory*.

Eric Lindland is a Senior Researcher with the FrameWorks Institute. Prior to joining FrameWorks, he taught anthropology at Emory University, Loyola University Chicago, and the University of Notre Dame, and before that was a high school teacher and administrator in Guatemala. As a cognitive anthropologist, his research has focused on how analogies are used in language, symbolism, and ethics to bridge meanings between differing cultural systems. In particular, he has engaged cultural modeling theory to explore the intersection of African and Western religious and medical systems. His ethnographic and historical research in Malawi centered on the challenges of therapeutic decision making in a pluralistic religious and medical culture, and on people's creative development of new models that combine and correlate magical, spiritual, and biomedical healing techniques. Lindland has a B.A. in Political Studies from Gordon College and an M.A. and Ph.D. in anthropology from Emory University.

Sujen M. Maharjan, M.A., completed his training in psychology at Tribhuvan University in Kirtipur, Nepal. He has worked for Transcultural Psychosocial Organization (TPO) Nepal conducting research with child soldiers. He directs the Nepalese Psychology Network and recently produced comprehensive bibliographies of mental health research conducted in Nepal. He operates a blog about psychology research in Nepal at http://sujenman.wordpress.com.

Neely Myers (neelymyers@gmail.com) is a psychological anthropologist working at the intersections of culture, neuroscience, and psychiatric disorders. She is currently completing a postdoctoral fellowship as a researcher on translational science teams at Georgetown University investigating meditation-based interventions for clinical use in reducing symptoms of PTSD, depression, stress reactivity, and cardiovascular risk. She is also directing research on the use of peer services in mental health treatment settings in New York. Dr. Myers is an Assistant Clinical Professor of Psychiatry at George Washington University School of Medicine and Behavioral Sciences.

Mary Skinner, B.A., is a filmmaker who, with Helena Hansen, is producing a feature-length visual documentary on race, class, and addiction pharmaceuticals. She served as a volunteer in Bellevue Hospital's Chemical Dependency Program in New York City for six years. She has produced six feature films, which have been screened at the Cannes, Milan International, and U.S. film markets. Prior to moving to New York City she was a partner in a film production company in Los Angeles, Shoreline Entertainment.

Damber Timsina, B.A., works for the refugee clinic at the International Medical Center of Grady Hospital in Atlanta, Georgia. He conducts trainings and provides psychosocial services for numerous resettlement agencies in Atlanta, Georgia.